Handbook of Oral Implantology

Handbook of Oral Implantology

Editor: Victor Martinez

AMERICAN
MEDICAL PUBLISHERS
www.americanmedicalpublishers.com

AMERICAN
MEDICAL PUBLISHERS
www.americanmedicalpublishers.com

Cataloging-in-Publication Data

Handbook of oral implantology / edited by Victor Martinez.
p. cm.
Includes bibliographical references and index.
ISBN 978-1-63927-773-5
1. Dental implants. 2. Dental implants--Complications. 3. Mouth--Surgery.
4. Implants, Artificial. 5. Dentures. 6. Dentistry. I. Martinez, Victor.
RK667.I45 H36 2023
617.693--dc23

American Medical Publishers,
41 Flatbush Avenue,
1st Floor, New York,
NY 11217, USA

ISBN 978-1-63927-773-5 (Hardback)

Contents

Preface

Oral implantology refers to the area of medicine which deals with the assessment of health and diseases of the supporting and investing structures of dental implants and natural teeth. It is also concerned with oral mucous membrane, along with the prevention and treatment of diseases. The major focus of oral implantology is not the surgical phase but the restorative phase. The oral environment keeps changing and it is not possible to have perfect conditions for healing. The complications related with implant procedures can be reduced through a comprehensive and through assessment of dental history, knowledge of head and neck anatomy, and radiographic survey. It also comprises knowledge of pharmacological, prosthetic, and surgical processes, along with principles of follow up care. The success of dental surgical procedures depends on the health of the person receiving the treatment, health condition of the tissues in the mouth, and the drugs which affect the probability of osseointegration. The aim of this book is to present researches that have transformed the discipline of oral implantology and aided its advancement. Its extensive content provides the readers with a thorough understanding of the subject.

After months of intensive research and writing, this book is the end result of all who devoted their time and efforts in the initiation and progress of this book. It will surely be a source of reference in enhancing the required knowledge of the new developments in the area. During the course of developing this book, certain measures such as accuracy, authenticity and research focused analytical studies were given preference in order to produce a comprehensive book in the area of study.

This book would not have been possible without the efforts of the authors and the publisher. I extend my sincere thanks to them. Secondly, I express my gratitude to my family and well-wishers. And most importantly, I thank my students for constantly expressing their willingness and curiosity in enhancing their knowledge in the field, which encourages me to take up further research projects for the advancement of the area.

Editor

1

Using Genipin to Immobilize Bone Morphogenetic Protein-2 on Zirconia Surface for Enhancing Cell Adhesion and Mineralization in Dental Implant Applications

Ying-Sui Sun [1,2], Yu-An Lin [3] and Her-Hsiung Huang [2,3,4,5,6,7,*]

1 School of Dental Technology, Taipei Medical University, Taipei 11031, Taiwan; yingsuisun@tmu.edu.tw
2 Department of Dentistry, National Yang-Ming University, Taipei 11221, Taiwan
3 Institute of Oral Biology, National Yang-Ming University, Taipei 11221, Taiwan; ukorose@gmail.com
4 Department of Bioinformatics and Medical Engineering, Asia University, Taichung 41354, Taiwan
5 Department of Medical Research, China Medical University Hospital, China Medical University, Taichung 40402, Taiwan
6 Department of Stomatology, Taipei Veterans General Hospital, Taipei 11217, Taiwan
7 Department of Education and Research, Taipei City Hospital, Taipei 10341, Taiwan
* Correspondence: hhhuang@gm.ym.edu.tw

Abstract: Our objective in this study was to promote cell responses through the immobilization of bone morphogenetic protein-2 (BMP-2) on roughened zirconia (ZrO_2) through using the natural cross-linker genipin in dental implant applications. Field emission scanning electron microscope, X-ray photoelectron spectroscopy, and attenuated total reflection-Fourier transform infrared spectroscopy were used to analyze the surface characterizations, including the topography, chemistry, and functional groups, respectively, of the test specimens. Human bone marrow mesenchymal stem cells (hMSCs) were used to detect cell responses (adhesion, proliferation, and mineralization). The surface characterizations analysis results revealed that genipin was effective in immobilizing BMP-2 on roughened zirconia surfaces. BMP-2 proved effective in promoting the adhesion and mineralization of hMSCs on roughened zirconia. The surface modification proposed has potential in zirconia dental implant applications.

Keywords: natural cross-linker genipin; bone morphogenetic protein-2 (BMP-2); human bone marrow mesenchymal stem cell; cell adhesion; cell mineralization

---

1. Introduction

Tooth loss is commonly dealt with using removable dentures or dental bridges; however, many patients are dissatisfied with their functionality and aesthetic appearance. Titanium (Ti) dental implant is highly biocompatible; nevertheless, its metallic gray color is not aesthetically pleasing and its corrosion product may induce allergic reactions in patients [1,2]. Zirconia (ZrO_2) is a viable alternative to Ti as an implant material due to its good mechanical properties, biocompatibility, corrosion resistance, tooth-like appearance, and low plaque affinity [3]. However, bioinert zirconia surfaces tend to hinder bonding between implant and bone. Previous studies have shown that the roughening of the surface via physical treatments (such as sandblasting) improves the mechanical interlocking of the dental implant with the surrounding bone [4] and the adhesion, metabolic activity, and proliferation of human osteoblast-like cells [5]. Treatments involving the immobilization of biologically active molecules on zirconia surfaces have also been shown to enhance the bioactivity (i.e., Ca/P formation ability) [6,7].

Basically, surface modification aiming at improving the bone cell response of bioinert zirconia surfaces still needs detailed investigations [8].

Bone morphogenetic protein-2 (BMP-2) belongs to the transforming growth factor beta superfamily of proteins [9]. It is a potent osseoinductive factor involved in a variety of biological functions associated with osteogenesis and osteogenic differentiation, including the maintenance of normal bone as well as bone regeneration [9–13]. BMP-2 has also been shown to reduce bone resorption and improve osseointegration in dental implant applications [14]. Note, however, that a high dose of BMP-2 may induce apoptosis and cytotoxicity in periodontal ligament cells [15]. Recombinant human bone morphogenetic protein-2 (rhBMP-2) has been approved by the U.S. Food and Drug Administration (FDA) to promote the formation of bone and cartilage through induced osteoblast differentiation [16,17]. The overexpression of adenoviral-mediated BMP-2 promotes the upregulation of osteogenic gene expression, such as alkaline phosphatase (ALP) and runt-related transcription factor 2 (RUNX2), in bone marrow stem cells (BMSCs) [18]. Thus, it is interesting to know how BMP-2 positively affects the bone cell response to a bioinert zirconia surface without causing biological side effects.

Genipin is a chemical compound extracted from the fruit of Gardenia jasminoides which acts as a natural cross-linker for proteins, collagen, gelatin, and chitosan [19]. Genipin can be used in a similar manner to glutaraldehyde, the latter of which is widely used in clinical settings to enhance the mechanical properties of biomaterials; however, genipin is superior to glutaraldehyde in terms of cell cytotoxicity, biocompatibility, mechanical properties, and resistance to enzyme degradation in vivo [20]. In traditional Chinese medicine, genipin serves as an inhibitor of uncoupled protein 2, which has been shown to promote the release of insulin in patients with diabetes mellitus type 2 [21]. The antioxidant and anti-inflammatory effects of genipin have also been shown to suppress liver apoptosis in mice [22]. Based on the abovementioned literature, in the current study we used genipin as a simple, cost-effective natural cross-linker to immobilize bioactive BMP-2 on bioinert zirconia surfaces to enhance the bone cell responses in dental implant applications.

2. Materials and Methods

2.1. Specimen Preparation

Biomedical-grade zirconia disks with diameters of 15 mm and thicknesses of 3 mm were used as test substrates (designated as Z). The Z specimens were sandblasted using aluminum oxide particles (size 120 μm) for 10 sec by a dental sandblaster (pressure 4 bar) at a 5 cm distance from the surface of the disk. The resulting sandblasted zirconia specimens were designated ZS. Several ZS specimens were subjected to alkaline immersion treatment in 5M of NaOH at 60 °C for 24 h to attract hydroxyl (OH) groups to the roughened surface. The same specimens were then immersed in phosphate-buffered saline (PBS) containing genipin (0.05%) at 37 °C for 24 h. Note that genipin binds to hydroxyl groups on the specimen surface via the aldehyde groups (CO). The resulting genipin-treated ZS specimens were designated ZSG. Several ZSG specimens were immersed in ddH_2O containing BMP-2 (10 ng/mL) at 37 °C for 24 h. The N-terminals of the proteins interact with genipin to form amide bonds leading to the immobilization of BMP-2 on the roughened zirconia surface. The resulting BMP-2-immobiblized ZSG specimens were designated ZSGB.

2.2. Surface Characterization

Field emission scanning electron microscope (FESEM, JEOL Ltd., Tokyo, Japan), X-ray photoelectron spectroscopy (XPS, ULVAC-PHI, Inc., Kanagawa, Japan), and attenuated total reflection-Fourier transform infrared spectroscopy (ATR-FTIR, PerkinElmer Inc., Waltham, MA, USA) were respectively used to analyze the surface morphology, chemical elements, and functional groups of the specimens.

2.3. *Cell Responses*

2.3.1. Cell Culture

hMSCs were cultured in Dulbecco's Modified Eagle's Medium-low glucose (DMEM-low glucose; Merck KGaA, Darmstadt, Germany) containing 10% fetal bovine serum (FBS; Thermo Fisher Scientific, San Jose, CA, USA), 1.5 g/L of sodium bicarbonate, and 1% penicillin/streptomycin and maintained at 37 °C under humidified air with 5% CO_2.

2.3.2. Cell Adhesion

hMSCs were seeded at a density of 1.5×10^4 cells/specimen on test specimens. Following incubation for 6 h, cells adhering to the test specimens were fixed using fixation buffer (2% glutaraldehyde + 4% paraformaldehyde) and then dehydrated in a series of ethanol (10–100%). After coating the specimens with a platinum film, the cell adhesion morphology was observed using FE-SEM.

2.3.3. Cell Proliferation

Human bone marrow mesenchymal stem cell (hMSCs) (passage 5–8) were seeded at a density of 1×10^4 cells/specimen on test specimens. Following incubation periods of 1, 3, and 5 d, the cell proliferation was evaluated by adding alamarBlue® reagent (Thermo Fisher Scientific, Waltham, MA, USA) to a final concentration of 10%, followed by incubation at 37 °C for 1, 3, and 5 d. The reducing environment of the cells in the alamarBlue assay was measured in terms of the conversion of resazurin (oxidized form) to resorufin (reduced form) and expressed as a percentage reduction in alamarBlue as a function of culture time.

2.3.4. Cell Mineralization

The extracellular matrix (ECM) produces calcium deposits in the mineralization stage of osteogenic differentiation. hMSCs were seeded at a density of 5×10^3 cells/specimen on test specimens, then were cultured in normal medium for 24 h and moved to an osteogenic medium containing DMED (Merck KGaA, Darmstadt, Germany) supplemented with 10^{-8} M of dexamethasone, 10 mM of ß-glycerophosphate, and 50 μg/mL of ascorbic acid. Afterwards, the osteogenic medium was changed every two days. Following incubation periods of 7 and 21 d, the cell mineralization was evaluated by adding 1% Alizarin red S in distilled water (pH 4.2) for 1 h at room temperature (RT) to detect calcium components following cell fixation using ice-cold 70% ethanol. The cells were subsequently rinsed using distilled water until the color disappeared. The stained cells were observed and imaged using a metallographic microscope. The quantification of stained cells was performed by adding 10% (*w/v*) cetylpyridinium chloride in 10 mM of sodium phosphate (pH 7.0) at RT for 1 h to extract Alizarin red S. The absorbance at 540 nm was measured using a microplate reader. A higher optical density (OD) represented a higher mineralization ability.

2.4. *Statistical Analysis*

The results of cell proliferation and mineralization were presented as mean with standard deviation (SD). Student's t-test was used for statistical analysis, with a p value < 0.05 as statistical significance.

3. Results and Discussion

3.1. *Surface Characterization*

Figure 1 presents FESEM micrographs showing the surface morphology of Z, ZS, ZSG, and ZSGB. The ZSG specimens presented a snowflake-like pattern with a random distribution. The ZSGB specimens presented an irregular flake layer and the BMP-2 was mixed with the genipin. Several biomaterials have been used to mimic different biological microenvironments, such as genipin-crosslinked chitosan [23]. The immobilization of genipin to produce a biomolecular surface on

Ti alloy has considerable potential for bone implant applications [24]. In this study, we immobilized the BMP-2 as an activator to improve bone cell responses, as will be discussed later.

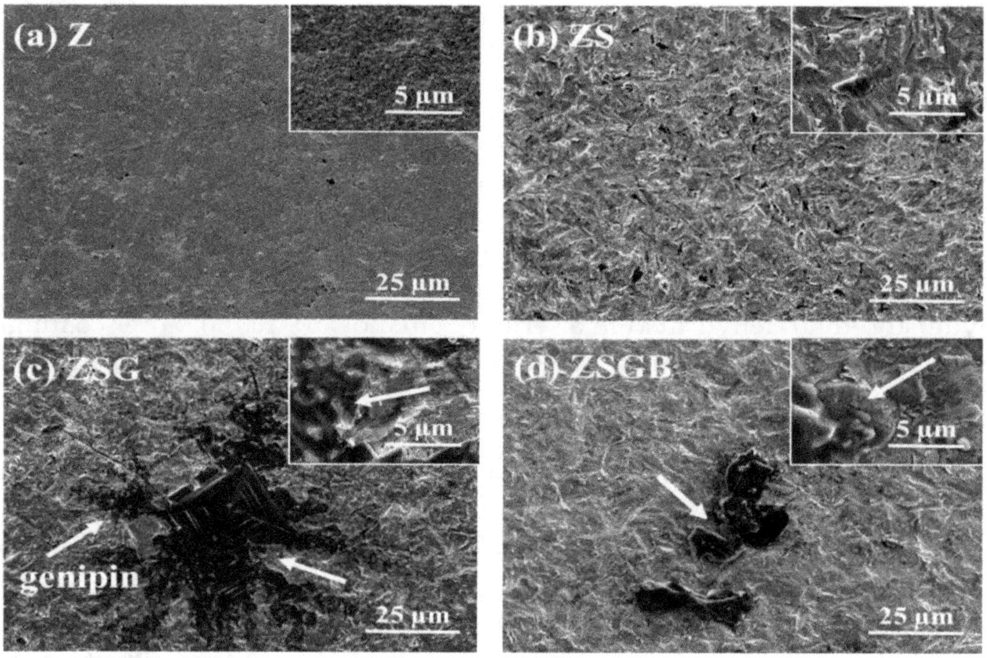

Figure 1. FESEM micrographs, showing the surface morphology of test specimens: (**a**) Z (untreated zirconia), (**b**) ZS (sandblasted Z), (**c**) ZSG (genipin-treated ZS), and (**d**) ZSGB (BMP-2-immobilized ZSG); the upper right corner of each figure is a partial enlarged view (arrows: genipin).

Figure 2 presents the XPS analysis results in terms of the N1s (1s orbital for nitrogen) spectra. According to the Thermo Scientific™ data system [25], the binding energy of N1s of amine groups (-NH2) is around 399–400 eV. The N1s intensity of ZSGB (attributable to the N-terminal of BMP-2 proteins) was higher than that of ZSG, indicating the successful immobilization of BMP-2. Figure 3 presents the typical ATR-FTIR spectra of test specimens. The ZSGB specimens revealed the C=O stretching vibrations of amide I (1600–1690 cm^{-1}), the C–N stretching and N–H bending vibrations of amide II (1480–1575 cm^{-1}), and the N–H stretching vibrations of amide A and B (3050–3700 cm^{-1}). This confirmed again the presence of BMP-2 in ZSGB specimens.

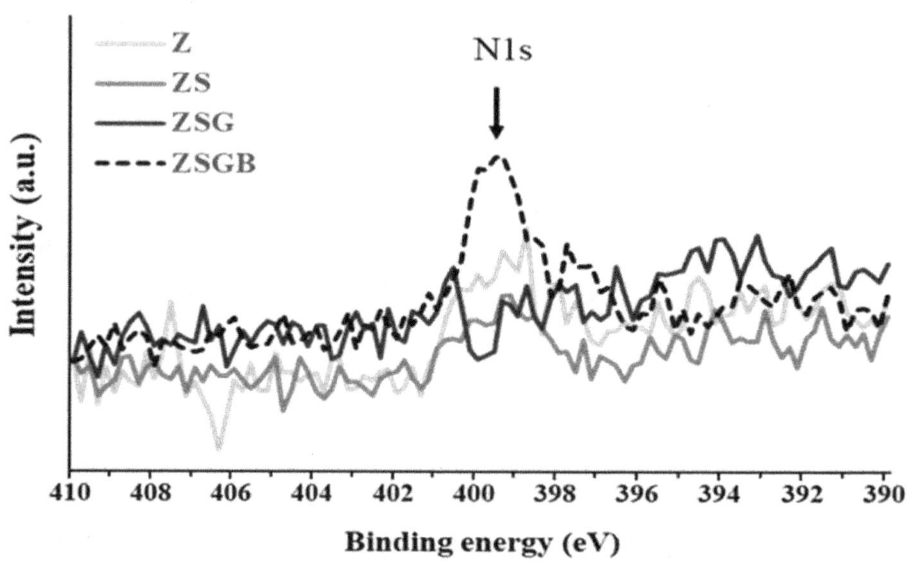

Figure 2. XPS analysis results, in terms of N1s (1s orbital for nitrogen) spectra, of test specimens.

The FTIR analysis results (Figure 3) indicated the successful immobilization of BMP-2 on roughened zirconia via amide groups between BMP-2 and genipin. Recently, BMP-2 has been successfully immobilized on porous Ti surfaces though genipin to enhance the bone cell response [26]. For future application potential, BMP-2 can be immobilized on ceramics as a local delivery growth factor [27].

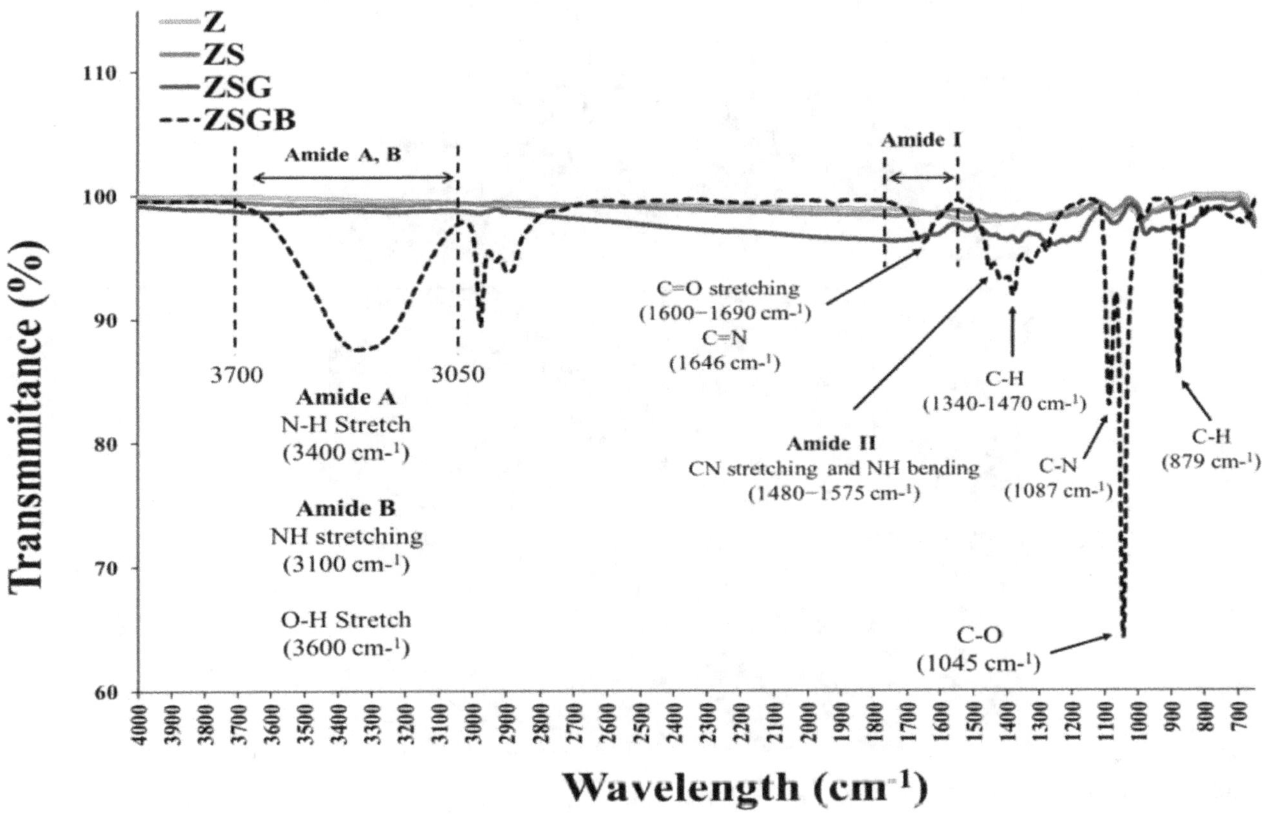

Figure 3. FTIR analysis results showing the function groups of test specimens.

3.2. Cell Responses

Figure 4 presents the FE-SEM analysis results of hMSCs following cell incubation for 6 h. The morphology of cells on BMP-2-immoblized specimens (ZSGB group) presented better spreading (flattening) morphology and cell–cell communication (as indicated by white arrows on the right micrograph) than that observed in the other specimens. Cell adhesion includes the propagation of a thin cell membrane, followed by the spreading of cell filopodia. The flattened cell morphology indicated a good cell adhesion, representing a good biocompatibility [28]. A research demonstrated that BMP-2 significantly alters the osteoblastic cytoskeletal and ECM organization and enhances the expressions of fibronectin and specific integrin receptor subunits, which contributes to downstream cellular responses that are important for bone cell growth [29].

Figure 5 illustrates the cell proliferation of hMSCs on test specimens throughout the 5-day cell incubation period. After 5 d of incubation, no statistically significant differences were observed among the test specimens in terms of cell proliferation. However, the average cell proliferation in the ZSG and ZSGB specimens was lower than that in the Z and ZS, indicating that BMP-2 had no positive effect on cell proliferation at day 3 and day 5. This result may imply that the hMSCs on ZSG and ZSGB surfaces proceeded faster to the later stage of cell growth—namely, the mineralization stage of osteogenic differentiation.

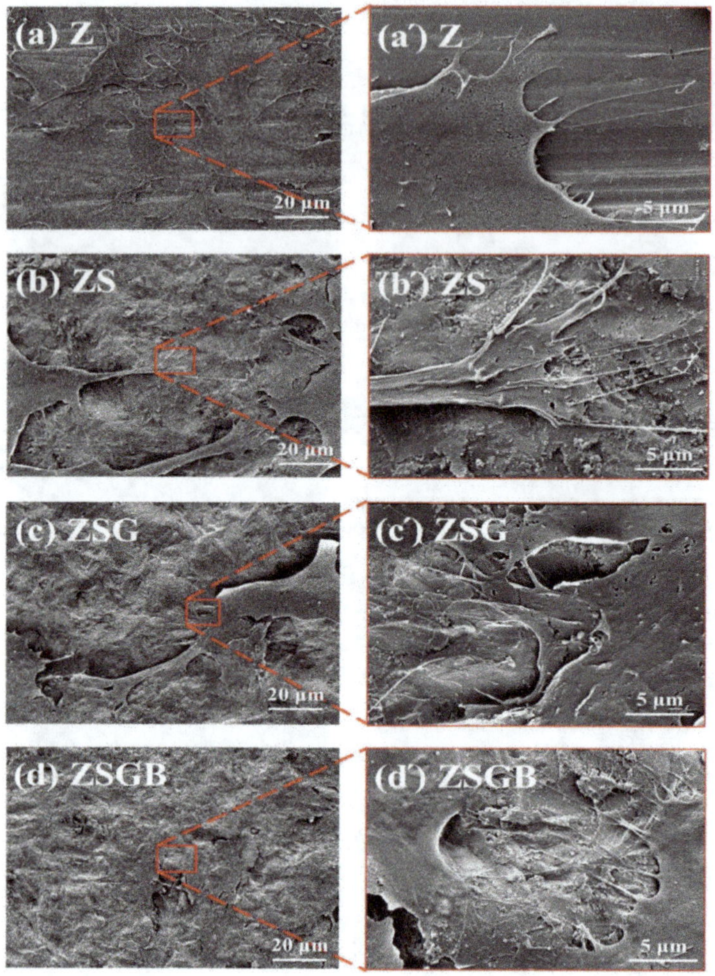

Figure 4. FESEM micrographs showing the cell morphology on test specimens after 6 h of incubation: (**a**) Z (untreated zirconia), (**b**) ZS (sandblasted Z), (**c**) ZSG (genipin-treated ZS), and (**d**) ZSGB (BMP-2-immobilized ZSG); the micrographs (**a′–d′**) are partial enlarged views of the micrographs (**a–d**), respectively.

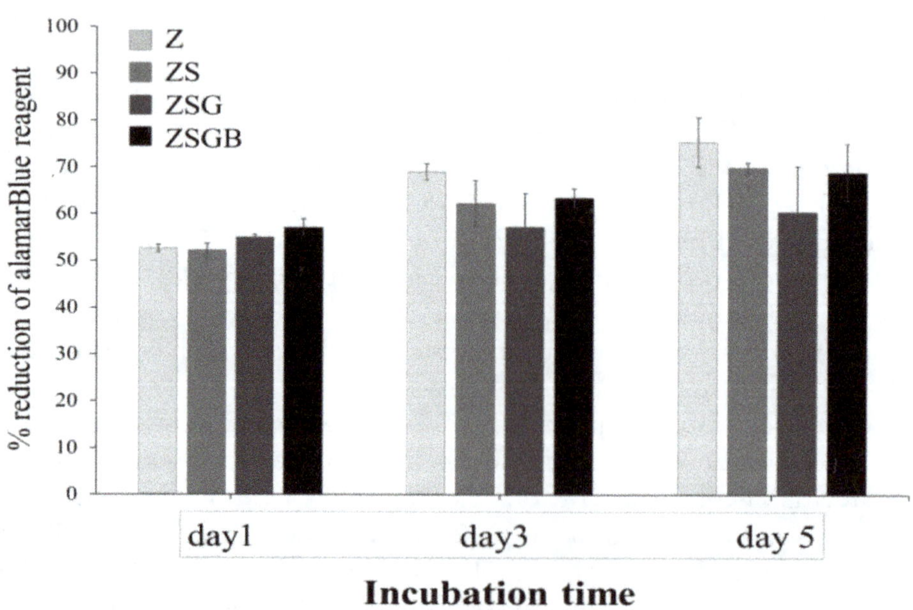

Figure 5. Cell proliferation of test specimens during the 5 d of incubation.

Figure 6 presents the cell mineralization analysis results, in terms of the Alizarin red S staining, of the test specimens after 7 d and 21 d of incubation. Based on the (a) qualitative and (b) quantitative data, no significant differences were observed in the mineralization ability at day 7, while ZSBG had the highest mineralization ability at day 21. It has been proved that the immobilization of BMP-2 on the porous Ti surface can considerably enhance the cell mineralization and biological activity, causing the surface of biomolecules to have excellent application potential in bone implantation [26]. In this study, Figure 6 shows that the cell mineralization on the roughened zirconia (TS) surfaces is significantly improved by the immobilization of BMP-2 (at day 21). This confirmed that the lower proliferation (day 5 in Figure 5) and faster mineralization (day 21 in Figure 6) of hMSCs on ZSGB surfaces advise that the immobilization of BMP-2 on roughened zirconia surfaces enhanced the bone cell growth. According this result, we suggest that the cross-linker genipin stabilized the immobilization of BMP-2 on roughened zirconia surfaces and reduced the degradation of BMP-2, resulting in the highest mineralization ability of ZSGB at day 21. However, this still needs further investigation.

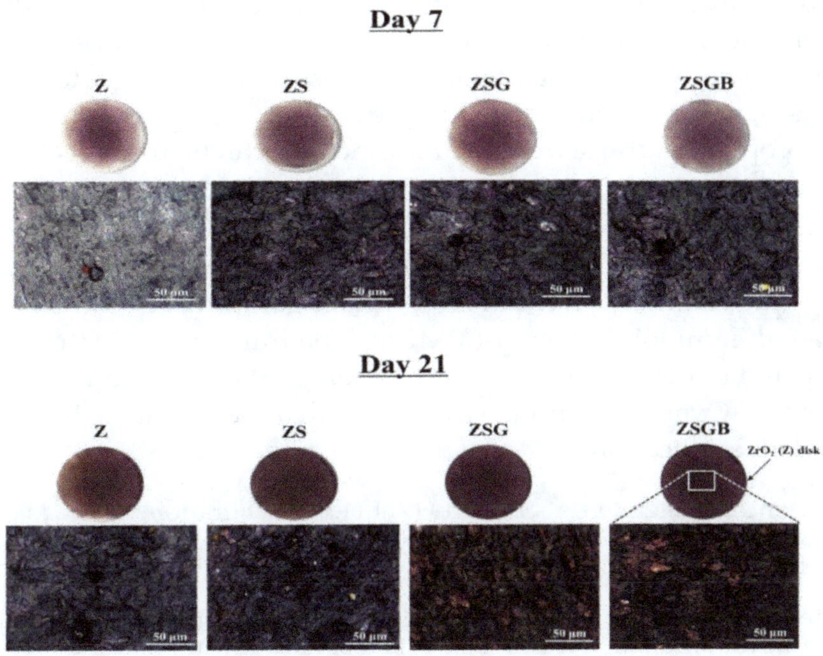

(a)

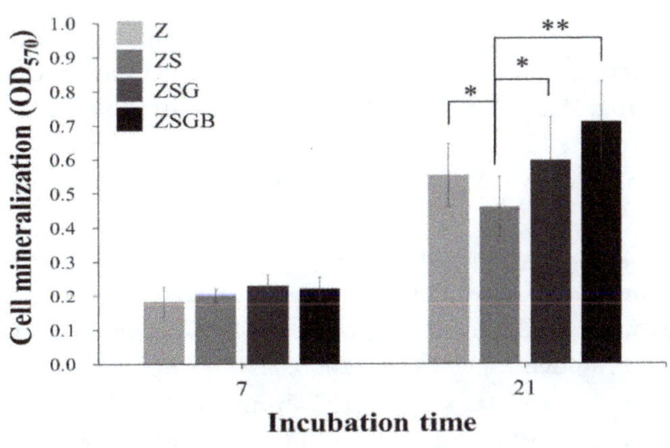

(b)

Figure 6. Cell mineralization analysis results, in terms of Alizarin red S staining, of the test specimens after 7 d and 21 d of incubation: (**a**) qualitative observation (upper row: zirconia disk; lower row: higher magnification of upper row); (**b**) quantitative analysis (* $p < 0.05$; ** $p < 0.01$).

According to a previous report, sandblasting can improve the adhesion and proliferation of human osteoblast-like cells on the surface of zirconia [5]. Note, however, that the rough ZS surface treated by sandblasting had a better cell adhesion morphology in terms of cell filopodia stretching (Figure 4), but a lower cell proliferation (Figure 5) and mineralization (Figure 6) as compared with the untreated smooth Z surface. A similar result has been reported, in that the patterned silicon nanowire surface can increase cell−substrate adhesion while limiting cell−cell communication [30]. Therefore, we speculate that the strong cell–substrate adhesion on the sandblasted rough ZS surface may limit cell–cell communication, leading to a subsequent reduction in cell proliferation and mineralization. The underlying mechanism, however, needs further investigation.

In this study, we immobilized BMP-2 on a zirconia surface using genipin as cross-linker. We comparrf our study with a previous report [23] which uses genipin to crosslink the chitosan nanoparticles to obtain hydrogels and scaffolds. We believe that both BMP-2 and chitosan contain the amine groups (–NH2) and carboxylic acid groups (–COOH) that can be cross-linked with genipin. However, in this study, the zirconia substrate after alkaline immersion treatment is believed to be chemically bonded with genipin through its surface OH groups. To our best of knowledge, there is very limited information about the use of the natural cross-linker genipin to crosslink biomolecules to zirconia surfaces. It is recommended that more detailed in vitro and in vivo biological tests be performed before the proposed surface treatment technology can be used in clinical applications.

4. Conclusions

This study reports a simple and cost-effective method for the immobilization of BMP-2 on a roughened zirconia surface using the natural cross-linker genipin. The natural cross-linker genipin was shown to facilitate the immobilization of BMP-2. The immobilization of BMP-2 on roughened zirconia surfaces triggered bone cell adhesion and mineralization, which was expected to accelerate the following osteogenesis. Overall, the proposed surface treatment scheme has considerable potential in zirconia dental implant applications.

Author Contributions: Conceptualization, Y.-S.S and H.-H.H.; Data curation, Y.-A.L.; Formal analysis, Y.-A.L.; Investigation, Y.-A.L.; Resources, H.-H.H.; Supervision, Y.-S.S. and H.-H.H.; Writing—original draft, Y.-S.S.; Writing—review and editing, H.-H.H. All authors have read and agreed to the published version of the manuscript.

Acknowledgments: The authors greatly acknowledge Shin-Hwa Chiou (Stem Cell Laboratory, Department of Medical Research and Education, Taipei Veterans General Hospital, Taiwan) for kindly providing us hMSCs.

References

1. Dunn, D.B. The use of a zirconia custom implant-supported fixed partial denture prosthesis to treat implant failure in the anterior maxilla: A clinical report. *J. Prosthet. Dent.* **2008**, *100*, 415–421. [CrossRef]
2. Sicilia, A.; Cuesta, S.; Coma, G.; Arregui, I.; Guisasola, C.; Ruiz, E.; Maestro, A. Titanium allergy in dental implant patients: A clinical study on 1500 consecutive patients. *Clin. Oral Implant. Res.* **2008**, *19*, 823–835. [CrossRef]
3. Huang, Y.S.; Huang, H.H. Effects of clinical dental implant abutment materials and their surface characteristics on initial bacterial adhesion. *Rare Met.* **2019**, *38*, 512–519. [CrossRef]
4. Shalabi, M.M.; Gortemaker, A.; Van't Hof, M.A.; Jansen, J.A.; Creugers, N.H. Implant surface roughness and bone healing: A systematic review. *J. Dent. Res.* **2006**, *85*, 496–500. [CrossRef] [PubMed]
5. Al Qahtani, W.M.; Schille, C.; Spintzyk, S.; Al Qahtani, M.S.; Engel, E.; Geis-Gerstorfer, J.; Rupp, F.; Scheideler, L. Effect of surface modification of zirconia on cell adhesion, metabolic activity and proliferation of human osteoblasts. *Biomed. Tech.* **2017**, *62*, 75–87. [CrossRef] [PubMed]
6. Trindade, R.; Albrektsson, T.; Tengvall, P.; Wennerberg, A. Foreign body reaction to biomaterials: On mechanisms for buildup and breakdown of osseointegration. *Clin. Implant Dent. Relat. Res.* **2016**, *18*, 192–203. [CrossRef] [PubMed]
7. Schickle, K.; Spitz, J.; Neuss, S.; Telle, R. Biomimetic in situ nucleation of calcium phosphates by protein immobilization on high strength ceramic materials. *J. Eur. Ceram. Soc.* **2018**, *38*, 271–277. [CrossRef]

8. Bächle, M.; Butz, F.; Hübner, U.; Bakalinis, E.; Kohal, R.J. Behavior of cal72 osteoblast—Like cells cultured on zirconia ceramics with different surface topographies. *Clin. Oral Implant. Res.* **2007**, *18*, 53–59. [CrossRef]
9. Chen, D.; Zhao, M.; Mundy, G.R. Bone morphogenetic proteins. *Growth Factors* **2004**, *22*, 233–241. [CrossRef]
10. Zhang, H.; Bradley, A. Mice deficient for BMP2 are nonviable and have defects in amnion/chorion and cardiac development. *Development* **1996**, *122*, 2977–2986.
11. Ducy, P.; Karsenty, G. The family of bone morphogenetic proteins. *Kidney Int.* **2000**, *57*, 2207–2214. [CrossRef] [PubMed]
12. Rosen, V. BMP2 signaling in bone development and repair. *Cytokine Growth Factor Rev.* **2009**, *20*, 475–480. [CrossRef]
13. Singh, A.P.; Castranio, T.; Scott, G.; Guo, D.; Harris, M.A.; Ray, M.; Harris, S.E.; Mishina, Y. Influences of reduced expression of maternal bone morphogenetic protein 2 on mouse embryonic development. *Sex. Dev.* **2008**, *2*, 134–141. [CrossRef]
14. Matin, K.; Senpuku, H.; Hanada, N.; Ozawa, H.; Ejiri, S. Bone regeneration by recombinant human bone morphogenetic protein-2 around immediate implants: A pilot study in rats. *Int. J. Oral Maxillofac. Surg.* **2003**, *18*, 211–217.
15. Muthukuru, M. Bone Morphogenic Protein–2 Induces Apoptosis and Cytotoxicity in Periodontal Ligament Cells. *J. Periodontol.* **2013**, *84*, 829–838. [CrossRef] [PubMed]
16. Schuckert, K.H.; Jopp, S.; Osadnik, M. The use of platelet rich plasma, bone morphogenetic protein-2 and different scaffolds in oral and maxillofacial surgery-literature review in comparison with own clinical experience. *J. Oral Maxillofac. Res.* **2011**, *2*, e2. [CrossRef] [PubMed]
17. Legendre, F.; Ollitrault, D.; Gomez-Leduc, T.; Bouyoucef, M.; Hervieu, M.; Gruchy, N.; Gerin, F.M.; Leclercq, S.; Demoor, M.; Galéra, P. Enhanced chondrogenesis of bone marrow-derived stem cells by using a combinatory cell therapy strategy with BMP-2/TGF-β1, hypoxia, and COL1A1/HtrA1 siRNAs. *Sci. Rep.* **2007**, *7*, 3406. [CrossRef]
18. Sharma, S.; Sapkota, D.; Xue, Y.; Sun, Y.; Finne-Wistrand, A.; Bruland, O.; Mustafa, K. Adenoviral mediated expression of BMP2 by bone marrow stromal cells cultured in 3D copolymer scaffolds enhances bone formation. *PLoS ONE* **2016**, *11*, e0147507. [CrossRef]
19. Bi, L.; Cao, Z.; Hu, Y.; Song, Y.; Yu, L.; Yang, B.; Mu, J.; Huang, Z.; Han, Y. Effects of different cross-linking conditions on the properties of genipin-cross-linked chitosan/collagen scaffolds for cartilage tissue engineering. *J. Mater. Sci. Mater. Med.* **2011**, *22*, 51–62. [CrossRef]
20. Peng, Z.; Li, Z.; Shen, Y. Influence of chemical cross-linking on properties of gelatin/chitosan microspheres. *Polym. Plast. Technol. Eng.* **2012**, *51*, 381–385. [CrossRef]
21. Zhang, C.; Parton, L.E.; Ye, C.P.; Krauss, S.; Shen, R.; Lin, C.T.; Porco, J.A.; Lowell, B.B. Genipin inhibits ucp2-mediated proton leak and acutely reverses obesity-and high glucose-induced β cell dysfunction in isolated pancreatic islets. *Cell Metab.* **2006**, *3*, 417–427. [CrossRef] [PubMed]
22. Yamamoto, M.; Miura, N.; Ohtake, N.; Amagaya, S.; Ishige, A.; Sasaki, H.; Komatsu, Y.; Fukuda, K.; Ito, T.; Terasawa, K. Genipin, a metabolite derived from th herbal medicine inchin-ko-to, and suppression of fas-induced lethal live apoptosis in mice. *Gastroenterology* **2000**, *118*, 380–389. [CrossRef]
23. Muzzarelli, R.A.; El Mehtedi, M.; Bottegoni, C.; Aquili, A.; Gigante, A. Genipin-crosslinked chitosan gels and scaffolds for tissue engineering and regeneration of cartilage and bone. *Mar. Drugs.* **2015**, *13*, 7314–7338. [CrossRef] [PubMed]
24. Sun, Y.S.; Huang, C.Y.; Chen, C.S.; Chang, J.H.; Hou, W.T.; Li, S.J.; Hao, Y.L.; Pan, H.; Huang, H.H. Bone cell responses to a low elastic modulus titanium alloy surface immobilized with the natural cross-linker genipin. *Surf. Coat. Technol.* **2018**, *350*, 918–924. [CrossRef]
25. Thermo Fisher Scientific Inc. *Thermo Scientific™ Avantage™ Data System for XPS*; Thermo Fisher Scientific Inc.: Waltham, MA, USA, 2020. Available online: https://xpssimplified.com/elements/nitrogen.php (accessed on 1 November 2020).
26. Sun, Y.S.; Chang, J.H.; Huang, H.H. Enhancing the biological response of titanium surface through the immobilization of bone morphogenetic protein-2 using the natural cross-linker genipin. *Surf. Coat. Technol.* **2016**, *303*, 289–297. [CrossRef]

27. Solorio, L.; Zwolinski, C.; Lund, A.W.; Farrell, M.J.; Stegemann, J.P. Gelatin microspheres crosslinked with genipin for local delivery of growth factors. *J. Tissue Eng. Regen. Med.* **2010**, *4*, 514–523. [CrossRef]
28. Orsini, G.; Assenza, B.; Scarano, A.; Piatelli, M.; Piattelli, A. Surface analysis of machined versus sandblasted and acid-etched titanium implants. *Int. J. Oral Maxillofac. Implants* **2000**, *15*, 779–784.
29. Shah, A.K.; Lazatin, J.; Sinha, R.K.; Lennox, T.; Hickok, N.J.; Tuan, R.S. Mechanism of BMP-2 stimulated adhesion of osteoblastic cells to titanium alloy. *Biol. Cell.* **1999**, *91*, 131–142. [CrossRef]
30. Qi, S.; Yi, C.; Ji, S.; Fong, C.-C.; Yang, M. Cell adhesion and spreading behavior on vertically aligned silicon nanowire arrays. *ACS Appl. Mater. Interfaces* **2009**, *1*, 30–34. [CrossRef]

2

Scientific Trends in Clinical Research on Zirconia Dental Implants: A Bibliometric Review

Felice Lorusso [1,2], Sammy Noumbissi [1,2], Inchingolo Francesco [3], Biagio Rapone [4], Ahmad G. A. Khater [5] and Antonio Scarano [1,2,*]

1 Department of Medical, Oral and Biotechnological Sciences, University of Chieti-Pescara, Via dei Vestini, 31, 66100 Chieti, Italy; drlorussofelice@gmail.com (F.L.); sammy@iaoci.com (S.N.)

2 Zirconia Implant Research Group (Z.I.R.G), International Academy of Ceramic Implantology, Silver Spring, MD 20910, USA

3 Department of Interdisciplinary Medicine, University of Bari Aldo Moro, 70121 Bari, Italy; f.inchingolo@icloud.com

4 Department of Basic Medical Sciences, Neurosciences and Sense Organs, University of Bari Aldo Moro, 70121 Bari, Italy; biagiorapone79@gmail.com

5 Faculty of Oral and Dental Medicine, Ahram Canadian University, 6th of October City, 8655 Giza, Egypt; ahmed.g.a.khater@gmail.com

* Correspondence: ascarano@unich.it

Abstract: Background: The clinical use of zirconia implants has been shown to increase steadily due to their biological, aesthetic, and physical properties; therefore, this bibliometric study aimed to review the clinical research and co-authors in the field of zirconia dental implant rehabilitation. Methods: We searched Scopus and Web of Science databases using a comprehensive search strategy to 5 October 2020, and independently paired reviewers who screened studies, and collected data with inclusion criteria restricted to clinical research only (either prospective or retrospective). Data on article title, co-authors, number of citations received, journal details, publication year, country and institution involved, funding, study design, marginal bone loss, survival rate, failure, follow-up, and the author's bibliometric data were collected and evaluated. Results: A total of 29 clinical studies were published between 2008 and 2020 as 41.4% were prospective cohort studies and 48.3% originated from Germany. Most of the included studies had been published in Clinical Oral Implant Research (n = 12), and the most productive institution was the Medical Center of University of Freiburg. The author with the largest number of clinical studies on zirconia implants was Kohal R.J. (n = 10), followed by Spies B.C. (n = 8). Conclusions: This study revealed that zirconia implants have been more prominent in the last ten years, which is a valuable option for oral rehabilitation with marginal bone loss and survival rate comparable to titanium dental implants.

Keywords: zirconia implant; bibliometrics; citations; scientometric

1. Introduction

The clinical application of dental implant rehabilitation represents consolidated effectiveness in the literature due to long-term predictability and high-level satisfactory functioning and aesthetics [1–4]. Titanium alloys are the most widely used biomaterials for dental implant fixtures due to their physical, chemical, and thermal properties, which produce the osseointegrating ability of the fixture placed to replace the natural teeth [2,5–12].

Recently, the use of zirconia as an implant material has become more prevalent due to its high aesthetic characteristics, particularly in the rehabilitation of the compromised anterior jaw area, where there is fine soft-tissue biotype and the metal sensibility of the patients [13–15].

In fact, the literature reports that the titanium ion dissolution related to the implant corrosion could alter the natural oral microbiome and the homeostatic functional balance of the oral tissues [16–20].

On the contrary, it has been shown in vitro that the zirconia surface can lead to a significant decrease in periodontal pathogen adhesion compared to the titanium surface [21], alongside similar bone–implant contact compared to the titanium fixture with an almost overlapping range [22].

Additionally, Scarano et al. reported in a rabbit study that zirconia implants had about 68.4% bone–implant contact with evidence of contact osteogenesis without fibrous tissue interposition [23].

Zirconia material is distinguished by its clear ivory appearance, which is very similar to the natural color of the teeth and is characterized by an intrinsic strength and physical resistance to the loading [24–26]; as a result, it has been introduced as a restorative material for dental crowns, bars, abutments, and specially designed drills and burs [26–34]. Therefore, zirconia has recently gained further attention in the scientific community by growing research activities to confirm the clinical effectiveness of zirconia as a dental implant material.

Although citations are not an infallible metric to determine whether research is beneficial to researchers and clinicians, citations and citation analysis can quantify an article's influence, author, subject of debate, country, journal, or a specialty [35,36]. Based on citation analysis, the bibliometric analysis aims to provide information about the trend in a research field and demonstrates its growth and development [37]; the number of citations received, researcher H-index, and journal impact factor are the most common bibliometric evaluation variables and considered as a scientific productivity score for the scientometric evaluation [38].

With the significant increase in the published articles on dental implants, recognizing trends and advances in a research field is critical and relevant to the needs of dental practitioners and researchers [39,40]. In this sense, bibliometric analysis is a useful tool for this purpose [41,42].

As far as we know, the trends and advances in zirconia dental implants have not been studied before; hence this study aimed to evaluate the bibliometric output of clinical research and co-authors in the field of zirconia dental implant rehabilitations.

2. Materials and Methods

We reported this bibliometric study in compliance with the Standards for Reporting Qualitative Research (SRQR) [43] and the Preferred Reporting Items for Systematic Reviews and Meta-Analyses (PRISMA) guidelines [44].

2.1. Search Strategy

An online literature search was conducted in Elsevier's Scopus and Clarivate Analytics' Web of Science (WoS) until 5 October 2020. We used the medical terms (MeSH) feature in the Cochrane Library to obtain the available synonyms for our search terms to create a detailed search strategy (Table 1).

Table 1. Search strategy used for each database.

Scopus	TITLE-ABS-KEY ("Zirconia" OR "Zirconium" OR "Zircon*") AND TITLE-ABS-KEY ("Dental implant" OR "Dental implants" OR "Oral implant" OR "Oral implants" OR "Implant dentistry" OR "Dental implantology" OR "Dental Implantation" OR "Osseointegrated" OR "Osseointegrated Dental Implantation") AND TITLE-ABS-KEY ("Intervention Study" OR "Clinical Trial" OR "Controlled Clinical Trial" OR "Randomized Controlled Trials OR "Non-Randomized Clinical Trial" OR "Nonrandomized Clinical Trial" OR "Quasi-Experimental" OR "Observational Study" OR "Prospective Study" OR "Prospective" OR "Retrospective Study" OR "Retrospective" OR "Comparative Study" OR "Multicenter Studies" OR "Epidemiologic Study" OR "Epidemiological Studies" OR "Cohort Study" OR "Case Studies" OR "Follow-Up Study" OR "Case-Control Study" OR "Case Report" OR "Case Series" OR "Pilot Study")

Table 1. *Cont.*

Web of Science	TS = ("Zirconia" OR "Zirconium" OR "Zircon*") AND TS = ("Dental implant" OR "Dental implants" OR "Oral implant" OR "Oral implants" OR "Implant dentistry" OR "Dental implantology" OR "Dental Implantation" OR "Osseointegrated" OR "Osseointegrated Dental Implantation") AND TS = ("Intervention Study" OR "Clinical Trial" OR "Controlled Clinical Trial OR "Randomized Controlled Trials" OR "Non-Randomized Clinical Trial" OR "Nonrandomized Clinical Trial" OR "Quasi-Experimental" OR "Observational Study" OR "Prospective Study" OR "Prospective" OR "Retrospective Study" OR "Retrospective" OR "Comparative Study" OR "Multicenter Studies" OR "Epidemiologic Study" OR "Epidemiological Studies" OR "Cohort Study" OR "Case Studies" OR "Follow-Up Study" OR "Case-Control Study" OR "Case Report" OR "Case Series" OR "Pilot Study") **Timespan:** All years. **Databases:** WOS, ARCI, BCI, KJD, MEDLINE, RSCI, SCIELO, ZOOREC. Search language = Auto.

2.2. Data Extraction and Bibliometric Parameters

We used a specially built Excel file (Microsoft, Redmond, WA, USA) to collect the findings of the literature search. The file contained the following information: abstracts, year of publication, indexed keywords, journal name, citations as well as all co-author bibliometric data (H-index, number of papers related to zirconia implant, the total number of papers, citation of paper regarding zirconia implant, and citation of paper regarding zirconia implant). Authors with the highest quantity of clinical studies regarding zirconia dental implants were evaluated and measured the average, the standard deviation, minimum and maximum of topic paper, total papers, topic citations, overall citations, and H-index. Moreover, we evaluated the scientific trend of the included study according to the year of publication and journal details (full title, the impact factor (IF), and rank) based on the Clarivate Analytics report for 2019 with selected categories: "Dentistry, Oral Surgery & Medicine", study design, number of citations received, marginal bone loss, survival rate, failure, and study follow-up.

2.3. Study Selection

We screened the literature search results in two steps, where the first phase was the screening of the title and abstract by paired reviewers separately. Then, the second phase was a full-text assessment by two expert reviewers (L.F and A.S). The reference list of the studies included in the full-text screening was hand-screened for potential additional studies. In this bibliometric study, inclusion criteria were only clinical studies (either prospective or retrospective) without time restrictions. Exclusion criteria were animal studies, in vitro studies, literature reviews, systematic reviews, short communications, personal opinion, letters, book chapters, and non-English studies.

2.4. Data Analysis

We used VOSviewer software (version 1.6.8; Leiden University, Leiden, The Netherlands) to visualize a term map analyzing keywords from the data obtained. "Create Map" function was used to analyze the data by using the "Citation" type and setting the unit of analysis as a "number of citations." In the keyword map, the node's size reflects the number of received citations, as the larger size indicates the author with the highest citations. Furthermore, keywords that often appeared together were classified as the same color in network visualization mode [45,46].

3. Results

3.1. Study Selection

A total of 1159 references were collected from electronic databases in which (n = 185) were omitted due to duplication. By title and abstract, 968 articles were screened and 841 excluded as irrelevant topics. By the full-text screening of 127 papers, 29 studies were included in this bibliometric study [47–75] excluding the remaining 98 articles because they did not meet our inclusion criteria (Figure 1).

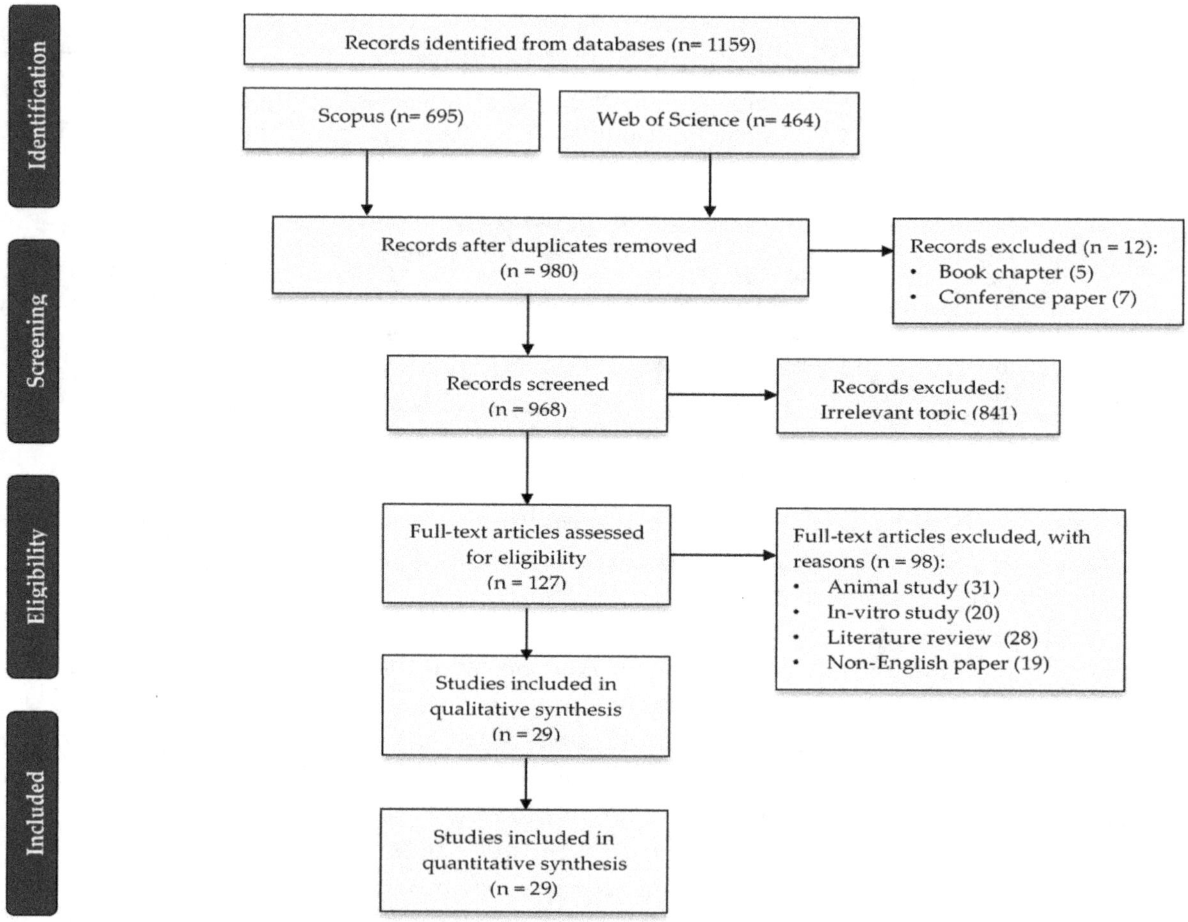

Figure 1. Preferred Reporting Items for Systematic Reviews and Meta-Analyses (PRISMA) flow chart demonstrates the process of literature search and study selection.

3.2. Study Characteristics

The included studies showed wide variability in the study design, presence/absence of a control group, experimental site, type of prosthetic rehabilitation, prosthetic connection (one-piece or two-piece), follow-up period, and different methods for evaluating the effectiveness of research. Although these differences exist, most studies reported favorable outcomes for the use of zirconia implants in oral rehabilitation. The main characteristics of the included studies are summarized in Table 2.

A total of 21 studies evaluated monolithic or one-piece zirconia implants [47–49,51–54,56–58,60, 62,64,66,70–74,76], two of which had titanium implants as their control and showed no significant difference in survival rate and marginal bone loss between groups ($p > 0.05$) [64,70]. Two studies evaluated the immediate loading of zirconia implants [53,64]: one study compared it to the non-occlusal loading procedure [64], while the other study compared it with the standard loading protocol [57]. Furthermore, 26 papers assessed the cylindrical microgeometry of zirconia implants [47–65,67,70–75], while three studies evaluated the root-analog zirconia implants obtained by a three-dimensional scan [66,68,69]. However, Akça et al. and Pirker et al. reported the lowest marginal bone loss after two years (0.31 ± 0.24 and 0.5 ± 0.7 mm, respectively), in which Akça et al. used specially designed titanium–zirconia alloy implants [47], and Pirker et al. used specially designed root-analog zirconia implants with a micro-retention surface in a fresh extraction socket [69].

Table 2. Main characteristics of the clinical research included (Zir: Zirconia implant group, Tit: Titanium implant group, IF: impact factor, RCT: Randomized controlled trial).

Authors (Year) [Ref]	Journal			Cited By	Study Design	Patients (Implants)	Test	Control	Marginal Bone Loss (Mean ± SD)	Survival Rate	Failure	Follow Up
	Full Title	Rank	IF									
Pirker et al. (2008) [68]	International Journal of Oral and Maxillofacial Surgery	33	2.068	50	Case report	1 (1 Implant)	Microretention and sandblasted root-analogue zirconia implant	-	-	100%	-	2 years
Pirker et al. (2009) [69]	International Journal of Oral and Maxillofacial Surgery	33	2.068	58	Prospective Case Series	18 (18 Implants)	Microretention and sandblasted root-analogue zirconia implants	Sandblasted root-analogue zirconia implants	0.5 ± 0.7 mm	Test: 92% Control: 0%	Test: 1 implant Control: All implants (6)	2 years
Cannizzaro et al. (2010) [54]	European Journal of Implantology	-	-	69	Multicenter RCT	40 (40 Implants)	Immediate occlusal loading zirconia Implants	Immediate non-occlusal loading zirconia Implants	Test: 0.90 ± 0.48 mm Control: 0.72 ± 0.59 mm	88.50%	5 implants (12.5%): Test: 3 Implants Control: 2 Implants	1 year
Borgonovo et al. (2011) [51]	Minerva Stomatologica	-	-	21	Prospective Case Series	16 (26 Implants)	One-piece yttrium stabilized zirconia implants	-	-	96.16%	1 Implant osseointegration failure	2 years
Payer et al. (2012) [66]	Clinical Oral Implants Research	8	3.723	61	Prospective Case Series	20 (20 Implants)	One-piece zirconia implants	-	1.29 ± 0.73 mm	95%	1 Implant osseointegration failure	2 years
Akça et al. (2013) [47]	International Journal of Oral and Maxillofacial Implants	24	2.32	8	Prospective Case Series	23 (52 Implants)	-	-	0.32 ± 0.24 mm	100%	No failure	2 years
Borgonovo et al. (2013) [52]	Minerva Stomatologica	-	-	10	Prospective Case Series	6 (14 Implants)	One-piece yttrium stabilized zirconia implants	-	0.67 ± 0.51 mm	100%	No failure	4 years
Kohal et al. (2013) [59]	Journal of Clinical Periodontology	2	5.241	47	Prospective Case Series	28 (56 Implants)	One-piece yttria-stabilized tetragonal zirconia implants	-	1.95 ± 0.65	98.20%	1 Implant osseointegration failure	1 year
Osman et al. (2013) [63]	International Journal of Prosthodontics	61	1.49	6	Pilot study	4 (28 Implants)	One-piece zirconia implants for ball abutment	-	-	85.70%	4 Implants	1 year
Osman et al. (2014) [64]	Clinical Oral Implants Research	8	3.723	34	RCT	19 (129 Implants)	One-piece zirconia implants for ball-abutment	One-piece titanium implants for ball-abutment	Zir: 0.42 ± 0.40 Tit: 0.18 ± 0.47	Zir: 90.9%Tit: 95.8%	Zir: 21Implants (3 fractured) Tit: 10Implants	1 year
Becker et al. (2015) [50]	Clinical Oral Implants Research	8	3.723	15	Prospective Cohort Study	52 (52 Implants)	Two-piece zirconia implants	-	-	95.80%	2 Implants	2 years
Cionca et al. (2015) [55]	Clinical Oral Implants Research	8	3.723	43	Prospective Case Series	32 (49 Implants)	Two-piece zirconia implants	-	-	87%	6 Implants	1 year

Table 2. *Cont.*

Authors (Year) [Ref]	Journal Full Title	Rank	IF	Cited By	Study Design	Patients (Implants)	Test	Control	Marginal Bone Loss (Mean ± SD)	Survival Rate	Failure	Follow Up
Jung et al. (2015) [56]	Clinical Oral Implants Research	8	3.723	27	Prospective Cohort Study	60 (71 Implants)	Immediate one-piece zirconia implants	-	0.78 ± 0.79 mm	98.30%	1 implant osseointegration failure	1 year
Payer et al. (2015) [67]	Clinical Oral Implants Research	8	3.723	41	RCT	22 (31 Implants)	Two-piece zirconia implants	Two-piece titanium implants	Zir: 1.48 ± 1.05 Tit: 1.43 ± 0.67	Zir: 93.3% Tit: 100%	Zir: 1 Implant Tit: No failure	2 years
Siddiqi et al. (2015) [70]	Clinical Implant Dentistry and Related Research	9	3.396	17	RCT	22 (150 Implants)	One-piece zirconia implants for ball-abutment	Titanium implants for one-piece ball-abutment	Zir: 2.23 ± 0.69 Tit: 1.59 ± 0.33	Zir: 67.6% Tit: 66.7%	Zir: 16 Implants Tit: 7 Implants	1 year
Spies et al. (2015) [73]	Journal of Dental Research	3	4.914	22	Prospective Cohort Study	40 (53 Implants)	One-piece alumina-toughened zirconia implant	-	0.79 ± 0.47 mm	94.2%	3 Implants osseointegration failure	3 years
Patankar et al. (2016) [65]	Journal of Maxillofacial and Oral Surgery	-	-	3	Case report	1 (1 Implant)	Microretention and sandblasted root-analogue zirconia implant	-	-	100%	-	1.5 year
Spies et al. (2016) [74]	Clinical Oral Implants Research	8	3.723	13	Prospective Cohort Study	27 (27 Implants)	Immediate one-piece alumina-toughened zirconia implant	-	0.77 ± 0.31 mm	88.90%	3 Implants osseointegration failure	1 year
Kniha et al. (2017) [58]	International Journal of Oral and Maxillofacial Surgery	33	2.068	9	Prospective Cohort Study	81 (105 Implants)	Zirconia implants	-	0.66 ± 0.33 mm	100%	No failure	3 years
Kniha et al. (2017) [57]	International Journal of Oral and Maxillofacial Surgery	33	2.068	9	Prospective Cohort Study	78 (82 Implants)	Immediate loading one-piece zirconia implants	Delayed one-piece zirconia implants	Immediate: 0.76 ± 1.13 mm Delayed: 0.83 ± 0.65 mm	Immediate: 100% Delayed: 100%	No failure	1 year
Spies et al. (2017) [71]	Journal of Dentistry	10	3.242	6	Prospective Case Series	60 (71 Implants)	One-piece zirconia oral implants	-	-	100%	No failure	3 years
Spies et al. (2017) [75]	Clinical Oral Implants Research	8	3.723	11	Prospective Case Series	13 (26 Implants)	One-piece zirconia implants	-	-	100%	No failure	5 years
Balmer et al. (2018) [49]	Clinical Oral Implants Research	8	3.723	11	Prospective Multicenter Cohort Study	60 (71 Implants)	One-piece immediate loading zirconia implants	-	0.70 ± 0.72 mm	98.50%	1 Implant osseointegration failure	3 years
Bormann et al. (2018) [53]	BMC Oral Health	38	1.911	7	Prospective Multicenter Cohort Study	44 (44 Implants)	Zirconia implants	-	0.97 ± 0.88 mm	97.50%	1 Implant	3 years
Kohal et al. (2018) [60]	Journal of Clinical Periodontology	2	5.241	5	Prospective Cohort Study	65 (65 Implants)	Immediate loading one-piece zirconia implants	-	1.45 ± 1.96 mm	90.80%	6 Implants	3 years

Table 2. *Cont.*

Authors (Year) [Ref]	Journal			Cited By	Study Design	Patients (Implants)	Test	Control	Marginal Bone Loss (Mean ± SD)	Survival Rate	Failure	Follow Up
	Full Title	Rank	IF									
Lorenz et al. (2019) [62]	Clinical Implant Dentistry and Related Research	9	3.396	4	Prospective Cohort Study	28 (83 Implants)	Zirconia implants	Natural teeth	1.2 ± 0.76 mm	100%	No failure one peri-implantitis resistant to therapies	7.8 years
Spies et al. (2019) [72]	Clinical Oral Implants Research	8	3.723	5	Prospective Multicenter Cohort Study	45 (45 Implants)	Zirconia implants	-	-	97.5 ± 2.47%.	Chipping (n = 19) occlusal roughness (n = 35)	5 years
Balmer et al. (2020) [48]	Clinical Oral Implants Research	8	3.723	4	Prospective Multicenter Cohort Study	60 (71 Implants)	Single crown one-piece zirconia implant	Multiple prostheses one-piece zirconia implant	0.7 ± 0.6 mm	98.4%	1 Implant	5 years
Koller et al. (2020) [61]	Clinical Oral Implants Research	8	3.723	0	Pilot RCT	22 (31 Implants)	Two-piece zirconia implants	Two-piece titanium implants	Zir: 1.38 ± 0.81 Tit: 1.17 ± 0.73 mm	Zir: 87.5%Tit: 93.3%	Zir: 2 Implants Tit: 1 Implant	6.67 years

3.3. Growth of Publications

In total, 29 clinical studies were published between 2008 and 2020, in which 19 papers (65.5%) were published in the last five years and ten papers published before 2015. The highest number of published studies was in 2015 ($n = 6$, 20.6%) followed by 2013 and 2017 ($n = 4$, 13.7% for each) (Figure 2).

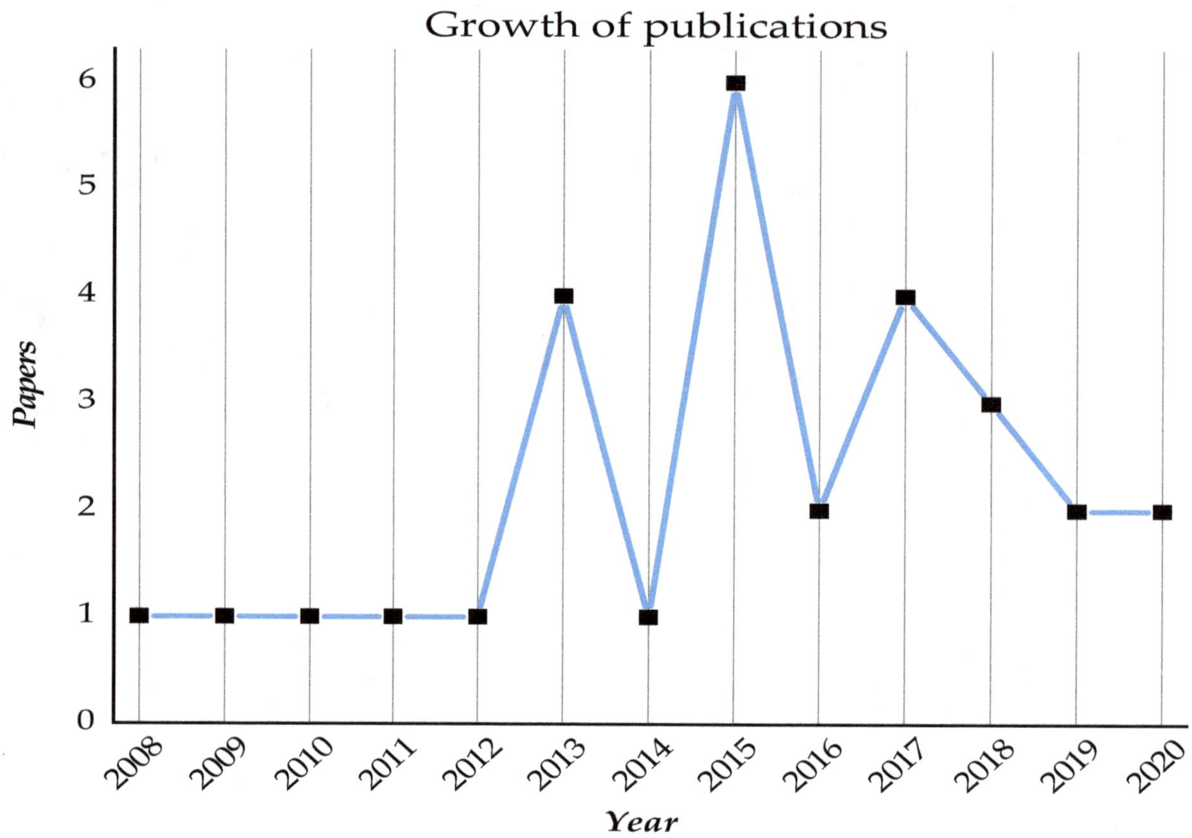

Figure 2. Publication trend of the clinical studies on the zirconia implants.

3.4. Journal of Publication

The clinical studies on the use of zirconia dental implants for oral rehabilitation were published across ten peer-reviewed journals. The journal with the largest number of publications was "Clinical Oral Implants Research" ($n = 12$, 41%), followed by "International Journal of Oral and Maxillofacial Surgery" ($n = 4$, 13.7%) (Figure 3).

The majority of publications were published in Q1 journals ($n = 25$, 86%), while the journal with the highest impact factor was "Journal of Clinical Periodontology" (IF = 5.241), which had two articles.

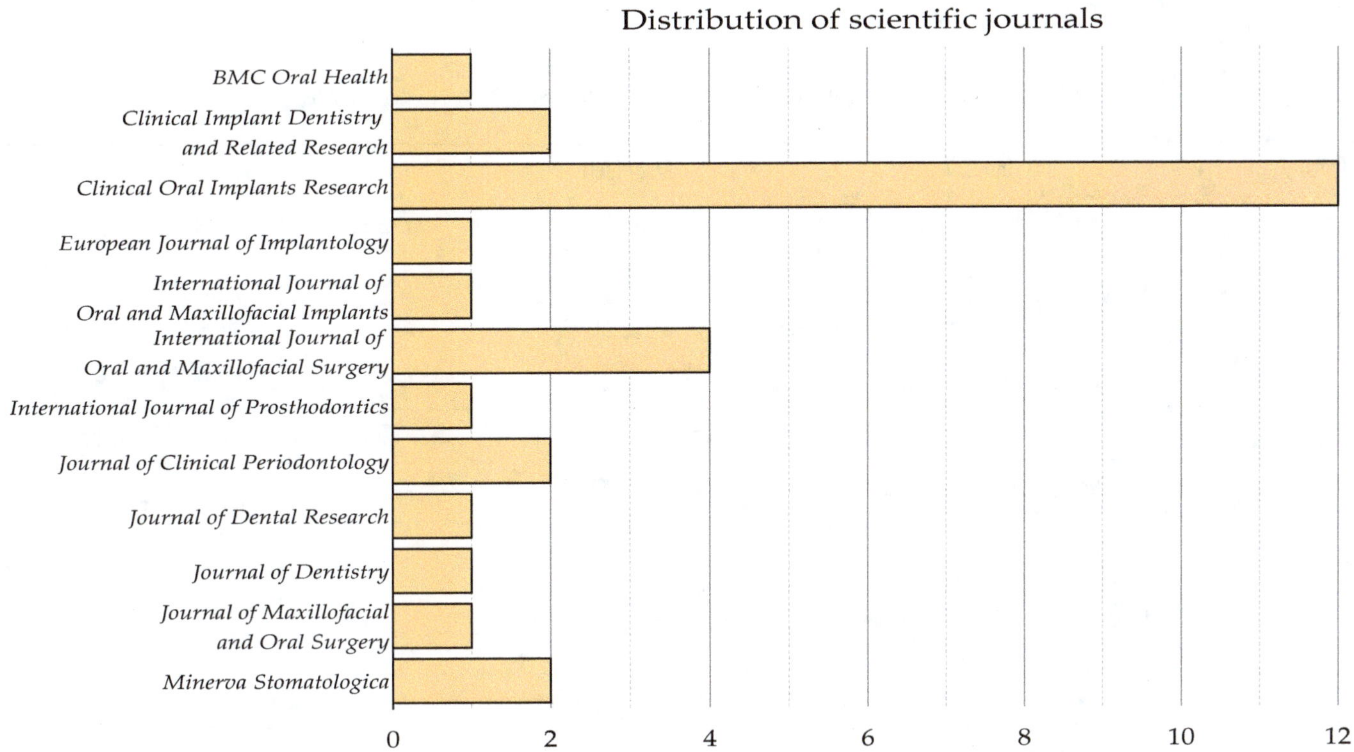

Figure 3. Contribution journals in clinical research on zirconia implants.

3.5. *Study Design and Level of Evidence*

All included studies were prospective, while the most common study design of clinical research on zirconia implants was cohort study (n = 12, 41.4%), followed by case series (n = 9, 31%), and RCT (n = 5, 17%). According to the hierarchy of evidence levels (Is) [77,78], the available evidence supporting the use of zirconia implants is 17% level II, 41.4% EL IV, and the remaining EL VI.

3.6. *Contribution of Countries and Institutions*

The majority of the studies originated from institutions in Germany (n = 14, 48.3%), followed by Switzerland, (n = 6, 20.7%), and Austria (n = 5, 17%), where the most productive institution was the Medical Center of University of Freiburg (n = 8, 27.6%), followed by the Center of Dental Medicine, University of Zürich (n = 5, 17%). While many of the included studies were funded, the most funding support for included research was provided by VITA Zahnfabrik—H. Rauter GmbH & Co. KG, Bad Säckingen, Germany (n = 5, 17%) (Table 3).

Table 3. Contribution of countries and institutions to clinical studies on zirconia implants.

Country	Institution	Study [Ref]	Funding
Germany	Universitätsklinikum Düsseldorf, Düsseldorf	Becker et al., 2015 [50]	ZV3 Zircon Vision GmbH, Wolfratshausen, Germany
	University Hospital Aachen, Aachen	Kniha et al., 2017 [57]	No Funding
	Friedrich-Alexander-University Erlangen-Nürnberg	Kniha et al., 2017 [58]	
	Johann-Wolfgang Goethe University, Frankfurt/Main	Lorenz et al., 2019 [62]	
	Hannover Medical School, Hannover	Bormann et al., 2018 [53]	Institut Straumann AG, Basel, Switzerland
	School of Dentistry, Albert-Ludwigs University, Freiburg	Kohal et al., 2013 [59]	Nobel Biocare AB, Göteborg, Sweden
	Medical Center of University of Freiburg, Freiburg	Kohal et al., 2018 [60]	
		Spies et al., 2015 [73]	Metoxit AG (Thayngen, Switzerland)
		Spies et al., 2016 [74]	
		Spies et al., 2017 [75]	Ivoclar Vivadent
Germany and Switzerland	Medical Center of University of Freiburg, Freiburg and Center of Dental Medicine, University of Zürich, Zürich	Spies et al., 2017 [71]	VITA Zahnfabrik—H. Rauter GmbH & Co. KG, Bad Säckingen, Germany
		Balmer et al., 2018 [49]	
		Spies et al., 2019 [72]	
		Balmer et al., 2020 [48]	
Switzerland	School of Dental Medicine, University of Geneva, Geneva	Cionca et al., 2015 [55]	Dentalpoint AG, Zürich, Switzerland
	Center of Dental Medicine, University of Zürich, Zürich	Jung et al., 2015 [56]	VITA Zahnfabrik—H. Rauter GmbH & Co. KG, Bad Säckingen, Germany
Austria	Alfred Kocher, Medical University Vienna, Vienna	Pirker et al., 2008 [68]	No Funding
		Pirker et al., 2009 [69]	
	School of Dentistry, Medical University Graz, Graz	Payer et al., 2012 [66]	Bredent medical GmbH, Senden, Germany
		Payer et al., 2015 [67]	Ziterion GmbH, Uffenheim, Germany
		Koller et al., 2020 [61]	
Italy	Private practice	Cannizzaro et al., 2010 [54]	Partially supported by Z-systems
	School of Dentistry, University of Milan, Milan	Borgonovo et al., 2011 [51]	Not reported
		Borgonovo et al., 2013 [52]	
New Zealand	Oral Implantology Research Group, Sir John Walsh Research Institute, School of Dentistry, University of Otago	Osman et al., 2013 [63]	Oral Implantology Research Group, Sir John Walsh Research Institute, School of Dentistry, University of Otago and Southern Implants
		Osman et al., 2014 [64]	
		Siddiqi et al., 2015 [70]	
India	BV Dental College and Hospital, Pune	Patankar et al., 2016 [65]	No Funding
Turkey	Faculty of Dentistry, Hacettepe University	Akça et al., 2013 [47]	No Funding

3.7. Bibliometric Assessment

A total of 29 articles with total citations$_{[Scopus]}$ ranged from 0 to 176 (mean 57.28 ± 42.18), while the number of citations$_{[Scopus]}$ received by each paper ranged from 0 to 69 (mean 21.3 ± 20). The top-cited study was the RCT of Cannizzaro et al. (2010) ($n_{[Scopus]}$ = 69) [54], followed by the prospective case series of Payer et al. (2012) ($n_{[Scopus]}$ = 61) [66], and Pirker et al. (2009) ($n_{[Scopus]}$ = 58) [69].

However, the author with the highest number of clinical research on zirconia implants was Kohal R.J. (n = 10), followed by Spies B.C. (n = 8) and Vach K. (n = 6), while the top-cited author of clinical studies on zirconia implants was Kohal R.J. ($n_{[WoS]}$ = 155), followed by Arnetzl G. ($n_{[WoS]}$ = 91), Koller M. ($n_{[WoS]}$ = 87), Payer M., and Jakse N. ($n_{[WoS]}$ = 86 for each) (Figures 4 and 5).

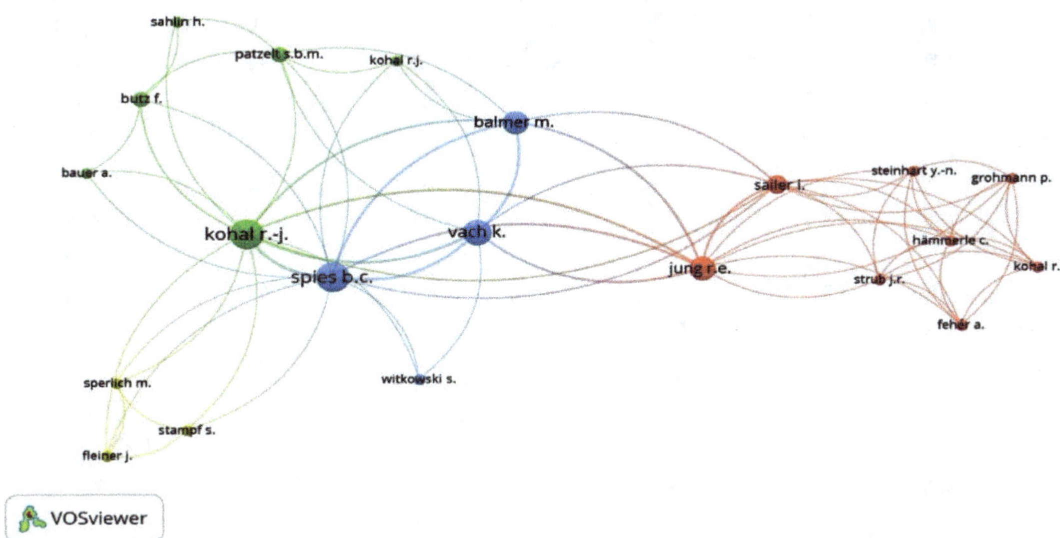

Figure 4. Network analysis of the authors with the largest number of clinical studies on zirconia implants.

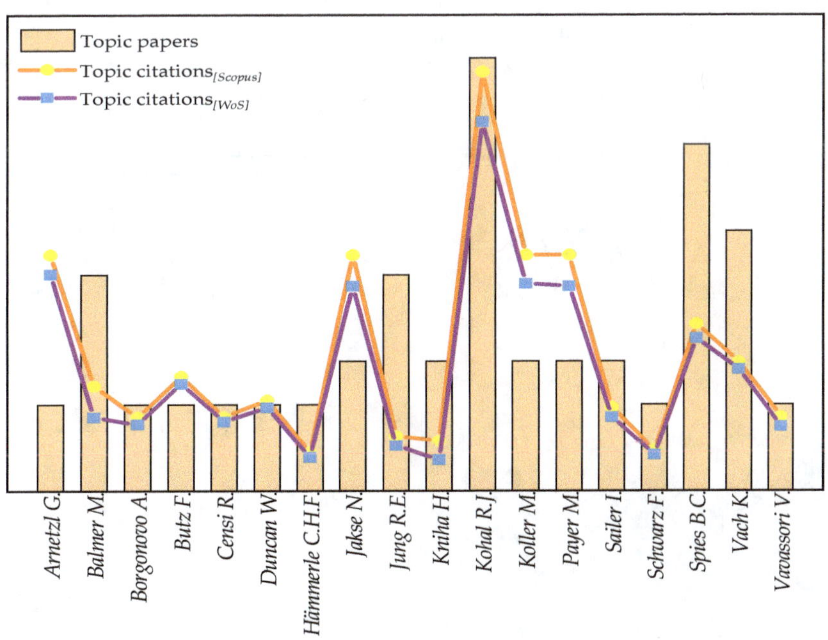

Figure 5. Bibliometric variables for authors with the highest number of topic papers.

The authors' H-index$_{Scopus}$ ranged from one to 79 (mean 22.67 ± 19.96), and the author with the most bibliometric characteristics was Hämmerle C.H.F., who had 364 publications (two of which were clinical studies on zirconia implants) with 8311 total citations and H-index$_{Scopus}$ = 79 (Table 4 and Figure 6).

Table 4. General bibliometric variables for authors with the largest number of topic papers.

Author	Topic Papers	Total Papers	Topic/Total Papers %	Topic Citations [Scopus]	Topic Citations [WoS]	Total Citations [Scopus]	Total Citation [WoS]	Topic/Total Citations % [Scopus-WoS]	H-index [Scopus]	H-index [WoS]
Kohal R.J.	10	109	9.17%	176	155	3053	2975	[5.76–5.21%]	30	29
Spies B.C.	8	47	17.02%	70	64	452	448	[15.49–14.29%]	14	14
Vach K.	6	73	8.22%	54	51	661	820	[8.17–6.21%]	15	16
Balmer M.	5	13	38.46%	44	31	256	130	[17.19–23.84%]	7	5
Jung R.E.	5	202	2.48%	23	19	8359	9126	[0.28–0.21%]	47	57
Jakse N.	3	70	4.29%	99	86	1114	981	[8.89–8.77%]	18	18
Kniha H.	3	28	10.71%	21	13	664	726	[3.16–1.779%]	11	13
Koller M.	3	9	33.33%	99	87	166	312	[59.64–27.88%]	5	5
Payer M.	3	48	6.25%	99	86	770	1484	[12.86–5.79%]	15	23
Sailer I.	3	113	2.65%	35	31	6027	5713	[0.58–0.54%]	34	33
Arnetzl G.	2	40	5.00%	99	91	437	183	[22.65–49.72%]	11	6
Butz F.	2	24	8.33%	48	45	1248	1441	[3.85–3.12%]	18	19
Censi R.	2	18	11.11%	31	29	169	95	[18.34–30.52%]	8	4
Duncan W.	2	87	2.30%	38	35	2163	1356	[1.76–2.58%]	20	19
Hämmerle C.H.F.	2	364	0.55%	16	14	18,311	16,032	[0.09–0.08%]	79	72
Schwarz F.	2	261	0.77%	17	15	9093	9169	[0.19–0.16%]	57	57
Vavassori V.	2	12	16.67%	31	27	136	96	[22.79–28.12%]	7	5
Borgonovo A.	2	51	3.92%	31	28	535	449	[5.79–6.23%]	12	11
Summary (Mean ± SD)	3.61 ± 2.33	87.17 ± 96.37	10.07 ± 0.11%	57.28 ± 42.18	50.39 ± 37.68	2978.56 ± 4750.05	2863.11 ± 4386.90	-	22.67 ± 19.96	22.56 ± 20.14

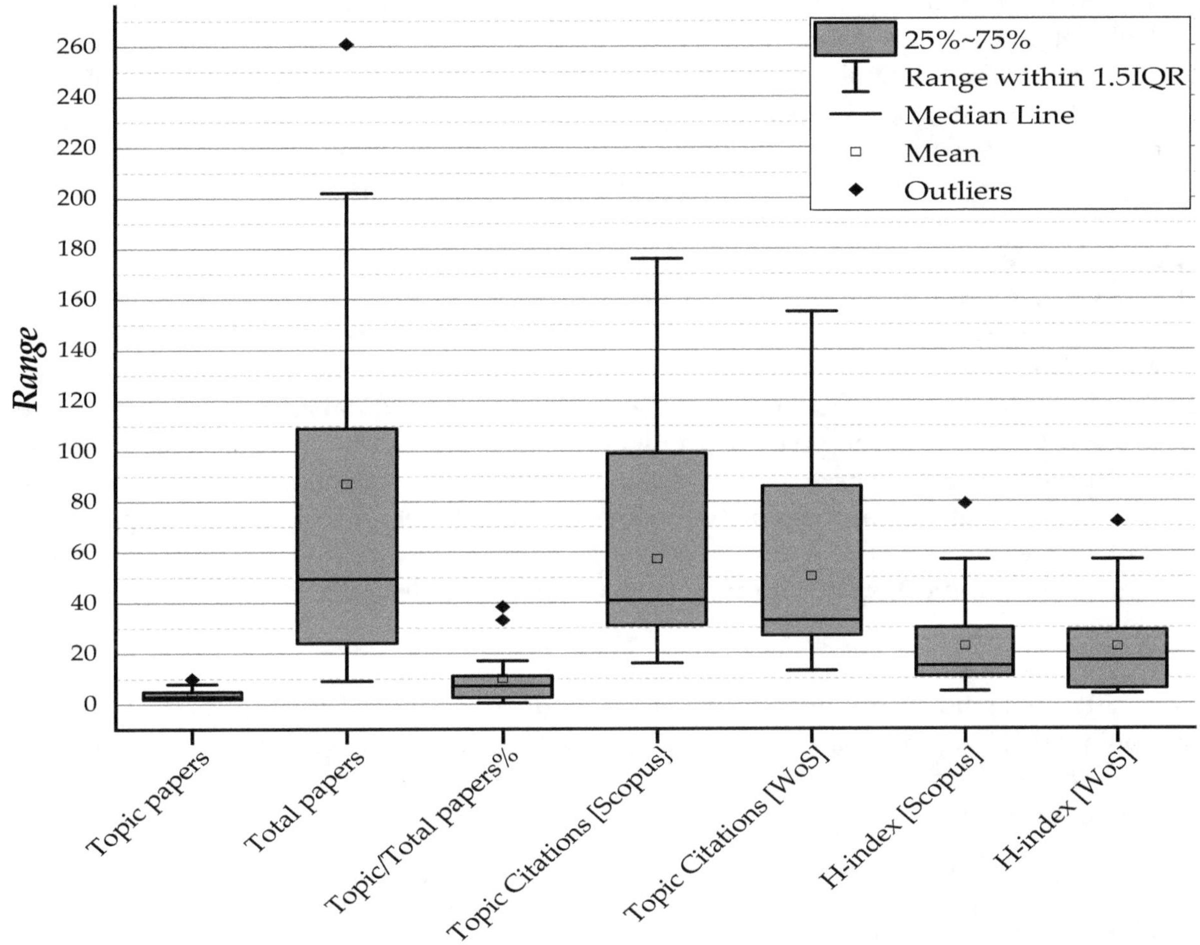

Figure 6. Box plots summarize the bibliometric variables of the authors with the largest number of studies.

4. Discussion

The present study carried out a bibliometric evaluation of clinical research on zirconia implant rehabilitation, highlighting the significant heterogeneity of the included studies, which revealed considerable variations in methodology, technical approaches, follow-up, and control group involvement. Our findings indicate that there is a trend for zirconia implants in oral rehabilitation as there has been an increase in about 180% of the studies published in the last five years.

The included studies reported a survival rate for zirconia implants ranging from 87% to 100% with follow-up periods from one to 7.8 years, while the least survival rate reported in RCT by Siddiqi et al. was 67.6% after one-year follow-up (i.e., 16 zirconia implants failed out of 68) [70]. This RCT aimed to study the effectiveness of zirconia vs. titanium implants restored with one-piece ball-abutment in mandibular and maxillary overdentures, while this high decrease in the survival rate was for both groups (i.e., 67.6% for zirconia implants and 66.7% for titanium implants); the outcomes of maxillary rehabilitation were worse than the mandible, while no mechanical fractures of the fixtures were reported [70].

Although one-piece and two-piece zirconia implants have been evaluated, the lower marginal bone loss and higher survival rates were observed in studies of one-piece zirconia implant rehabilitation on a single tooth or three element prosthetic rehabilitation [59,61]. However, the studies did not report any differences in the marginal bone loss and survival rate between the single crown and the fixed multiple zirconia implant recovery, while the prosthetic connection appears to have no apparent effect on these parameters [48]. Additionally, Lorenz et al. showed no significant difference in marginal bone loss with a total of 83 zirconia implants compared to natural teeth after 7.8 years of function [47], and the marginal bone loss was similar in the other studies, which was less than 1 mm in the first year and stabilized in subsequent functional loading [47–49,52,56–58,64,69,73,74]. Moreover, the prospective study by Kniha et al. contained the largest sample size of the included studies involving 81 patients with 105 implants for fixed rehabilitation, who reported a significant decrease of 0.66 ± 0.30 mm with a survival rate of 100% after three years [58].

However, the most common complication (70%) was the failure of implant osseointegration as 17 studies reported a loss of at least one implant in the first six months [48–51,53–56,59–61,63,64,66,67, 69,70,72–74].

As previously reported for titanium dental implant threads, microgeometry appears to have a significant effect on the osseointegration of zirconia implants [79,80], whereas a more retentive surface resulted in an increased survival rate compared to a sandblasted surface only [68,69].

Although all clinical research included in this analysis was screened and selected from the Scopus and Web of Science databases, which may avoid restriction in each database [39,81], our investigation has further limitations. First, the year of publication, which is a reliable indicator of the number of citations received, as older papers receive more citations than recent publications because there is more time to cite them, regardless of their impact [82,83]. Second, open access policies have a significant influence on the citations received in the evaluated papers [84–86], as a result, we found large heterogeneity in Topic/Total Citations% and co-authors' H-index.

5. Conclusions

This was the first study highlighting bibliometric output of clinical research and co-authors in the field of zirconia dental implants and shows a strong interest in the development of research into the clinical application of zirconia dental implants, as evidenced by the increase in the number of scientific papers published in the last ten years.

Author Contributions: Conceptualization, F.L. and A.S.; Methodology, F.L. and A.G.A.K.; Software, F.L.; Validation, F.L. and A.S.; Formal analysis, F.L. and A.G.A.K.; Investigation, A.S., F.L. and B.R.; Data curation, F.L., A.G.A.K. and A.S.; Writing—original draft preparation, F.L. and A.S.; Writing—review and editing, F.L., A.G.A.K. and S.N.; Visualization, A.S., B.R. and I.F.; Supervision, A.S. and I.F. All authors have read and agreed to the published version of the manuscript.

References

1. Albrektsson, T.; Wennerberg, A. On osseointegration in relation to implant surfaces. *Clin. Implant Dent. Relat. Res.* **2019**, *21* (Suppl. 1), 4–7. [CrossRef]
2. Buser, D.; Janner, S.F.M.; Wittneben, J.-G.; Brägger, U.; Ramseier, C.A.; Salvi, G.E. 10-Year Survival and Success Rates of 511 Titanium Implants with a Sandblasted and Acid-Etched Surface: A Retrospective Study in 303 Partially Edentulous Patients. *Clin. Implant Dent. Relat. Res.* **2012**, *14*, 839–851. [CrossRef] [PubMed]
3. Degidi, M.; Piattelli, A. A 7-year Follow-up of 93 Immediately Loaded Titanium Dental Implants. *J. Oral Implantol.* **2005**, *31*, 25–31. [CrossRef] [PubMed]
4. Scarano, A.; Inchingolo, F.; Murmura, G.; Traini, T.; Piattelli, A.; Lorusso, F. Three-Dimensional Architecture and Mechanical Properties of Bovine Bone Mixed with Autologous Platelet Liquid, Blood, or Physiological Water: An In Vitro Study. *Int. J. Mol. Sci.* **2018**, *19*. [CrossRef] [PubMed]
5. Barros, R.R.M.; Degidi, M.; Novaes, A.B.; Piattelli, A.; Shibli, J.A.; Iezzi, G. Osteocyte Density in the Peri-Implant Bone of Immediately Loaded and Submerged Dental Implants. *J. Periodontol.* **2009**, *80*, 499–504. [CrossRef]
6. Gehrke, S.; Mazón, P.; Del Fabbro, M.; Tumedei, M.; Aramburú Júnior, J.; Pérez-Díaz, L.; De Aza, P. Histological and Histomorphometric Analyses of Two Bovine Bone Blocks Implanted in Rabbit Calvaria. *Symmetry* **2019**, *11*, 641. [CrossRef]
7. Scarano, A.; Carinci, F.; Lorusso, F.; Festa, F.; Bevilacqua, L.; Santos de Oliveira, P.; Maglione, M. Ultrasonic vs Drill Implant Site Preparation: Post-Operative Pain Measurement Through VAS, Swelling and Crestal Bone Remodeling: A Randomized Clinical Study. *Mater. Basel* **2018**, *11*, 2516. [CrossRef]

8. Scarano, A.; Crincoli, V.; Di Benedetto, A.; Cozzolino, V.; Lorusso, F.; Podaliri Vulpiani, M.; Grano, M.; Kalemaj, Z.; Mori, G.; Grassi, F.R. Bone Regeneration Induced by Bone Porcine Block with Bone Marrow Stromal Stem Cells in a Minipig Model of Mandibular "Critical Size" Defect. *Stem. Cells Int.* **2017**, *2017*, 9082869. [CrossRef]
9. Scarano, A.; De Oliveira, P.S.; Traini, T.; Lorusso, F. Sinus Membrane Elevation with Heterologous Cortical Lamina: A Randomized Study of a New Surgical Technique for Maxillary Sinus Floor Augmentation without Bone Graft. *Mater. Basel* **2018**, *11*, 1457. [CrossRef]
10. Piattelli, A.; Scarano, A.; Piattelli, M. Detection of alkaline and acid phosphatases around titanium implants: A light microscopical and histochemical study in rabbits. *Biomaterials.* **1995**, *16*, 1333–1338. [CrossRef]
11. Comuzzi, L.; Tumedei, M.; Piattelli, A.; Iezzi, G. Short vs. Standard Length Cone Morse Connection Implants: An In Vitro Pilot Study in Low Density Polyurethane Foam. *Symmetry* **2019**, *11*, 1349. [CrossRef]
12. Tumedei, M.; Savadori, P.; Del Fabbro, M. Synthetic Blocks for Bone Regeneration: A Systematic Review and Meta-Analysis. *Int. J. Mol. Sci.* **2019**, *20*, 4221. [CrossRef] [PubMed]
13. Afrashtehfar, K.I.; Del Fabbro, M. Clinical performance of zirconia implants: A meta-review. *J. Prosthet. Dent.* **2020**, *123*, 419–426. [CrossRef] [PubMed]
14. Hanawa, T. Zirconia versus titanium in dentistry: A review. *Dent. Mater. J.* **2020**, *39*, 24–36. [CrossRef] [PubMed]
15. Hashim, D.; Cionca, N.; Courvoisier, D.S.; Mombelli, A. A systematic review of the clinical survival of zirconia implants. *Clin. Oral Investig.* **2016**, *20*, 1403–1417. [CrossRef]
16. Cantore, S.; Mirgaldi, R.; Ballini, A.; Coscia, M.F.; Scacco, S.; Papa, F.; Inchingolo, F.; Dipalma, G.; De Vito, D. Cytokine gene polymorphisms associate with microbiogical agents in periodontal disease: Our experience. *Int. J. Med. Sci.* **2014**, *11*, 674–679. [CrossRef]
17. Noronha Oliveira, M.; Schunemann, W.V.H.; Mathew, M.T.; Henriques, B.; Magini, R.S.; Teughels, W.; Souza, J.C.M. Can degradation products released from dental implants affect peri-implant tissues? *J. Periodontal Res.* **2017**, *53*, 1–11. [CrossRef]
18. Noumbissi, S.; Scarano, A.; Gupta, S. A Literature Review Study on Atomic Ions Dissolution of Titanium and Its Alloys in Implant Dentistry. *Mater. Basel* **2019**, *12*, 368. [CrossRef]
19. Ottria, L.; Lauritano, D.; Andreasi Bassi, M.; Palmieri, A.; Candotto, V.; Tagliabue, A.; Tettamanti, L. Mechanical, chemical and biological aspects of titanium and titanium alloys in implant dentistry. *J. Biol. Regul. Homeost. Agents* **2018**, *32* (Suppl. 1), 81–90.
20. Rodrigues, D.C.; Valderrama, P.; Wilson, T.G.; Palmer, K.; Thomas, A.; Sridhar, S.; Adapalli, A.; Burbano, M.; Wadhwani, C. Titanium Corrosion Mechanisms in the Oral Environment: A Retrieval Study. *Mater. Basel* **2013**, *6*, 5258–5274. [CrossRef]
21. Scarano, A.; Piattelli, M.; Caputi, S.; Favero, G.A.; Piattelli, A. Bacterial Adhesion on Commercially Pure Titanium and Zirconium Oxide Disks: An In Vivo Human Study. *J. Periodontol.* **2004**, *75*, 292–296. [CrossRef] [PubMed]
22. Mihatovic, I.; Golubovic, V.; Becker, J.; Schwarz, F. Bone tissue response to experimental zirconia implants. *Clin. Oral Investig.* **2016**, *21*, 523–532. [CrossRef] [PubMed]
23. Scarano, A.; Di Carlo, F.; Quaranta, M.; Piattelli, A. Bone Response to Zirconia Ceramic Implants: An Experimental Study in Rabbits. *J. Oral Implantol.* **2003**, *29*, 8–12. [CrossRef]
24. Agustín-Panadero, R.; Serra-Pastor, B.; Roig-Vanaclocha, A.; Fons-Font, A.; Solá-Ruiz, M.F. Fracture resistance and the mode of failure produced in metal-free crowns cemented onto zirconia abutments in dental implants. *PLoS ONE* **2019**, *14*, e0220551. [CrossRef] [PubMed]
25. Bethke, A.; Pieralli, S.; Kohal, R.-J.; Burkhardt, F.; von Stein-Lausnitz, M.; Vach, K.; Spies, B.C. Fracture Resistance of Zirconia Oral Implants In Vitro: A Systematic Review and Meta-Analysis. *Mater. Basel* **2020**, *13*, 562. [CrossRef] [PubMed]
26. Sailer, I.; Asgeirsson, A.G.; Thoma, D.S.; Fehmer, V.; Aspelund, T.; Özcan, M.; Pjetursson, B.E. Fracture strength of zirconia implant abutments on narrow diameter implants with internal and external implant abutment connections: A study on the titanium resin base concept. *Clin. Oral Implant. Res.* **2018**, *29*, 411–423. [CrossRef]

27. Cao, Y.; Yu, C.; Wu, Y.; Li, L.; Li, C. Long-Term Survival and Peri-Implant Health of Titanium Implants with Zirconia Abutments: A Systematic Review and Meta-Analysis. *J. Prosthodont.* **2019**, *28*, 883–892. [CrossRef]
28. Fanali, S.; Tumedei, M.; Pignatelli, P.; Inchingolo, F.; Pennacchietti, P.; Pace, G.; Piattelli, A. Implant primary stability with an osteocondensation drilling protocol in different density polyurethane blocks. *Comput. Methods Biomech. Biomed. Eng.* **2020**, 1–7. [CrossRef]
29. Fujiwara, S.; Kato, S.; Bengazi, F.; Urbizo Velez, J.; Tumedei, M.; Kotsu, M.; Botticelli, D. Healing at implants installed in osteotomies prepared either with a piezoelectric device or drills: An experimental study in dogs. *Oral Maxillofac. Surg.* **2020**. [CrossRef]
30. Kermanshah, H.; Geramy, A.; Ebrahimi, S.F.; Bitaraf, T. IPS-Empress II inlay-retained fixed partial denture reinforced with zirconia bar: Three-dimensional finite element andin-vitrostudies. *Acta Odontol. Scand.* **2012**, *70*, 569–576. [CrossRef]
31. Kotsu, M.; Urbizo Velez, J.; Bengazi, F.; Tumedei, M.; Fujiwara, S.; Kato, S.; Botticelli, D. Healing at implants installed from ~ 70- to <10-Ncm insertion torques: An experimental study in dogs. *Oral Maxillofac. Surg.* 2020. [CrossRef]
32. Scarano, A.; Di Carlo, F.; Piattelli, A. Effect of sterilization and cleansing on implantology drills: Zirconia vs steel. *Ital. Oral Surg.* **2008**, *3*, 61–72.
33. Scarano, A.; Valbonetti, L.; Marchetti, M.; Lorusso, F.; Ceccarelli, M. Soft Tissue Augmentation of the Face with Autologous Platelet-Derived Growth Factors and Tricalcium Phosphate. Microtomography Evaluation of Mice. *J Craniofac. Surg.* **2016**, *27*, 1212–1214. [CrossRef] [PubMed]
34. Scarano, A.; Piattelli, A.; Quaranta, A.; Lorusso, F. Bone Response to Two Dental Implants with Different Sandblasted/Acid-Etched Implant Surfaces: A Histological and Histomorphometrical Study in Rabbits. *BioMed Res. Int.* **2017**, *2017*, 8724951. [CrossRef] [PubMed]
35. Ibrahim, G.M.; Carter Snead, O.; Rutka, J.T.; Lozano, A.M. The most cited works in epilepsy: Trends in the "Citation Classics". *Epilepsia* **2012**, *53*, 765–770. [CrossRef]
36. Parker, J.N.; Lortie, C.; Allesina, S. Characterizing a scientific elite: The social characteristics of the most highly cited scientists in environmental science and ecology. *Scientometrics* **2010**, *85*, 129–143. [CrossRef]
37. Park, K.M.; Park, B.S.; Park, S.; Yoon, D.Y.; Bae, J.S. Top-100 cited articles on headache disorders: A bibliometric analysis. *Clin. Neurol. Neurosurg.* **2017**, *157*, 40–45. [CrossRef]
38. Lorusso, F.; Inchingolo, F.; Scarano, A. Scientific Production in Dentistry: The National Panorama through a Bibliometric Study of Italian Academies. *BioMed Res. Int.* **2020**, *2020*, 3468303. [CrossRef]
39. Jayaratne, Y.S.N.; Zwahlen, R.A. The evolution of dental journals from 2003 to 2012: A bibliometric analysis. *PLoS ONE* **2015**, *10*, e0119503. [CrossRef]
40. Pommer, B.; Valkova, V.; Ubaidha Maheen, C.; Fürhauser, L.; Rausch-Fan, X.; Seeman, R. Scientific Interests of 21st Century Clinical Oral Implant Research: Topical Trend Analysis. *Clin. Implant Dent. Relat. Res.* **2015**, *18*, 850–856. [CrossRef]
41. Gutiérrez-Vela, M.M.; Díaz-Haro, A.; Berbel-Salvador, S.; Lucero-Sánchez, A.; Robinson-García, N.; Cutando-Soriano, A. Bibliometric analysis of research on regenerative periodontal surgery during the last 30 years. *J. Clin. Exp. Dent.* **2012**, *4*, e112–e118. [CrossRef] [PubMed]
42. Tetè, S.; Zizzari, V.L.; De Carlo, A.; Lorusso, F.; Di Nicola, M.; Piattelli, A.; Gherlone, E.; Polimeni, A. Characterizing scientific production of Italian Oral Surgery professionals through evaluation of bibliometric indices. *Ann. Di Stomatol.* **2014**, *5*, 23. [CrossRef]
43. O'Brien, B.C.; Harris, I.B.; Beckman, T.J.; Reed, D.A.; Cook, D.A. Standards for Reporting Qualitative Research. *Acad. Med.* **2014**, *89*, 1245–1251. [CrossRef] [PubMed]
44. Liberati, A.; Altman, D.G.; Tetzlaff, J.; Mulrow, C.; Gøtzsche, P.C.; Ioannidis, J.P.A.; Clarke, M.; Devereaux, P.J.; Kleijnen, J.; Moher, D. The PRISMA statement for reporting systematic reviews and meta-analyses of studies that evaluate health care interventions: Explanation and elaboration. *PLoS Med.* **2009**, *6*, e1000100. [CrossRef]
45. Van Eck, N.J.; Waltman, L. Software survey: VOSviewer, a computer program for bibliometric mapping. *Scientometrics* **2010**, *84*, 523–538. [CrossRef]
46. Van Eck, N.J.; Waltman, L. VOSviewer manual. *Leiden Univeristeit Leiden* **2013**, *1*, 1–53.
47. Akça, K.; Cavusoglu, Y.; Uysal, S.; Cehreli, M.C. A Prospective, Open-Ended, Single-Cohort Clinical Trial on Early Loaded Titanium-Zirconia Alloy Implants in Partially Edentulous Patients: Up-to-24-Month Results. *Int. J. Oral Maxillofac. Implant.* **2013**, *28*, 573–578. [CrossRef]

48. Balmer, M.; Spies, B.C.; Kohal, R.J.; Hämmerle, C.H.F.; Vach, K.; Jung, R.E. Zirconia implants restored with single crowns or fixed dental prostheses: 5-year results of a prospective cohort investigation. *Clin. Oral Implant. Res.* **2020**, *31*, 452–462. [CrossRef]
49. Balmer, M.; Spies, B.C.; Vach, K.; Kohal, R.-J.; Hämmerle, C.H.F.; Jung, R.E. Three-year analysis of zirconia implants used for single-tooth replacement and three-unit fixed dental prostheses: A prospective multicenter study. *Clin. Oral Implant. Res.* **2018**, *29*, 290–299. [CrossRef]
50. Becker, J.; John, G.; Becker, K.; Mainusch, S.; Diedrichs, G.; Schwarz, F. Clinical performance of two-piece zirconia implants in the posterior mandible and maxilla: A prospective cohort study over 2 years. *Clin. Oral Implant. Res.* **2015**, *28*, 29–35. [CrossRef]
51. Borgonovo, A.; Censi, R.; Dolci, M.; Vavassori, V.; Bianchi, A.; Maiorana, C. Use of endosseous one-piece yttrium-stabilized zirconia dental implants in premolar region: A two-year clinical preliminary report. *Minerva. Stomatol.* **2011**, *60*, 229–241. [PubMed]
52. Borgonovo, A.; Vavassori, V.; Censi, R.; Calvo, J.; Re, D. Behavior of endosseous one-piece yttrium stabilized zirconia dental implants placed in posterior areas. *Minerva. Stomatol.* **2013**, *62*, 247–257. [PubMed]
53. Bormann, K.-H.; Gellrich, N.-C.; Kniha, H.; Schild, S.; Weingart, D.; Gahlert, M. A prospective clinical study to evaluate the performance of zirconium dioxide dental implants in single-tooth edentulous area: 3-year follow-up. *BMC Oral Health* **2018**, *18*, 181. [CrossRef] [PubMed]
54. Cannizzaro, G.; Torchio, C.; Felice, P.; Leone, M.; Esposito, M. Immediate occlusal versus non-occlusal loading of single zirconia implants. A multicentre pragmatic randomised clinical trial. *Eur. J. Oral Implant.* **2010**, *3*, 111–120.
55. Cionca, N.; Müller, N.; Mombelli, A. Two-piece zirconia implants supporting all-ceramic crowns: A prospective clinical study. *Clin. Oral Implant. Res.* **2015**, *26*, 413–418. [CrossRef]
56. Jung, R.E.; Grohmann, P.; Sailer, I.; Steinhart, Y.-N.; Fehér, A.; Hämmerle, C.; Strub, J.R.; Kohal, R. Evaluation of a one-piece ceramic implant used for single-tooth replacement and three-unit fixed partial dentures: A prospective cohort clinical trial. *Clin. Oral Implant. Res.* **2015**, *27*, 751–761. [CrossRef]
57. Kniha, K.; Kniha, H.; Möhlhenrich, S.C.; Milz, S.; Hölzle, F.; Modabber, A. Papilla and alveolar crest levels in immediate versus delayed single-tooth zirconia implants. *Int. J. Oral Maxillofac. Surg.* **2017**, *46*, 1039–1044. [CrossRef]
58. Kniha, K.; Schlegel, K.A.; Kniha, H.; Modabber, A.; Hölzle, F.; Kniha, K. Evaluation of peri-implant bone levels and soft tissue dimensions around zirconia implants—A three-year follow-up study. *Int. J. Oral Maxillofac. Surg.* **2017**, *47*, 492–498. [CrossRef]
59. Kohal, R.-J.; Patzelt, S.B.M.; Butz, F.; Sahlin, H. One-piece zirconia oral implants: One-year results from a prospective case series. 2. Three-unit fixed dental prosthesis (FDP) reconstruction. *J. Clin. Periodontol.* **2013**, *40*, 553–562. [CrossRef] [PubMed]
60. Kohal, R.-J.; Spies, B.C.; Bauer, A.; Butz, F. One-piece zirconia oral implants for single-tooth replacement: Three-year results from a long-term prospective cohort study. *J. Clin. Periodontol.* **2018**, *45*, 114–124. [CrossRef] [PubMed]
61. Koller, M.; Steyer, E.; Theisen, K.; Stagnell, S.; Jakse, N.; Payer, M. Two-piece zirconia versus titanium implants after 80 months: Clinical outcomes from a prospective randomized pilot trial. *Clin. Oral Implant. Res.* **2020**, *31*, 388–396. [CrossRef] [PubMed]
62. Lorenz, J.; Giulini, N.; Hölscher, W.; Schwiertz, A.; Schwarz, F.; Sader, R. Prospective controlled clinical study investigating long-term clinical parameters, patient satisfaction, and microbial contamination of zirconia implants. *Clin. Implant Dent. Relat. Res.* **2019**, *21*, 263–271. [CrossRef] [PubMed]
63. Osman, R.B.; Payne, A.; Duncan, W.; Ma, S. Zirconia implants supporting overdentures: A pilot study with novel prosthodontic designs. *Int. J. Prosthodont.* **2013**, *26*, 277–281. [CrossRef]
64. Osman, R.B.; Swain, M.V.; Atieh, M.; Ma, S.; Duncan, W. Ceramic implants (Y-TZP): Are they a viable alternative to titanium implants for the support of overdentures? A randomized clinical trial. *Clin. Oral Implant. Res.* **2014**, *25*, 1366–1377. [CrossRef] [PubMed]
65. Patankar, A.; Kshirsagar, R.; Patankar, S.; Pawar, S. Immediate, non submerged root analog zirconia implant in single rooted tooth replacement: Case report with 2 years follow up. *J. Maxillofac. Oral Surg.* **2016**, *15*, 270–273. [CrossRef]

66. Payer, M.; Arnetzl, V.; Kirmeier, R.; Koller, M.; Arnetzl, G.; Jakse, N. Immediate provisional restoration of single-piece zirconia implants: A prospective case series-results after 24 months of clinical function. *Clin. Oral Implant. Res.* **2012**, *24*, 569–575. [CrossRef]
67. Payer, M.; Heschl, A.; Koller, M.; Arnetzl, G.; Lorenzoni, M.; Jakse, N. All-ceramic restoration of zirconia two-piece implants—A randomized controlled clinical trial. *Clin. Oral Implant. Res.* **2015**, *26*, 371–376. [CrossRef]
68. Pirker, W.; Kocher, A. Immediate, non-submerged, root-analogue zirconia implant in single tooth replacement. *Int. J. Oral Maxillofac. Surg.* **2008**, *37*, 293–295. [CrossRef]
69. Pirker, W.; Kocher, A. Immediate, non-submerged, root-analogue zirconia implants placed into single-rooted extraction sockets: 2-year follow-up of a clinical study. *Int. J. Oral Maxillofac. Surg.* **2009**, *38*, 1127–1132. [CrossRef]
70. Siddiqi, A.; Kieser, J.A.; De Silva, R.K.; Thomson, W.M.; Duncan, W.J. Soft and Hard Tissue Response to Zirconia versus Titanium One-Piece Implants Placed in Alveolar and Palatal Sites: A Randomized Control Trial. *Clin. Implant Dent. Relat. Res.* **2015**, *17*, 483–496. [CrossRef]
71. Spies, B.C.; Balmer, M.; Jung, R.E.; Sailer, I.; Vach, K.; Kohal, R.-J. All-ceramic, bi-layered crowns supported by zirconia implants: Three-year results of a prospective multicenter study. *J. Dent.* **2017**, *67*, 58–65. [CrossRef] [PubMed]
72. Spies, B.C.; Balmer, M.; Jung, R.E.; Sailer, I.; Vach, K.; Kohal, R.J. All-ceramic single crowns supported by zirconia implants: 5-year results of a prospective multicenter study. *Clin. Oral Implant. Res.* **2019**, *30*, 466–475. [CrossRef] [PubMed]
73. Spies, B.C.; Balmer, M.; Patzelt, S.B.M.; Vach, K.; Kohal, R.J. Clinical and Patient-reported Outcomes of a Zirconia Oral Implant: Three year Results of a Prospective Cohort Investigation. *J. Dent. Res.* **2015**, *94*, 1385–1391. [CrossRef] [PubMed]
74. Spies, B.C.; Sperlich, M.; Fleiner, J.; Stampf, S.; Kohal, R.-J. Alumina reinforced zirconia implants: 1-year results from a prospective cohort investigation. *Clin. Oral Implant. Res.* **2016**, *27*, 481–490. [CrossRef] [PubMed]
75. Spies, B.C.; Witkowski, S.; Vach, K.; Kohal, R.J. Clinical and patient-reported outcomes of zirconia-based implant fixed dental prostheses: Results of a prospective case series 5 years after implant placement. *Clin. Oral Implant. Res.* **2017**, *29*, 91–99. [CrossRef] [PubMed]
76. Borgonovo, A.-E.; Fabbri, A.; Vavassori, V.; Censi, R.; Maiorana, C. Multiple teeth replacement with endosseous one-piece yttrium-stabilized zirconia dental implants. *Med. Oral Patol. Oral Cir. Bucal.* **2012**, *17*, e981–e987. [CrossRef] [PubMed]
77. Greenhalgh, T. How to read a paper: Getting your bearings (deciding what the paper is about). *BMJ* **1997**, *315*, 243–246. [CrossRef]
78. Guyatt, G.H.; Sackett, D.L.; Sinclair, J.C.; Hayward, R.; Cook, D.J.; Cook, R.J.; Bass, E.; Gerstein, H.; Haynes, B.; Holbrook, A. Users' guides to the medical literature: IX. A method for grading health care recommendations. *JAMA* **1995**, *274*, 1800–1804. [CrossRef]
79. Scarano, A.; Crocetta, E.; Quaranta, A.; Lorusso, F. Influence of the thermal treatment to address a better osseointegration of Ti6Al4V dental implants: Histological and histomorphometrical study in a rabbit model. *BioMed Res. Int.* **2018**. [CrossRef]
80. Scarano, A.; Degidi, M.; Perrotti, V.; Degidi, D.; Piattelli, A.; Iezzi, G. Experimental Evaluation in Rabbits of the Effects of Thread Concavities in Bone Formation with Different Titanium Implant Surfaces. *Clin. Implant Dent. Relat. Res.* **2013**, *16*, 572–581. [CrossRef]
81. Van Eck, N.J.; Waltman, L. Accuracy of citation data in Web of Science and Scopus. *arXiv* **2019**, arXiv:1906.07011.
82. Feijoo, J.F.; Limeres, J.; Fernández-Varela, M.; Ramos, I.; Diz, P. The 100 most cited articles in dentistry. *Clin. Oral Investig.* **2014**, *18*, 699–706. [CrossRef] [PubMed]
83. Ugolini, D.; Neri, M.; Cesario, A.; Bonassi, S.; Milazzo, D.; Bennati, L.; Lapenna, L.M.; Pasqualetti, P. Scientific production in cancer rehabilitation grows higher: A bibliometric analysis. *Supportive Care Cancer* **2012**, *20*, 1629–1638. [CrossRef] [PubMed]
84. Davis, P.M. Open access, readership, citations: A randomized controlled trial of scientific journal publishing. *FASEB J.* **2011**, *25*, 2129–2134. [CrossRef] [PubMed]

85. Gargouri, Y.; Hajjem, C.; Larivière, V.; Gingras, Y.; Carr, L.; Brody, T.; Harnad, S. Self-selected or mandated, open access increases citation impact for higher quality research. *PLoS ONE* **2010**, *5*, e13636. [CrossRef] [PubMed]
86. Hua, F.; Shen, C.; Walsh, T.; Glenny, A.-M.; Worthington, H. Open Access: Concepts, findings, and recommendations for stakeholders in dentistry. *J. Dent.* **2017**, *64*, 13–22. [CrossRef] [PubMed]

3

Healing Pattern Analysis for Dental Implants Using the Mechano-Regulatory Tissue Differentiation Model

Ming-Jun Li †, Pei-Ching Kung †, Yuan-Wei Chang and Nien-Ti Tsou *

Department of Materials Science and Engineering, National Chiao Tung University, Hsin-chu 30010, Taiwan; a0916986941@gmail.com (M.-J.L.); peggygong1014@gmail.com (P.-C.K.); aone.chang@gmail.com (Y.-W.C.)

* Correspondence: tsounienti@nctu.edu.tw

† These authors contributed equally to this work.

Abstract: (1) Background: Our aim is to reveal the influence of the geometry designs on biophysical stimuli and healing patterns. The design guidelines for dental implants can then be provided. (2) Methods: A two-dimensional axisymmetric finite element model was developed based on mechano-regulatory algorithm. The history of tissue differentiation around eight selected implants can be predicted. The performance of the implants was evaluated by bone area (BA), bone-implant contact (BIC); (3) Results: The predicted healing patterns have very good agreement with the experimental observation. Many features observed in literature, such as soft tissues covering on the bone-implant interface; crestal bone loss; the location of bone resorption bumps, were reproduced by the model and explained by analyzing the solid and fluid biophysical stimuli and (4) Conclusions: The results suggested the suitable depth, the steeper slope of the upper flanks, and flat roots of healing chambers can improve the bone ingrowth and osseointegration. The mechanism related to solid and fluid biophysical stimuli were revealed. In addition, the model developed here is efficient, accurate and ready to extend to any geometry of dental implants. It has potential to be used as a clinical application for instant prediction/evaluation of the performance of dental implants.

Keywords: dental implants; mechano-regulatory; tissue differentiation; healing chamber

1. Introduction

Dental implants have been widely used to restore tooth function and esthetics. The success of surgeries is affected by the design of implant shapes, loading conditions, and bone/tissue differentiation around the implant [1]. The healing chamber is defined as the space between the adjacent threads [2]. Proper healing chamber design improves the osseointegration around the implant, and reduces the healing period. Beutel et al. [3] discovered that implants with a trapezoidal healing chamber had the best osseointegration among the cases they considered. Marin et al. [2] designed healing chambers with simple geometrical design, and compared the resulting bone ingrowth through histomorphologic evaluation.

The appropriate design of the healing chamber may vary with the implantation position and the health condition of the patient. Thus, customization, computer-aided design, and additive manufacturing have become important in the dental and healthcare industries. Many new configurations of implants have been proposed in the literature, such as porous [4], gyroid [5], and eagle-beak [6] shapes. It was shown, either experimentally or numerically, that these highly complex shapes performed better than implants manufactured by traditional machining techniques. However, designs are typically based on trial-and-error, and the relationship between the geometry of an implant and osseointegration is still subtle.

The history of bone ingrowth and tissue differentiation after insertion surgery is difficult to be observed experimentally. Thus, numerical methods are used to analyze the healing pattern in the initial stage of fracture healing [7,8]. The mechano-regulatory theory [9–12] is a well-accepted approach to predicting the osseointegration and tissue differentiation around implants [13]. Based on clinical experiments, Pauwels [14] first proposed that the formation of fibrous tissue and cartilage is characterized by the biophysical stimuli due to the distribution of bone elongation and hydrostatic pressure. Prendergast et al. [10] adopted deviatoric strain and fluid velocity as the biophysical stimuli. Lacroix and Prendergast [15] further improved the model, using poroelasticity material properties to simulate the mechanical behavior of bone tissue. The detailed healing pattern in the fractured bones were predicted accurately. Chou et al. [16] adopted an axisymmetric model to predict the length of the bone-implant contact and the bone volume formed in the healing callus around a set of implants using different micro-motions, healing callus size, and implant thread design. The results suggest that implant thread design is the most important factor of tissue differentiation.

In order to investigate the effect of implant geometry on the osseointegration and healing process, eight dental implants with distinct healing chamber designs were simulated by using the mechano-regulatory model in this work. Both the distribution of bones/tissues around the implants, and the solid/fluid stimuli will be analyzed and discussed. Moreover, the predicted bone ingrowth and performance of the implants will also be compared in the following sections.

2. Results

In order to validate the current model, we firstly reproduced the result of bone healing around a given implant shown in Chou et al. [16], which is a well-accepted research work using mechano-regulation algorithm. Here, all the settings used were following their works. The healing pattern on 28 day showed high similarity to Chou's result as shown in Figure S1 in the supplementary. Then, our models were further validated by comparing the history of bone ingrowth and cell differentiation around implants A and B (i.e., No. 1 and 3 implants used by Marin et al. [2]) with those in the animal test. Figure 1a shows the results of implant A. On the 4th day, the bones maturated from both sides, resulting in a thin band of the immature bones connecting all the threads of the implant. This feature shows good agreement with results found in the literature [17]. The resorption firstly appeared on the top surface of the callus region around the neck of the implant. This corresponds to the common feature of crestal bone loss in dental implants. Note that, although the mature and immature bones were present on the 4th day, Young's modulus of these regions was still close to the granulation tissue, based on Equation (3). This was due to the low concentration of the mesenchymal stem cells at the early stage of cell migration. On the 21st day, immature bones were only found in the regions under the implant and the crest of the top threads. Resorption became significant with time, especially in the lower six healing chambers. There was no significant change in the distribution of the cell phenotypes after the 21st day. Young's modulus of the mature and immature bones reached their maximum values on the 35th day, as the cell migration was completed.

Implant B had a similar bone ingrowth pattern to implant A, as shown in Figure 1b. However, mild resorption was found around the root of the healing chambers in the upper eight threads on the 21st day. Bone resorption became severe and extended to almost every implant thread by the 35th day.

As mentioned above, implants A and B corresponded to No. 1 and 3 implants used in the animal tests done by Marin et al. [2]. The wound-healing pattern they observed around implant A in beagle dogs, from the 21st and 35th day, are shown in Figure 2a,b, respectively. The predicted results generated by the current model are shown in Figure 2c,d, which are the enlarged images of the focused regions marked within the red rectangle in Figure 1a. Some instances of healing were also revealed in the simulations. For example, the resorption length was approximately half of the chamber length [2]; there were resorption bumps located at the middle of the lower flank of the healing chambers; and resorption typically formed at the upper left corner of the healing chambers, as shown in Figure 2c,d. Details about the formation of resorption bumps will be examined later in the Discussion. In the case of implant B, mild bone resorption on the 21st day could be both observed experimentally and numerically, as shown in Figure 2e,g. The feature of resorption bumps was also revealed. On the 35th day, more bone resorption was discovered, and the resorption length was also half of the chamber length, as shown in Figure 2f,h. It is remarkable that the experimental and numerical results had very good agreement. Thus, the accuracy of the current model is verified.

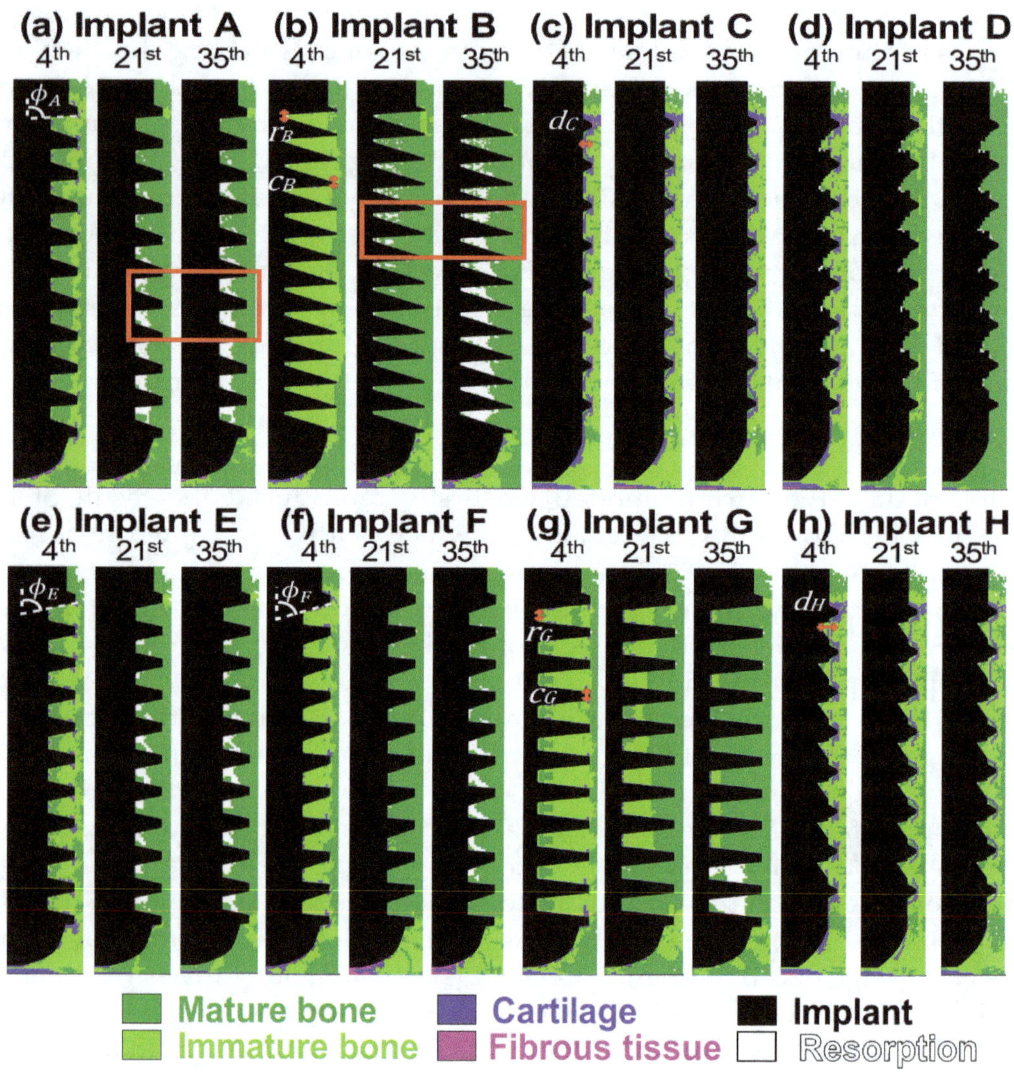

Figure 1. (**a–h**) The predicted history of the bone ingrowth and cell differentiation around implant A to H.

Figure 1c shows the predicted healing pattern around implant C. On the 4th day, the granulation tissues which attached to the implant body differentiated into soft tissues. These soft tissues were surrounded by immature bones, and the mature bones filled in the rest of the callus region. Similar to the other implants, the resorption was initiated around the neck of implant C, on the 4th day. Although there was relatively less mature bone around the implant, bone resorption was absent in the healing chambers of implant C. It is of interest to note that the distribution of the phenotypes of cells remained consistent throughout the entire healing progress in this case, and only the material properties altered with the stem cell concentration due to the cell migration.

Implant D is an addictive-manufactured dental implant with eagle-beak shaped healing chambers designed by Lee et al. [6]. Since the design was modified from implant C [6], the healing patterns in the early stages were similar (see the patterns for the 4th day in Figure 1c,d). However, the non-uniform roots of implant D suppressed the formation of soft tissues. Similar to implant A, the mature bones grew from both sides, i.e., the cells origin and the healing chamber roots, during the 4th to 21st day. There were almost no immature bones or soft tissues left at the end of the healing process. In addition, the resorption regions in all healing chambers were so small, with a dimension of only two to three elements.

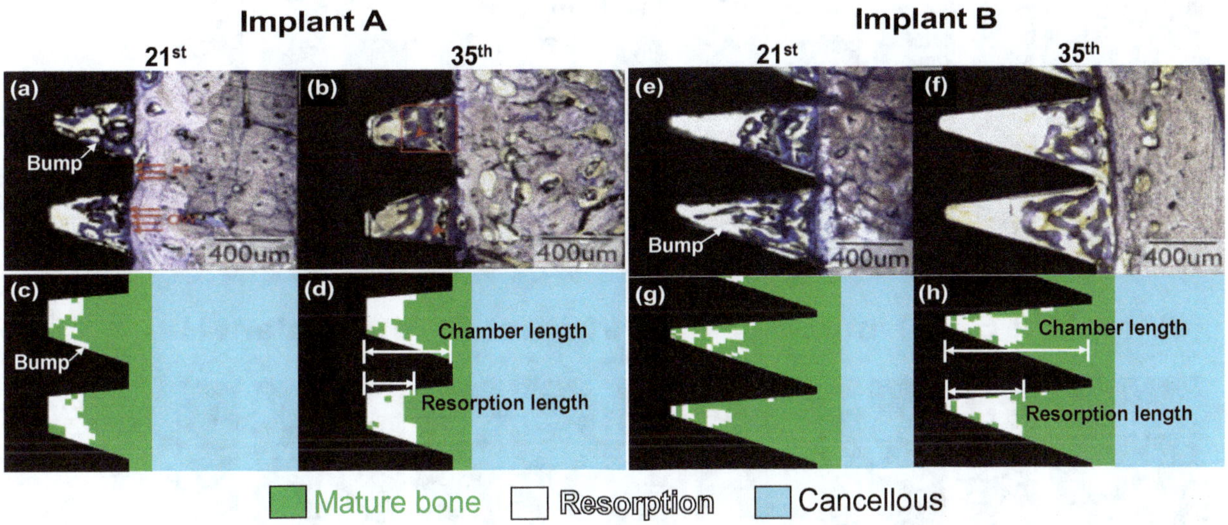

Figure 2. The wound-healing pattern around (**a**,**b**) implants A and (**e**,**f**) implant B on the 21st and 35th day observed in the animal experimental done by Marin et al. [2]. Zoom-in on the region marked in red in Figure 1, showing the predicted patterns of (**c**,**d**) implant A and (**g**,**h**) implant B.

Now consider the performance of implants A through D by examining their bone-implant contact (BIC) and bone area (BA) on the 35th day, as shown in Table 1. The other four implants E to H will be discussed in the following section. Implant D gave the highest BIC and BA values among the four implants, 74% and 95%, respectively. The BIC value of implant C (64%) was higher than that of implants A (58%) and B (60%). However, the situation reversed when looking at BA values of implants A, B (74%, 71%), and C (68%). It is worth noting that the BIC and BA levels of implant C were mainly contributed to immature bones, while those of implants A, B and D were contributed to mature bones. Thus the osteointegration results of implant C might be overestimated, since the value of Young's modulus of immature bone is six times lower than the value of mature bone. The results showed that implant D had the best osseointegration, and that healing chamber design can significantly affect the osseointegration and performance of dental implants.

Table 1. The values of BA and BIC of implants A to H.

Implant	A	B	C	D	E	F	G	H
Bone Area (BA%)	74	71	68	95	80	84	86	85
Bone implant contact (BIC%)	58	60	64	74	69	71	75	85

3. Discussion

We next examine how the biophysical stimuli affect the healing pattern and tissue differentiation around implants. Figures 3 and 4 show the contour plots of solid and fluid stimuli (the first and second terms in Equation (1), respectively) for implants A through H on the 4th, 21st, and 35th day. In general, high solid and fluid stimuli were observed in the regions under the tip of implant due to the vertical loading. In most cases, both stimuli decreased with time, and thus, bone resorption ($S \leq 0.010$) primarily occurred later on.

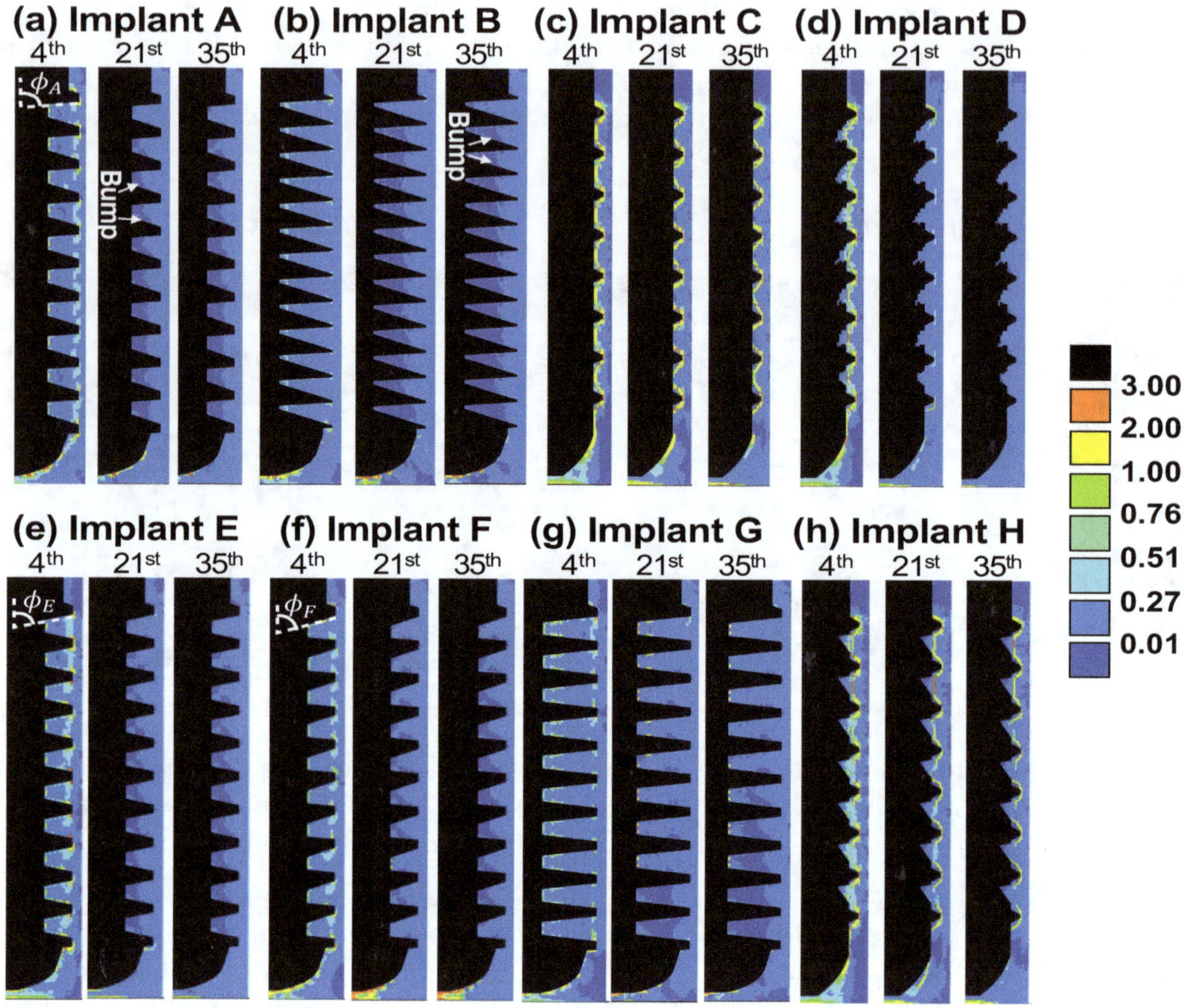

Figure 3. (**a**–**h**) The contour plots of solid stimulus for implants A to H, on the 4th, 21st, and 35th day.

As for implant A, the healing was dominated by solid stimulus, since the pattern of soft tissues, the thin band of immature bone on the 4th day, and the resorption regions on the 21st and 35th day (see Figure 1a) were in accordance with that of the solid stimulus, as shown in Figure 3a. By contrast, the healing around implant B was dominated by fluid stimulus. It can be observed in Figure 4b that the pattern of fluid stimulus matched the immature bone regions on the 4th day, and the resorption regions on the 21st and 35th day (see Figure 1b).

Both implants A and B led to severe bone resorption. This was caused by the healing chambers' poor design and relatively greater depth. From the perspective of solid stimulus, the thread crests provided the major fixation of the implant against the applied vertical load. Thus, the regions near the root of the healing chambers were less strained, leading to a low solid stimulus (see the bumps in dark blue on the 21st day in Figure 3a,b). The shape of the over-sized healing chambers resulted in undesired resorption and poor osseointegration.

It is significant that implant C lead to the most stable healing pattern among all the cases. Implant C had the smallest healing chambers in the current study. This allowed the fluid to flow into the entire chambers, resulting in high fluid stimulus ranging from 0.27 to 3.0, as shown in Figure 4c. In addition, high solid stimulus (greater than 1.0) can be found in Figure 3c due to the stress concentrated at the small threads. Both high stimuli lead to immature bones and soft tissues covering the implant. The feature of soft tissues covering the bone-implant interface was also found in the literature [18]. Moreover, the large amount of immature bones occurred around the implant, reducing the strength of the entire implantation system, as the Young's modulus of immature bones was only one sixth the value of the mature bones.

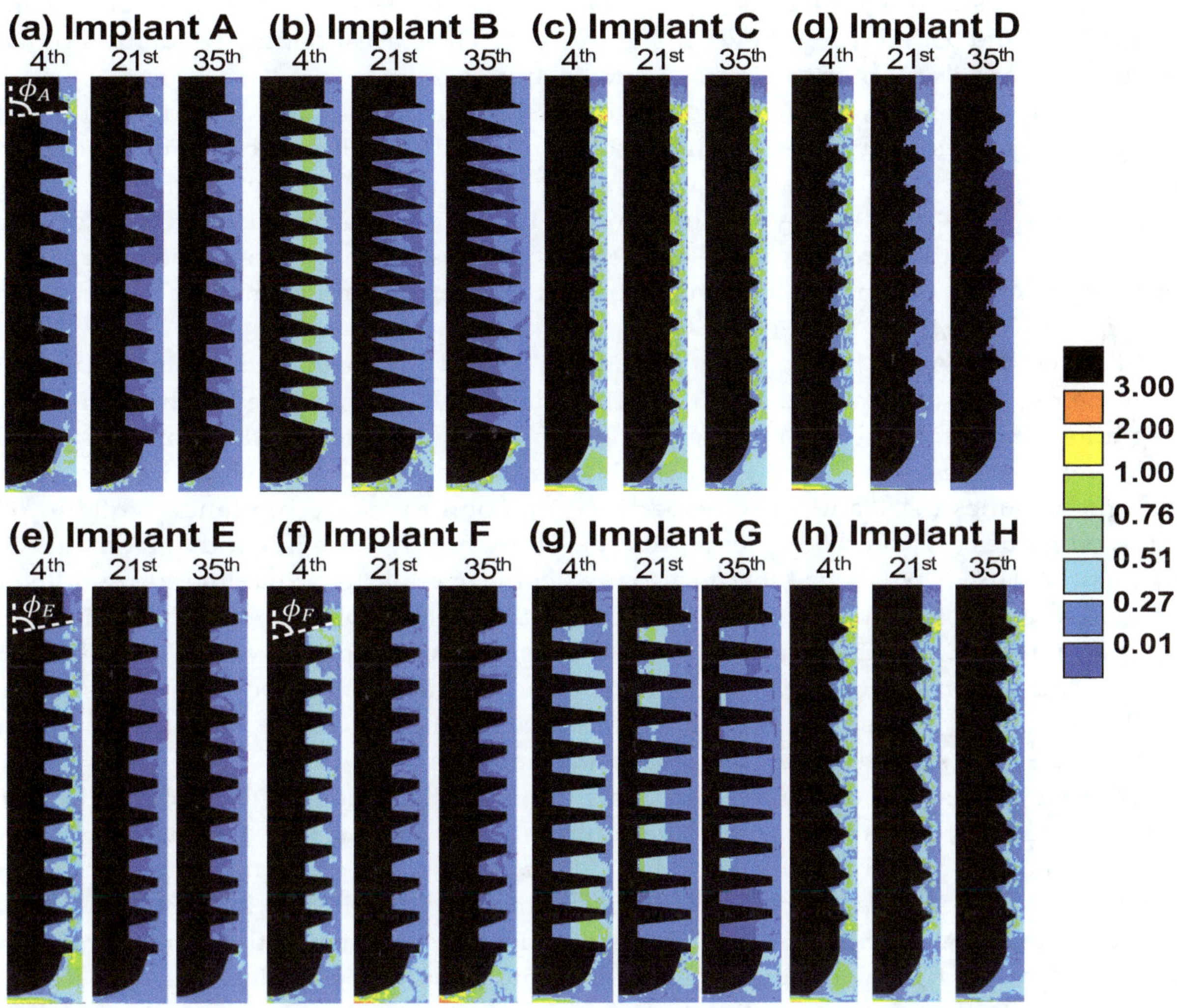

Figure 4. (**a**–**h**) The contour plots of fluid stimulus for implants A to H, on the 4th, 21st, and 35th day.

The depth of the healing chambers of implant D was relatively greater than that of implant C, but shallower than that of implant A. The values and contours of both stimuli of implant D were similar to those of implant C on the 4th day, as shown in Figures 3c,d and 4c,d. However, the healing pattern of implant D became similar to that of implant A on the 21st day, e.g., the cartilage and fibrous tissues were absent. On the 35th day, both stimuli of implant D, in most of the healing chambers, decreased to suitable values ranging from 0.01 to 0.27. Therefore, no severe bone resorption occurred, resulting in the formation of mature bones. This healing chamber design [6], with its adequate depth and eagle-beak shape, significantly improves the resulting BA and BIC, and provides for better osseointegration of the implant.

In order to understand the influence of the design of healing chambers on solid, fluid stimuli, and osseointegration, we will now discuss the performance of implants E to H, which were modified from implants A to D. In this section, the implants will be divided into three groups to reveal the influence of the slope of flank (Group1: A, E, F), the length of root and crest (Group2: B, G), and the depth of healing chamber (Group3: C, D, H) on the performance of implants, as shown in Figure 1.

Implants E and F were based on implant A, and yet, showed increasing slopes of the upper flanks of each healing chamber (i.e., $\phi_A > \phi_E > \phi_F$). The slopes on the upper and lower flanks of implant E were the same, while implant F had steeper upper flanks than its lower flanks. The depth of healing chambers in implant G were similar to that of implant B, however, the roots (r) and crests (c) of implant

G were flat (i.e., $r_B < r_G$, $c_B < c_G$). Finally, implant H had a greater depth in the upper half of the healing chambers compared with implant C (i.e., $d_C < d_H$). This also had inverse eagle-beak shaped healing chambers (upside down to the design of implant D). The tissue differentiation of implants E to H on the 4th, 21st, and 35th day are shown in Figure 1e–h. The corresponding solid and fluid stimuli of implants E to H are also shown in Figures 3 and 4e–h, respectively.

Now consider implants A, E, F. It was found that in the 35th day, steeper slopes in the upper flanks (i.e., $\phi_F < \phi_E < \phi_A$) generally resulted in higher solid and fluid stimuli, especially in the region under implants (please see Figures 3a,e,f and 4a,e,f. This was because the smaller the angle of ϕ, the less fixation and resistance is provided by the surrounding bones (ϕ is the angle between the orientations of the upper flanks and the direction of the applied force) Thus, there was less bone resorption in the lower healing chambers, and more immature bones in the region under implant F on the 35th day (as shown in Figure 1a,e,f).

Table 1 shows the BA and BIC values of implants A, E, and F. Note that, the calculation of BA/BIC focuses on the region we concerned about (ROI), which mainly contributes to the performance of osseointegration near threads. It can be observed that implants with steeper slopes in the upper flanks (ϕ) provide greater values of BA and BIC in 35th day, leading to better osseointegration, e.g., implant F had the highest values (84% and 71%, respectively) among the three implants, while implant A had the lowest values (74% and 58%, respectively). These findings are in good agreement with the reported literature [16]. Next, the model can also predict the overall strength of the surrounding bones, the averaged Young's modulus evolution process for the eight implants were shown in Figure 5a. Although the values of BA/BIC of implant F were the highest in Group1, the overall averaged Young's modulus in callus region showed with an opposite trend. As mentioned above, this is caused by the relatively higher biophysical stimulus, leading to the exist of fibrous tissue, cartilage and immature bone with lower Young's modulus in the region under implant F.

By comparing the shape of healing chambers in implants B and G, the effect of the roots and crests can be revealed. It can be observed that implant G maintains a greater value (>0.27) of the fluid stimulus in most of the regions until the 21st day, as shown in Figure 4g. Due to the high biophysical stimulus, there was less bone resorption in implant G on the 21st and 35th day (Figure 1g), giving great values of BA and BIC (86% and 75%, respectively), compared to that of implant B. Thus, in the cases of implants with similar depths, the flat roots and crests of the healing chambers led to better osseointegration. Furthermore, according to Figure 5a, bone tissue maturated faster in the case of implant B (orange line) than it of implant G (black line), leading to to overall higher Young's modulus in the surrounding bones.

Now consider implant H, which has a greater depth in the upper half of the healing chambers, compared with implant C. It is of interest to note that, such differences do not seem to alter the contours of the healing pattern, the solid stimuli, or the fluid stimuli of implant H, compared to those of implant C, as shown in Figures 1, 3 and 4c,h. By contrast, the shape of implant D (inverse of implant H) has a greater depth in the lower half of the healing chambers compared with implant C, and the history of the healing pattern was dramatically changed, as is mentioned in the Results. Thus, it can be concluded that in the cases of the considered implants which were subjected to vertical loading, the influence of the depth of the lower half of the healing chambers is relatively more significant than the depth of the upper half of the healing chambers.

Although the healing patterns of implants C and H were similar, the BA and BIC numerical data of implant H were improved, as shown in Table 1. This indicates that the depth (d) of the healing chamber is crucial for the performance of implants. Furthermore, when comparing the cases of implant D with H, it can be seen that implant D resulted in a greater value of BA, and had more mature bone implant contact. Next, by examine the averaged Young's modulus evolution in Group3 (see Figure 5a), it was observed that the averaged Young's modulus of implant D was also the highest among the eight implants. Moreover, Figure 5b shows the averaged Young's modulus distribution of each elements in callus region for implants C, D and H. The results showed that values of the most of the elements in implant C and H were in the range of 0 to 2 MPa, while those in implant D were in the range of 4 to 6 MPa. This shows that although implant H has high BA/BIC values, the overall strength of the surrounding bone of implant H was still relatively lower than it of implant D. This confirms, once again, that implants with steeper upper flanks lead to better osseointegration, as mentioned above.

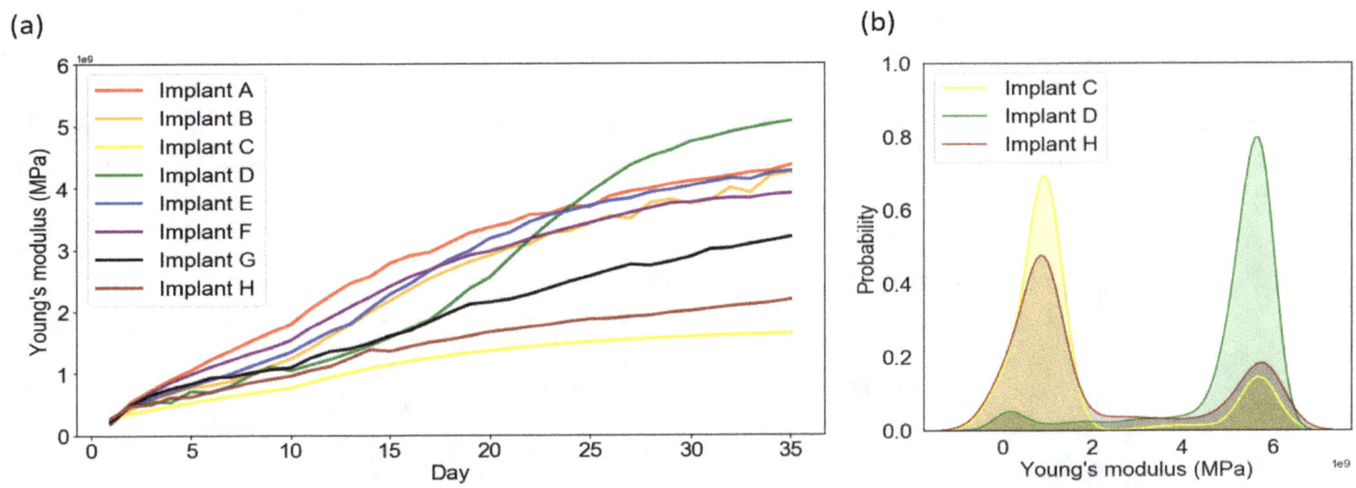

Figure 5. (**a**) The overall averaged Young's modulus evolution in the callus region for implant A–H. (**b**) The Young's modulus distribution of each element in the callus region for implants C, D, H.

It has been proved by in vivo and in vitro animal test that thread design has a great influence on the osseointegration [19–21]. Scarano et al. [22,23] found that vessel formed in the concavities of the threads (i.e., inside the healing chambers) rather than the convexities, and this was positively correlated with bone formation rate. Bone healing of this type was also reproduced in the current study, where implants A, E, and G resulted in the initiation of mature bones from the root of the healing chambers in the early stage (Day 4) of bone healing, as shown in Figure 1a,e,g. Moreover, several simulation studies have focused on the biomechanical stimulus of bones, in order to eliminating stress concentration and reducing bone resorption around implants [24–27]. However, uniform material properties of bones around the implants were typically assumed; cell differentiation and fluid stimulus was also ignored. Thus, the current study resolved these problems and gave a direct analysis for osseointegration.

The current study reproduced the bone healing features of the work done by Marin et al. [2], and provided possible design guideline for the geometry of the healing chamber of implants. However, only vertical applied force can be considered since a simplified 2D axisymmetric model was used in the current work. This simplification was necessary as mechano-regulation algorithm was typically computationally demanding, and many design parameters in healing chambers should be processed. This issue can be resolved by incorporating 3D FEM model and regarded as the future work.

4. Materials and Methods

The current model was built in two-dimensional axisymmetry using the commercial finite element (FE) package, ANSYS. It consisted of a Ti-6Al-4V implant, a cortical layer, cancellous bones, and callus. The geometrical detail is shown in Figure 6a. The implant was meshed by 2D four-node solid structure elements, with the ANSYS built-in element type, PLANE42. The remaining parts of the geometry, e.g., the calluses, cortical bones, and cancellous bones, were meshed by 2D four-node coupled pore-pressure mechanical solid element, with the element type CPT212. Elements of this type enable the calculation of the fluid velocity and pressure in the pores of the bones while under external mechanical loads. A mesh size of 0.05 mm was set to allow for an accurate and stable solution, while the detail of the complex configuration could also be captured.

An average displacement of 8 μm along the $-y$ axis was applied at nodes on the top surface of the implant. This value corresponded to the displacement resulting from the biting force (≈100 N) of beagle dogs [28], and thus, our simulation results could be validated by the data obtained from the animal tests done by Marin et al. [2] (the trial followed the approval of the bioethics committee for animal experimentation at the Universidade Federal de Santa Catarina, Brazil) The displacement degree of freedom along the y axis at the bottom nodes and along the x axis in the bottom-left node were constrained, as shown in Figure 6a. The axisymmetric boundary condition was set at the nodes lying on the y axis, marked as a dot-dashed line. The callus region located around the implant was where the bone/tissue differentiation occurred. The boundary, marked with a dashed line, shows the cells' origin, and is defined as the source of diffusion of the mesenchymal stem cells, i.e., the stem cell concentration was set as 100%. The interface between the implant and callus was set to allow sliding with a friction coefficient of 0.3 [29]. The material properties used in the current study are shown in Table 2 [16].

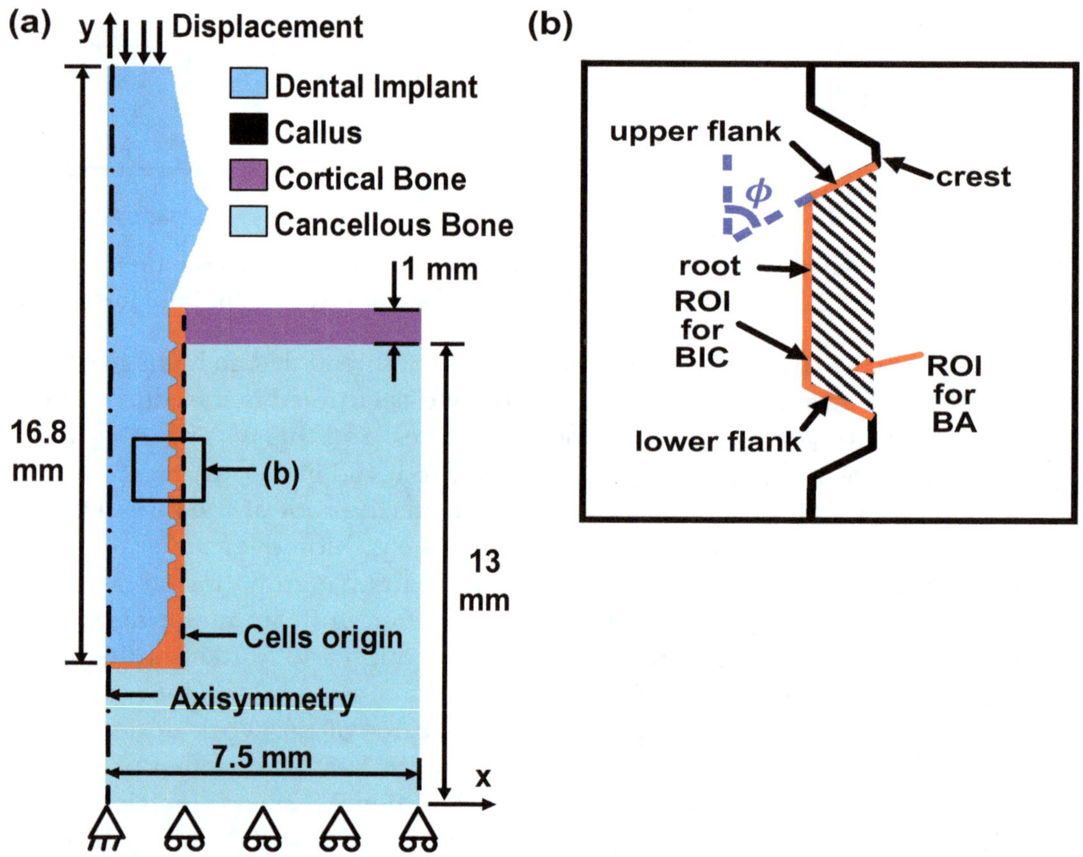

Figure 6. The schematic plots of (**a**) the model with boundary conditions and (**b**) ROI of BIC and BA in one of the threads.

Table 2. The material properties used in the current work [11,30–35].

Tissue Phenotype	Young's Modulus (MPa)	Poisson's Ratio	Permeability (m^4/Ns)
Granulation tissue	1	0.17	1×10^{-14}
Fibrous tissue	2	0.17	1×10^{-14}
Cartilage	10	0.17	5×10^{-15}
Immature bone	1000	0.30	1×10^{-13}
Mature bone	6000	0.30	3.7×10^{-13}
Cortical bone	20,000	0.30	1×10^{-17}
Cancellous bone	6000	0.30	3.7×10^{-13}
Ti-6Al-4V	113,000	0.30	N/A

There were a total of 35 iterations in the simulation, corresponding to the healing period in the animal tests [2]. In the current study, each iteration represented one healing day. The iterative procedure was based on the procedure of Chou et al. [16]. A MATLAB user-defined function was developed to automate the modification of the FE model.

The solid and fluid stimuli considered in the mechano-regulation model corresponds to two important values [10]: the octahedral shear strain γ and the relative fluid/solid velocity $\nu = \sqrt{\nu_x^2 - \nu_y^2}$, where ν_x and ν_y are the fluid velocity in the transverse and normal directions. The phenotype of the cells of each element in the callus region for the next step, i.e., $(i+1)$th iteration, was determined by the cell stimulus factor S, which is related to γ and ν, such that

$$S = \frac{\gamma}{a} + \frac{\nu}{b} \tag{1}$$

where solid stimulus constant $a = 0.0375$ and fluid stimulus constant $b = 3$ μm/s [36]. The ranges of the value of S and the corresponding phenotypes of cell, including fibrous tissue ($S > 3$), cartilage ($3 \geq S > 1$), immature bone ($1 \geq S > 0.266$), mature bone ($0.266 \geq S > 0.010$), and resorption ($0.010 \geq S$), can be specified. Each phenotype has a set of material properties, such as Young's modulus, Poisson's ratio and permeability, as shown in Table 2 [16,30]. Thus, the material settings in each element in the callus region were required to be updated for the next iteration.

Two issues needed to be considered when updating the material settings for the next step, the $(i+1)$th iteration. The first issue was the mesenchymal stem cell migration [11], which is related to the level of transition from the granulation tissue to cells of different phenotypes. It was modeled as a random anisotropic diffusion [15]. The concentration of stem cells n increased in each successive step of iterations, governed by

$$\frac{dn}{dt} = D\nabla^2 n \tag{2}$$

where t is time; D is the diffusion coefficient with the unit of square meter per day. Here, the diffusion coefficient D was determined so that the entire healing callus reached the maximal cell concentration after 35 day [2,12]. The effective material property X_{mix} in the next iteration, such as Young's modulus, Poisson's ratio and permeability, depended on the concentration of the stem cells n_i in the ith iteration, that is

$$X_{mix} = \frac{n_{max} - n_i}{n_{max}} X_g + \frac{n_i}{n_{max}} X_d \tag{3}$$

where n_{max} is the maximum concentration of cells; X_g and X_d are the material property of the granulation tissue and the differentiated tissue, respectively. With this linear combination, the progress of tissue transition could be modeled.

The second issue when updating the material settings for the next iteration was the application of the smoothing procedure. The material property X_{mix} obtained in Equation (3) needed to be averaged with those in the previous nine iterations in order to avoid numerical instability and sudden changes. The material properties for the next iteration could be written as

$$X_i = \frac{1}{N}(X_{mix} + X_{i-1} + X_{i-2} + \cdots + X_{i-(N-1)}) \tag{4}$$

where i is the number of iteration. For the iteration of $i < 9$, the average was made from the ith iteration to the first.

In the current study, four implants labeled A to D were considered first. Implants A and B corresponded to No. 1 and 3 implants used in the animal test done by Marin et al. [2]. Implant C was similar to the commercial ITI (Institute Straumann AG, Waldenburg, Switzerland) solid cylindrical screwed implant, number 033.512S. The healing chambers of implant D were eagle-beak shaped, which were modified from implant C in the author's previous work [6]. Such complex configuration was expected to promote osseointegration. Next, implants E to H, which were modified from implants A to D, were also discussed to reveal the influence of healing chamber geometry on osseointegration.

Two parameters were defined for the histomorphometric evaluation of the performance of implants: bone-implant contact (BIC), and bone area (BA). The region of interest (ROI) of BIC is the total length of upper/lower flank and the root of all the threads in the implant. ROI of BIC in one of the threads are illustrated with red solid lines in Figure 6b. BIC is defined as the percentage of the total length of the interface between the implant elements and the mature/immature bone elements in the ROI. Similarly, ROI for BA is the total area between all the threads (illustrated as shaded area). The definition of BA is the percentage of the total area of the mature/immature bone elements in the ROI. It is expected that the higher the BIC and BA values, the better the osseointegration of an implant [16].

5. Conclusions

In the current study, a 2D axisymmetric finite element model with a mechano-regulatory algorithm was developed to study the bone ingrowth and tissue differentiation around eight dental implants, A to H, each with different healing chamber designs. The predicted healing patterns in implants A and B were verified by the data obtained in the animal test done by Marin et al. [2], showing very good agreement. The performance of the implants was then evaluated by bone area (BA) and bone-implant contact (BIC). The results showed that severe bone resorption occurred due to the over-sized and sharp configuration of the healing chambers. The commercial ITI implant (implant C) with small healing chambers led to high solid and fluid stimuli retention, immature bones and soft tissue covering the implant, moreover, resulting in the most steady healing pattern with no significant change on the phenotype of cells. Implant D, which was suitable for additive manufacturing, had eagle-beak shaped healing chambers, and showed remarkable osseointegration, based its BA and BIC values.

Additional implants were discussed to reveal the influence of the designs of the healing chamber on both the stimuli and the healing patterns. Implants A, E, and F showed that steeper upper flanks result in less resorption and better osseointegration. The results of implants B and G revealed that flat roots of healing chambers lead to better osseointegration. The cases of implants C, D and H show that the depth of the upper half of the healing chambers has a significant effect on the healing pattern. The healing chamber design of implant D matched all the design criteria mentioned above, such as steep upper flanks, relatively flat roots, and adequate depth. Thus, implant D led to the best osseointegration among all the implants considered in the current work.

The mechano-regulatory tissue differentiation model developed in the current work is rapid, accurate, and customizable for any given dental implant with an axisymmetric cross-section. The results generated here can also serve as design guidelines and our model is able to provide "possible trends" for improving the performance of dental implants under the specific boundary conditions considered in the current work.

Author Contributions: Conceptualization, M.-J.L. and N.-T.T.; methodology, M.-J.L. and P.-C.K.; software, M.-J.L. and P.-C.K.; validation, M.-J.L. and P.-C.K.; formal analysis, M.-J.L.; investigation, M.-J.L.; resources, M.-J.L. and N.-T.T.; data curation, M.-J.L. and N.-T.T.; writing–original draft preparation, Y.-W.C. and P.-C.K.; writing–review and editing, P.-C.K. and N.-T.T.; visualization, M.-J.L. and P.-C.K.; supervision, Y.-W.C. and N.-T.T.; project administration, N.-T.T.; funding acquisition, N.-T.T. All authors have read and agreed to the published version of the manuscript.

Acknowledgments: The authors would like to thank Yun-Yi Chu and Tzu-Han Ma for their assistance on editing the manuscript and generating the figures of the implants.

References

1. Javed, F.; Romanos, G.E. The role of primary stability for successful immediate loading of dental implants. A literature review. *J. Dent.* **2010**, *38*, 612–620. [CrossRef]

2. Marin, C.; Granato, R.; Suzuki, M.; Gil, J.N.; Janal, M.N.; Coelho, P.G. Histomorphologic and histomorphometric evaluation of various endosseous implant healing chamber configurations at early implantation times: A study in dogs. *Clin. Oral Implant. Res.* **2010**, *21*, 577–583. [CrossRef]
3. Beutel, B.G.; Danna, N.R.; Granato, R.; Bonfante, E.A.; Marin, C.; Tovar, N.; Suzuki, M.; Coelho, P.G. Implant design and its effects on osseointegration over time within cortical and trabecular bone. *J. Biomed. Mater. Res. Part Appl. Biomater.* **2016**, *104*, 1091–1097. [CrossRef]
4. Traini, T.; Mangano, C.; Sammons, R.L.; Mangano, F.; Macchi, A.; Piattelli, A. Direct laser metal sintering as a new approach to fabrication of an isoelastic functionally graded material for manufacture of porous titanium dental implants. *Dent. Mater.* **2008**, *24*, 1525–1533. [CrossRef]
5. Stübinger, S.; Mosch, I.; Robotti, P.; Sidler, M.; Klein, K.; Ferguson, S.J.; von Rechenberg, B. Histological and biomechanical analysis of porous additive manufactured implants made by direct metal laser sintering: A pilot study in sheep. *J. Biomed. Mater. Res. Part Appl. Biomater.* **2013**, *101*, 1154–1163. [CrossRef]
6. Lee, H.C.; Tsai, P.I.; Huang, C.C.; Chen, S.Y.; Chao, C.G.; Tsou, N.T. Numerical Method for the Design of Healing Chamber in Additive-Manufactured Dental Implants. *Biomed Res. Int.* **2017**, *2017*, 1970680. [CrossRef]
7. van der Stok, J.; Koolen, M.; Jahr, H.; Kops, N.; Waarsing, J.; Weinans, H.; Van der Jagt, O. Chondrogenically differentiated mesenchymal stromal cell pellets stimulate endochondral bone regeneration in critical-sized bone defects. *Eur. Cells Mater.* **2014**, *27*, 137–48. [CrossRef]
8. Hendrikson, W.J.; van Blitterswijk, C.A.; Rouwkema, J.; Moroni, L. The use of finite element analyses to design and fabricate three-dimensional scaffolds for skeletal tissue engineering. *Front. Bioeng. Biotechnol.* **2017**, *5*, 30. [CrossRef]
9. Carter, D.; Blenman, P.; Beaupre, G. Correlations between mechanical stress history and tissue differentiation in initial fracture healing. *J. Orthop. Res.* **1988**, *6*, 736–748. [CrossRef]
10. Prendergast, P.; Huiskes, R.; Søballe, K. Biophysical stimuli on cells during tissue differentiation at implant interfaces. *J. Biomech.* **1997**, *30*, 539–548. [CrossRef]
11. Claes, L.; Heigele, C. Magnitudes of local stress and strain along bony surfaces predict the course and type of fracture healing. *J. Biomech.* **1999**, *32*, 255–266. [CrossRef]
12. Lacroix, D.; Prendergast, P.; Li, G.; Marsh, D. Biomechanical model to simulate tissue differentiation and bone regeneration: Application to fracture healing. *Med. Biol. Eng. Comput.* **2002**, *40*, 14–21. [CrossRef]
13. Isaksson, H.; Wilson, W.; van Donkelaar, C.C.; Huiskes, R.; Ito, K. Comparison of biophysical stimuli for mechano-regulation of tissue differentiation during fracture healing. *J. Biomech.* **2006**, *39*, 1507–1516. [CrossRef]
14. Pauwels, F. Eine neue Theorie über den Einfluß mechanischer Reize auf die Differenzierung der Stützgewebe. *Zeitschrift für Anat. Und Entwicklungsgeschichte* **1960**, *121*, 478–515. [CrossRef]
15. Lacroix, D.; Prendergast, P. A mechano-regulation model for tissue differentiation during fracture healing: Analysis of gap size and loading. *J. Biomech.* **2002**, *35*, 1163–1171. [CrossRef]
16. Chou, H.Y.; Müftü, S. Simulation of peri-implant bone healing due to immediate loading in dental implant treatments. *J. Biomech.* **2013**, *46*, 871–878. [CrossRef]
17. Kuzyk, P.R.; Schemitsch, E.H. The basic science of peri-implant bone healing. *Indian J. Orthop.* **2011**, *45*, 108. [CrossRef]
18. Schatzker, J.; Horne, J.; Sumner-Smith, G. The effect of movement on the holding power of screws in bone. *Clin. Orthop. Relat. Res.* **1975**, *111*, 257–262. [CrossRef]
19. Gehrke, S.A.; Eliers Treichel, T.L.; Pérez-Díaz, L.; Calvo-Guirado, J.L.; Aramburú Júnior, J.; Mazón, P.; de Aza, P.N. Impact of Different Titanium Implant Thread Designs on Bone Healing: A Biomechanical and Histometric Study with an Animal Model. *J. Clin. Med.* **2019**, *8*, 777. [CrossRef]
20. Falco, A.; Berardini, M.; Trisi, P. Correlation Between Implant Geometry, Implant Surface, Insertion Torque, and Primary Stability: In Vitro Biomechanical Analysis. *Int. J. Oral Maxillofac. Implants* **2018**, *33*, 824–830. [CrossRef]
21. Di Stefano, D.A.; Arosio, P.; Perrotti, V.; Iezzi, G.; Scarano, A.; Piattelli, A. Correlation between Implant Geometry, Bone Density, and the Insertion Torque/Depth Integral: A Study on Bovine Ribs. *J. Dent.* **2019**, *7*, 25. [CrossRef]

22. Scarano, A.; Perrotti, V.; Artese, L.; Degidi, M.; Degidi, D.; Piattelli, A.; Iezzi, G. Blood vessels are concentrated within the implant surface concavities: A histologic study in rabbit tibia. *Odontology* **2014**, *102*, 259–266. [CrossRef] [PubMed]
23. Scarano, A.; Degidi, M.; Perrotti, V.; Degidi, D.; Piattelli, A.; Iezzi, G. Experimental evaluation in rabbits of the effects of thread concavities in bone formation with different titanium implant surfaces. *Clin. Implant Dent. Relat. Res.* **2014**, *16*, 572–581. [CrossRef]
24. Calì, M.; Zanetti, E.M.; Oliveri, S.M.; Asero, R.; Ciaramella, S.; Martorelli, M.; Bignardi, C. Influence of thread shape and inclination on the biomechanical behaviour of plateau implant systems. *Dent. Mater.* **2018**, *34*, 460–469. [CrossRef]
25. Oswal, M.M.; Amasi, U.N.; Oswal, M.S.; Bhagat, A.S. Influence of three different implant thread designs on stress distribution: A three-dimensional finite element analysis. *J. Indian Prosthodont. Soc.* **2016**, *16*, 359. [CrossRef]
26. Paracchini, L.; Barbieri, C.; Redaelli, M.; Di Croce, D.; Vincenzi, C.; Guarnieri, R. Finite Element Analysis of a New Dental Implant Design Optimized for the Desirable Stress Distribution in the Surrounding Bone Region. *Prosthesis* **2020**, *2*, 225–236. [CrossRef]
27. Pirmoradian, M.; Naeeni, H.A.; Firouzbakht, M.; Toghraie, D.; Darabi, R. Finite element analysis and experimental evaluation on stress distribution and sensitivity of dental implants to assess optimum length and thread pitch. *Comput. Meth. Prog. Biol.* **2020**, *187*, 105258. [CrossRef]
28. Barbier, L.; Sloten, J.V.; Krzesinski, G.; Van Der Perre, E.S. Finite element analysis of non-axial versus axial loading of oral implants in the mandible of the dog. *J. Oral Rehabil.* **1998**, *25*, 847–858. [CrossRef]
29. Winter, W.; Klein, D.; Karl, M. Micromotion of dental implants: Basic mechanical considerations. *J. Med. Eng.* **2013**, *2013*, 265412. [CrossRef]
30. Mukherjee, K.; Gupta, S. Bone ingrowth around porous-coated acetabular implant: A three-dimensional finite element study using mechanoregulatory algorithm. *Biomech. Model. Mechanobiol.* **2016**, *15*, 389–403. [CrossRef]
31. Hori, R.; Lewis, J. Mechanical properties of the fibrous tissue found at the bone-cement interface following total joint replacement. *J. Biomed. Mater. Res.* **1982**, *16*, 911–927. [CrossRef] [PubMed]
32. Jurvelin, J.; Buschmann, M.; Hunziker, E. Optical and mechanical determination of Poisson's ratio of adult bovine humeral articular cartilage. *J. Biomech.* **1997**, *30*, 235–241. [CrossRef]
33. Armstrong, C.; Mow, V. Variations in the intrinsic mechanical properties of human articular cartilage with age, degeneration, and water content. *J. Bone Jt. Surgery. Am. Vol.* **1982**, *64*, 88–94. [CrossRef]
34. Ochoa, J.; Hillberry, B. Permeability of bovine periodontal ligament after application of orthodontic force cancellous bone. In Proceedings of the 38th Annual Meeting, Orthopaedic Research Society, Washington, DC, USA, 17–20 February 1992; Volume 162, p. 165.
35. Cowin, S.C. Bone poroelasticity. *J. Biomech.* **1999**, *32*, 217–238. [CrossRef]
36. Huiskes, R.; Van Driel, W.; Prendergast, P.; Søballe, K. A biomechanical regulatory model for periprosthetic fibrous-tissue differentiation. *J. Mater. Sci. Mater. Med.* **1997**, *8*, 785–788. [CrossRef]

4

Evaluation of the Cortical Deformation Induced by Distal Cantilevers Supported by Extra-Short Implants: A Finite Elements Analysis Study

Enrique Fernández-Bodereau [1,*], Viviana Yolanda Flores [2], Rafael Arcesio Delgado-Ruiz [3], Juan Manuel Aragoneses [4] and José Luis Calvo-Guirado [5]

1 Department of Fixed Prosthodontics, Faculty of Dentistry, Universidad Nacional de Córdoba, Córdoba 5000, Argentine
2 Department of Oral Biology, Faculty of Dentistry, Universidad Nacional de Córdoba, Córdoba 5000, Argentine; vivyflores@gmail.com
3 Department of Prosthodontics, School of Dental Dental Medicine, Stony Brook, NY 1103, USA; Rafael.Delgado-Ruiz@stonybrookmedicine.edu
4 Department of Dental Research in Universidad Federico Henríquez y Carvajal (UFHEC), Santo Domingo 10107, Dominicana Republic; jmaragoneses@gmail.com
5 Department of Oral and Implant Surgery, Faculty of Health Sciences, Universidad Católica San Antonio de Murcia (UCAM), Murcia 30002, Spain; jlcalvo@ucam.edu
* Correspondence: fernandezenrique5@gmail.com

Abstract: Background: The aim of the study was to analyze the distribution of stresses caused by an axial force in a three-dimensional model with the finite element method in the implant-supported fixed partial denture with distal overhang (PPFIVD) on short dental implants in the posterior edentulous maxilla. Methods: geometrical models of the maxilla with a bone remnant of 9 and 5 mm were created. Straumann SP® (Base, Switzerland) implants were placed in the premolar area. Two groups with subgroups were designed. Group A (GA): PPFIVD on two implants (GA1: 4.1 × 8 mm and GA2: 4.1 × 4 mm); Group B (GB): PPFIVD on the single implant (GB1: 4.1 × 8 mm and GB2: 4.1 × 4 mm). It was applied to a static force of 100 N to 30°. Results: PPFIVD on two implants reached the maximum tension in GA2 with respect to GA1; the difference was not significant in implants. In the maxilla GA2 was lower in relation to GA1; the difference was not significant. In PPFIVD over an implant, the stress was greater in GB2 with respect to GB1; the difference was significant in maxilla and implants. Peri-implant bone micro deformations and prosthesis-implant displacements were observed. Conclusions: PPFIVD over short splinted implants could be viable in the maxilla with reduced bone height, being an option when lifting the floor of the maxillary sinus. The rehabilitation with unitary implant (4 mm) did not provide adequate results. The dominant tensions evidenced bone micro-distortions with a displacement of the prosthesis-implant set. The real statement of this paper was to define that short splinted implants can be used in soft bone with high success rate in reducing bending forces.

Keywords: short dental implant; finite element analysis; distal cantilever; implant-supported partial fixed prosthesis; microdeformations; displacements; geometric model; maxilla

1. Introduction

The Brånemark system defined osseointegration as the direct bonding between titanium implants and the surrounding bone, maintained during functional loads [1,2]. After extraction of the teeth in the posterior edentulous maxilla, the resorption of the bony crest, the pneumatization of the maxillary sinus, or the combination of both are evidenced, which reduces the possibility of placing fixings of standard length and is generally accompanied by complex surgical procedures [3,4]. In general, these surgical treatments include: maxillary floor elevation and grafts, other procedures combine grafting and the use of membranes [5,6]. An alternative technique to complex surgical procedures is the use of short implants (implants with lengths of ≤8 mm) [7,8].

Recently, extra-short implants of 4 mm in length have emerged. Extra-short implants are destined to zones with noticeable bony resorption unable to support a short implant, thus, avoiding the use invasive techniques, potential reduction of the time of healing and the financial burden for the patients. In the case of using extra-short implants, the crown/implant ratio can be of 2–3:1 varying with the prosthetic space [9,10].

During the mechanical load of the implant restoration, adaptive processes occur at the peri-implant supporting tissues that influence the healing, remodeling, and resorption of the surrounding bone [11,12]. Physiological bone deformation happens between 1000 $\mu\varepsilon$ and 1500 $\mu\varepsilon$ ($\mu\varepsilon$ = microstrains) in the normal bite [13–15]. However, in extra-short implants, these values may increase, affecting bone healing and regeneration. [14,16].

Indeed, measurements of static bite force indicate that magnitude is in average 100–150 N in adult men [17,18]; the location of the implants in the edentulous maxilla determines the force intensity, being the posterior areas those with the higher registered forces [19]. Of preference, a balanced occlusion can grant a better distribution of forces [20].

Important parameters were established for the use of cantilevers with standard and long implants [21]. However, there is a lack of information of the long-term effects cantilevers supported by extra-short implants [22–24]. Finite element analysis (FEA) has been used to evaluate the biomechanics of extra-short implants under axial forces [2,14,15].

The hypothesis of the present study is that that the forces generated during the mastication in the posterior region of the maxilla transmitted through the prosthetic restoration with a distal cantilever to the standard and extra-short implants could affect the osseous tissue in a similar fashion.

The objective of the present research was to analyze with FEA, the distribution of tensions produced by an axial force applied to the fixed partial prosthesis with distal cantilever, supported by extra-short implants of 4 mm length in the posterior sector of the partially edentulous maxilla.

2. Materials and Methods

For this experimental FEA study, the following variables considered: Standard Plus® (Straumann, Basel, Switzerland) implants with a diameter of 4.1 mm by 8 mm in length and extra-short implant with a diameter of 4.1 mm by 4 mm in length.

The behavior of the bone and the prosthesis under simulated static load was evaluated. The distribution of the tensions was studied as per ISO 14801:2003 and ISO 1942-1 standards. The geometric model of a unilateral edentulous maxilla was generated using Abaqus®, 6.4 Version (Abaqus Inc., Providence, RI, USA) through the use of optical scanners [25].

The distribution of the tensions in bone when applying an axial force on the fixed partial prosthesis was also evaluated. The geometry of a partially edentulous maxillary segment was determined with a frontal cut around the first premolar; dimensions in the three axes of the space were registered.

The dimensions of the implant, abutment, and prosthetic components were settled down with a digital caliper; a representative average with the projection of the profiles was registered, using a TAF003 profilometer from Mitutoyo® (Tokyo, Japan).

The coefficient and modulus of elasticity (e) of Poisson (V) were assigned as follows: Cortical bone (E13700 MPa; V0.3), trabecular bone (E13700 MPa; V0.3), titanium implants (E110000 MPa; V0.3), and chromium-nickel prosthesis (E171000 MPa; V0.3) did not include the cement because its modulus of elasticity is low with respect to the used materials [13,26]. The geometric model was characterized as a trabecular core surrounded by a cortical layer that resembles the characteristics of a partially toothless maxilla [27].

Available bone heights were 9 and 5 mm. In the edentulous section of the first and second premolar and first molar, short and extra-short implants were inserted, a connection of the abutments to the fixed partial denture with the distal cantilever (PPFIVD) was simulated. The mesiodistal distance of each cantilever averages 7 mm.

Two groups were analyzed: group A (GA) constituted by two subgroups: GA1, two short implants of 4.1 × 8 mm; and GA2, two extra-short implants of 4.1 × 4 mm. Group B (GB), also had two subgroups: GB1, a short implant of 4.1 × 8 mm, and GB2, with an extra short implant of 4.1 × 4 mm.

The osseous tissue was modeled in close relation with the implant threads to accentuate the precision of the results (Table 1) with a mechanically ideal interface and assuming 100% of bone-to-implant contact.

Table 1. Numeric detail geometric patterns made for this investigation.

Models	Amount of Elements	Number of Nodes	Types of Elements	Bone Height (mm)	Implants Dimensions (mm)
Two implants	321,066	65,826	Tetrahedron	9	4.1 × 8
Two implants	424,672	85,442	Tetrahedron	5	4.1 × 4
An implant	199,443	40,776	Tetrahedron	9	4.1 × 8
An implant	264,076	53,261	Tetrahedron	5	4.1 × 4

Algorithmic calculations were applied to define the geometry, to generate the mesh, the load conditions, and the properties of the materials. Afterward, a set of n-equations and n-incognito were solved with an algorithm for the system [26]. Linear homogeneous and isotropic equations were applied. With all the registered data, magnitudes derived from the nodes were calculated (Table 1).

A physiological static load of 100 N (Newton) with an angulation of 30° was applied [18,19] by means of a standard circular piece whose purpose was to distribute the load uniformly. The application point was standardized for all the models in mesial of the triangular crest of the palatal peak.

The present investigation was completed on the base of the criterion of three-dimensional tensions of Von Mises, expressed in the following formula:

σ_ (VM √ (((σ_1 〖σ〗_2) ^2 (σ_ (2) - σ_3) ^2 (σ_3 σ_1) ^2)/2))

where σVM is the tension of Von Mises and σ1; σ2; σ3 the principal stresses.

3. Results

3.1. Distribution of the Tensions in the Implant

In GA1 and GA2, the load applied in the crown it distributed the principal stresses in the cervical third of both implants; in the cantilever area, the tension increased at the cervical third of both implants, also including the middle third the second implant located at the level of the second premolar.

GA2 was greater with respect to GA1, but without significant difference. The distribution of the tensions in GB1 and GB2 was observed in the cervical third of both implants in the cantilever, the principal stresses included the cervical third and middle in both sub-groups. GB2 was greater in relation to GB1 (Table 2; Figures 1–3).

Table 2. Distribution of the principal stresses in ultrashort implants.

Models	Crown (MPa)	Cantilever (MPa)	Load (N)	Implant Dimensions (mm)
A Two implants	183.7	173.9	100	4.1 × 8
	170	205.4	100	4.1 × 4
B An implant	330.2	334	100	4.1 × 8
	321.6	381.4	100	4.1 × 4

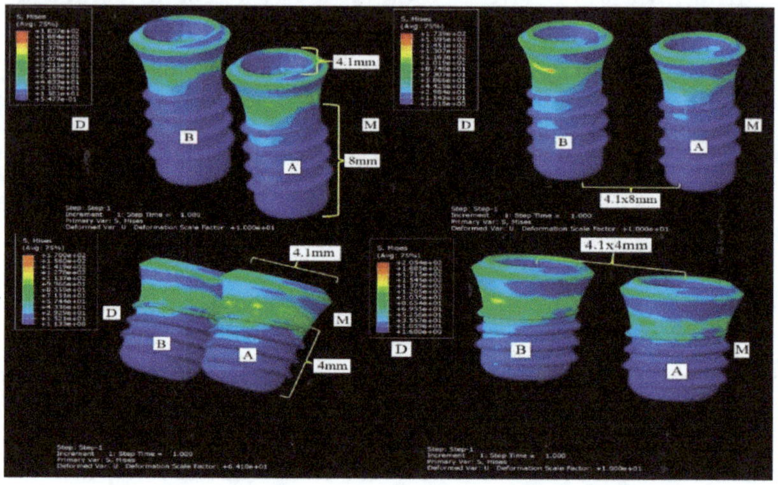

Figure 1. Distribution of the main stresses in short implants. On the left of the figure, the load on the crown of the implant-supported fixed partial prosthesis on two implants of 4.1 × 8 mm (top) and 4.1 × 4 mm (below) observed. To the right of the figure, the load in the cantilever is observed. A. Implant located at the level of the first upper premolar and B at the level of the second upper premolar. Cervical tensions are observed in both A and B.

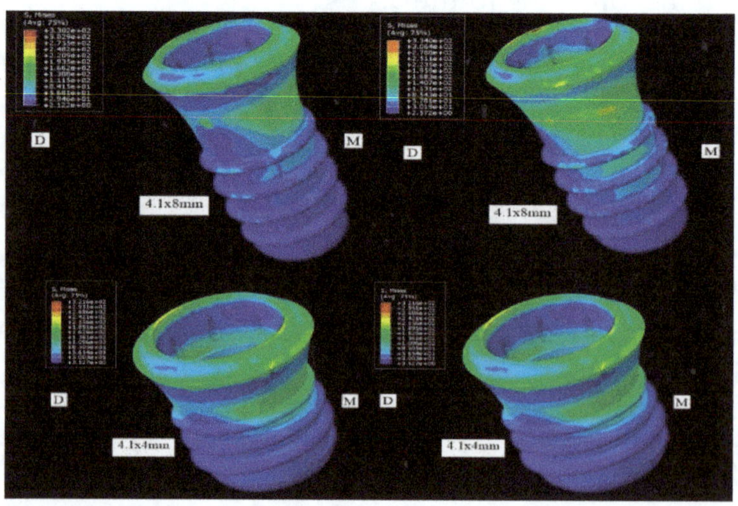

Figure 2. Distribution of the main tensions in the short implants located at the level of the first upper premolar. On the left of the figure, the load on the crown of the implant-supported fixed partial prosthesis is observed on an implant of 4.1 × 8 mm (on top) and 4.1 × 4 mm (below). To the right of the figure, the load in the cantilever is observed. Tensions are observed in the cervical and middle third.

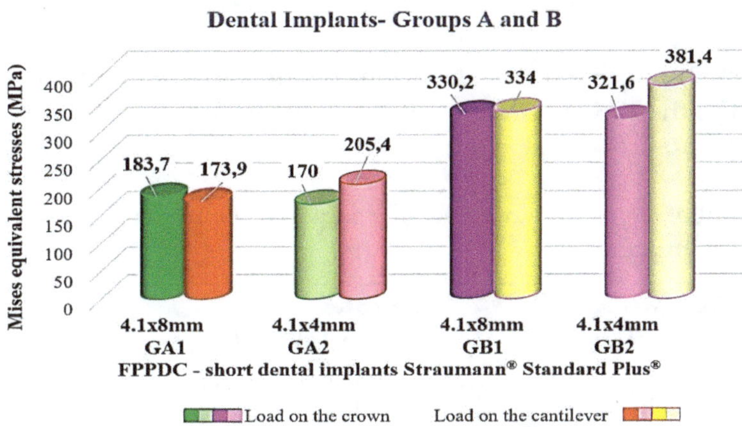

Figure 3. Distribution principal stresses in implants. Fixed partial prosthesis with distal cantilever, supported by ultrashort implants -FPPDC-.

3.2. Distribution of the Tensions in the Solid Model

The load in the crown distributed the tensions in the cervical third of GA1 and GA2; in the cantilever, tensions were observed in the cervical third corresponding to the first premolar, and in the cervical and middle third of the second premolar, in both sub-groups. GA1 was greater with respect to GA2, without significant difference among them.

In GB1 and GB2 the distribution of the principal stresses was demonstrated in the cervical third; in the cantilever, increased tensional values were observed in the cervical and middle third, in both sub-groups. GB2 was larger than GB1, with significant differences among them, marking a critical situation on a map for GB2 (Table 3; Figure 4).

Table 3. Distribution of the principal stresses in the maxillary.

Models	Crown (MPa)	Cantilever (MPa)	Load (N)	Implant Dimensions (mm)
A Two implants	57.55	86.26	100	4.1 × 8
	58.61	78.42	100	4.1 × 4
B An implant	96.83	128.5	100	4.1 × 8
	101.3	168.5	100	4.1 × 4

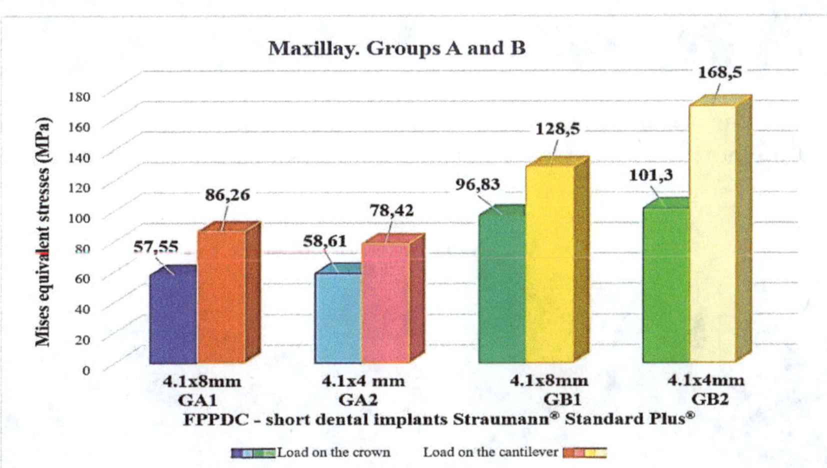

Figure 4. Distribution principal stresses in maxillary. Fixed implant-supported partial prosthesis with distal cantilever -FPPDC-.

3.3. Bone Behavior

The high tensions brought bone micro deformations in a proportional way (higher tensions then more deformation). In GB2 there were higher values with respect to GB1, with significant differences (Table 4 and Figures 5–9).

Table 4. Distribution of the microstrain in the solid model. Fixed partial prosthesis with distal cantilever, supported by ultrashort implants.

Models	Crown (Maximum Tensile) με	Cantilever (Maximum Tensile) με	Load (N)	Implants Dimensions (mm)
A Two implants	3.439	6.983	100	4.1 × 8
	6.648	5.990	100	4.1 × 4
B An implant	5.777	8.553	100	4.1 × 8
	6.538	9.253	100	4.1 × 4

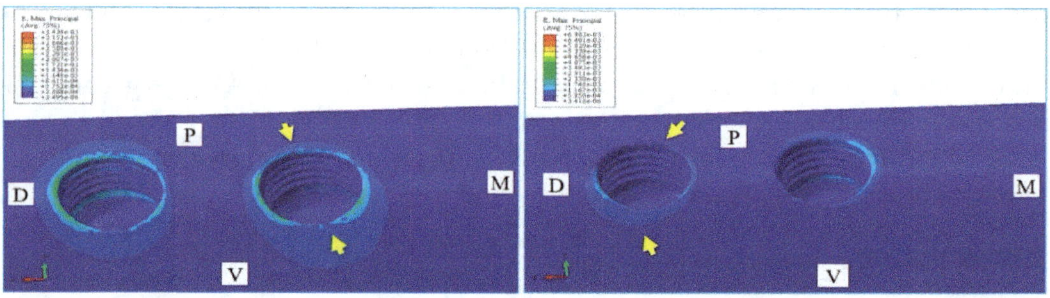

Figure 5. Microdeformations in the maxillary. Load on the crown (**left**) and the cantilever (**right**) of PPDC supported by two ultrashort implants of 4.1 × 8 mm. Arrows indicate microstrain in the bone crest.

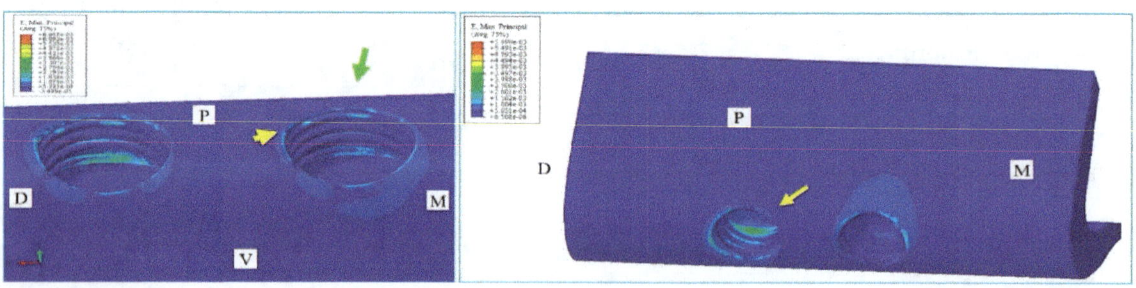

Figure 6. Microstrain in the maxillary. Load on the crown (**left**) and the cantilever (**right**) of the PPFIVD supported by two ultrashort implants of 4.1 × 4 mm. Arrows indicate microstrain in the bone crest.

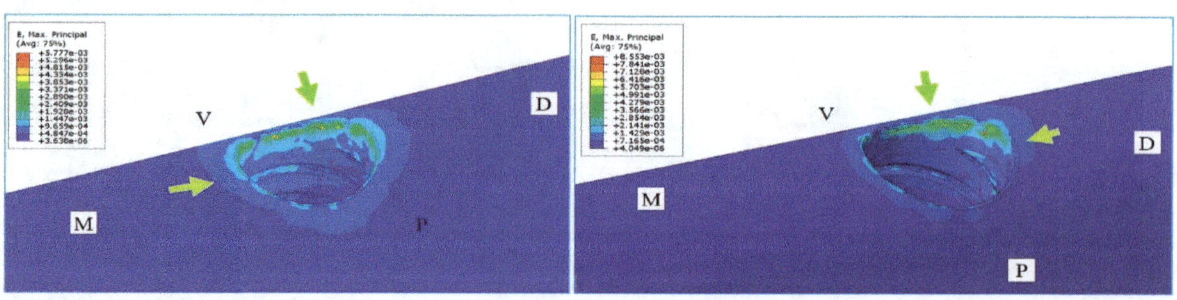

Figure 7. Microdeformations in the maxilla. Load on the crown (**left**) and on the cantilever (**right**) of the PPFIVD supported by an ultrashort implant of 4.1 × 8 mm. Arrows indicate microstrain in the bone crest.

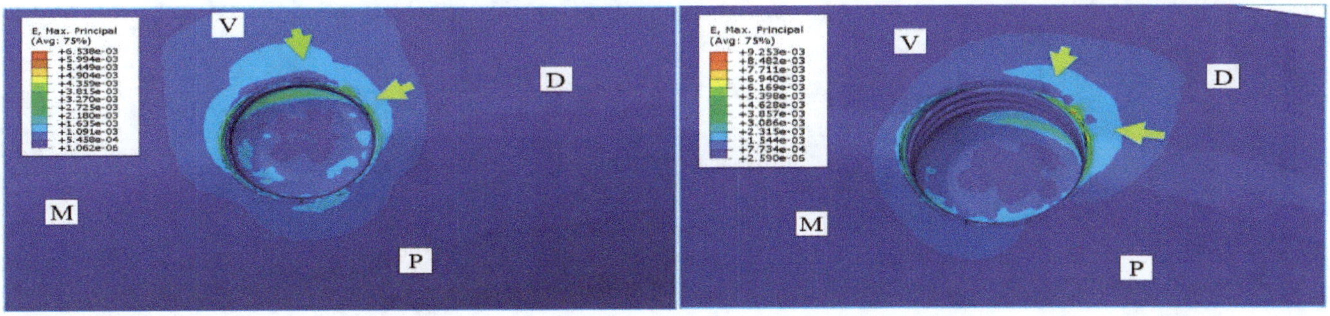

Figure 8. Microdeformations in the maxilla. Load on the crown (**left**) and the cantilever (**right**) of the PPFIVD supported by an ultrashort 4.1 × 4mm. Arrows indicate microstrain in the bone crest.

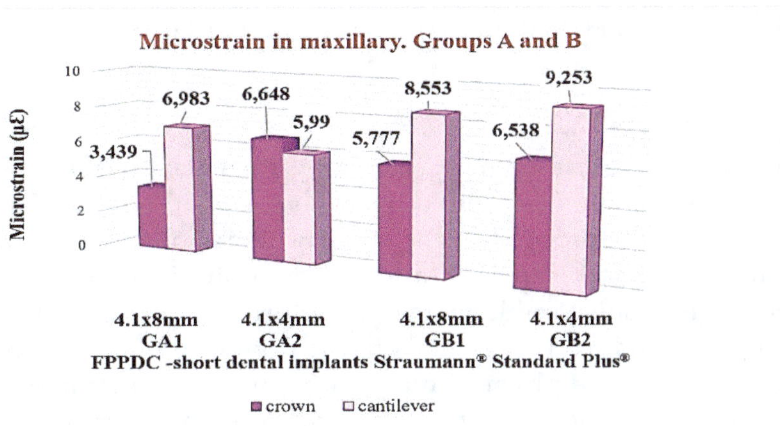

Figure 9. Microstrain in maxillary. Fixed partial prosthesis with distal cantilever, supported by ultrashort implants -FPPDC-.

3.4. Prosthesis Behavior

The micro-deformations facilitated the displacement of the joint prosthesis-implant. In GA1 and GA2 it was oriented through the buccal side. In GB1 and GB2 the displacement was in the buccal-distal direction. GB2 was a major that GB1, with significant difference (Table 5; Figure 10).

Table 5. Displacements of the fixed partial prosthesis with distal cantilever supported by ultrashort implants.

Models	Displacement Crown (mm)	Displacement Cantilever (mm)	Load (N)	Implant Dimensions (mm)
A Two short implants	0.02897	0.04072	100	4.1 × 8
	0.02896	0.04045	100	4.1 × 4
B A short implant	0.05933	0.00728	100	4.1 × 8
	0.06705	0.08347	100	4.1 × 4

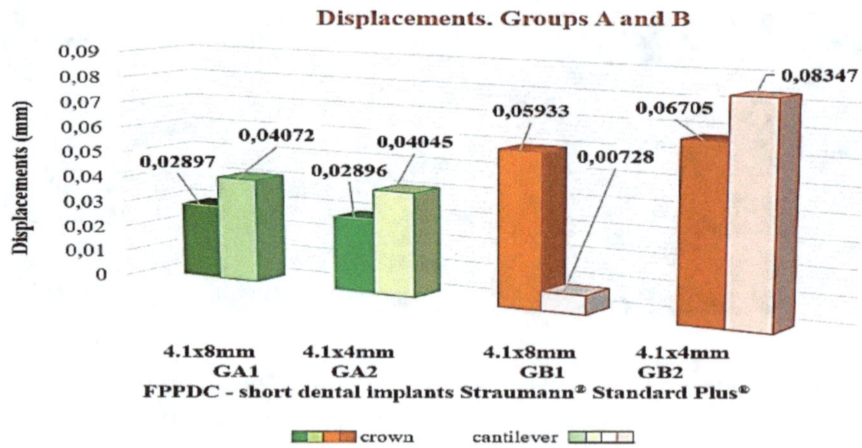

Figure 10. Displacements of the fixed partial prosthesis with distal cantilever, supported by ultrashort implants -FPPDC-.

4. Discussion

The obtained data were described in agreement with a Ceá hypothesis, the error committed in the approach of an exact solution was limited by the error of approach of the obtained solution [27]. The approach error depended crucially on the size and amount of the elements and the equality of other factors that caused this to be smaller, and it was limited to the error of the solution of finite elements. The distribution of short implants in the posterior sector of the maxilla is a challenge when the available bony height is reduced and is next to the floor of the maxillary sinus.

The tension of Von Mises is a physical magnitude of the distortion energy, and is a compound tension that indicates to the average level of tension whose maximum value indicates the possibility of damage occurring. The variables can be manipulated; the software eliminates the variation of the resulting probability of the error of the sample. The initial deformation of the majority of solids is elastic, which implies that the deformation is reversible when stopping applying the tension, and the reason why the solid recovers its initial form.

In the majority of cases, and in agreement with the Hooke's Law, the relation tension-deformation in the elastic regime is linear, and it expresses $\sigma = E \cdot \varepsilon$, where σ is the tension expressed in MPa and is the Young's modulus or modulus of elasticity, and ε is the deformation. If the modulus of elasticity is sprightly, the following formula is obtained whose obtained value indicates that the piece in the study can reconstitute its original form: $E = \sigma/\varepsilon$. However, when the maximum tensional values surpass the reversible capacity of the material it produces a permanent dimensional change. The deformation formula can be established simply: $\varepsilon = \sigma/E$. However, the three-dimensional resolution is more complex.

Sotto Maior et al. [28], described the stress concentration in short single implants of 5 mm in diameter by 7 mm in length in 32 partially-edentulous atrophic jaws. They simulated traumatic occlusion and a crown-implant relation of 2:1 or 2.5:1. The crown created high bending stresses which produced a peri-implant bone loss. Bolle et al. [29] used implants 4 mm in diameter and 10 mm in length over the mandibular channel with and without bone augmentation. Additionally, the inserted implants were 4 to 5 mm in length below the maxillary sinus with and without sinus elevation. After one year of load, the short implants obtained similar results compared to implants of conventional lengths (10 mm). They concluded that short implants could be an option to the surgical procedures since the treatment is less invasive, faster, and economical.

Toti et al. [30] inserted short implants in the posterior atrophic zone of partially-edentulous jaws, and their results showed better compared with implants of standard length placed in the augmented bone. Additionally, the short implants presented less crestal bone loss. Tabrizi et al. [31] evaluated the bone loss in 65 short implants in the jaw. There were no significant differences in the marginal bone loss between the three groups analyzed. However, the authors found that increasing the number of short implants reduced the percentages of crestal bone loss given a better force distribution. Gastaldi et al. [32] compared prosthesis on short implants of 5 × 5 mm or of 5 × 10 mm. inserted in atrophic jaws with augmented bone and maxillary bilateral sinus elevation. After three years of load, short implants obtained results similar to standard implants. They concluded that short implants can be a preferable option to the vertical bone augmentation.

Chou et al. [33], compared the stress distribution around the peri-implant bone of narrow implants with standard length (3.5 mm wide by 10.7 mm length) compared with short and wide implants (5 mm diameter by 7 mm length) in the mandible. It was demonstrated that the development of tension in the cervical region is inevitable, with more uniform distributions in the peri-implant tissue in the short and wide implants. Sahrmann et al. [34], compared implants 6 and 10 mm in length through X-rays. Higher mineralization percentages were observed around short implants compared to standard implants. This was related to the capacity of bone adaptation.

Peixoto et al. [35] used digital images to calculate the deformations of the prosthesis supported by splinted short dental implants during an occlusal load of 250 N. It was found that the veneering material did not influence the distribution of the deformation. Esfahrood et al. [36] performed a prospective study comparing the fixed prosthesis with overdentures supported by short implants (<10 mm). The cumulative success in the implant with rough surfaces was higher than in implants with machined surfaces. The survival of short implants in edentulous maxilla was high when the implants were placed under strict clinical protocols. Therefore, the authors consider the short implants as a safe and predictable technique.

On the other hand, Lemos et al. [37] compared short implants (≤8 mm) with standard implants (>8 mm) placed in the posterior regions of the maxilla and the mandible and found that shorter implants >8 mm presented a greater risk of failure. Block et al. [38] analyzed the level of bone deformation when changing the prosthetic design and different occlusal schemes. It was found that the restorations with splinted implants reduced the levels of deformation in the area of the neck of the implants and provide a better deformation distribution under cyclic load. De Souza Batista et al. [39] compared the influence of the pontic designs and the effect of mesial and distal cantilevers in prostheses supported by standard implants (4 × 10 mm). Axial forces of 400 N and of 200 N were applied in an oblique direction. In the group with two implants supporting a distal cantilever, an unfavorable biomechanical behavior with higher stresses was observed.

In the present work, there were no observed differences between GA1 and GA2 implants. The tensions in GB2 were, principally, greater than those of GB1. However, GB2 (4.1 × 4 mm) exerted higher tensions, an unpredictable situation for implants of short height. Ormianer et al. [40] studied the marginal bone loss related to implants of different designs, (different threads, thread direction, and apical design). In the long-term, there was minor bone loss in implants with greater interthread distances, deep apical turns, and narrow cores. Their results favored a single-piece implant design with a "V" thread design. Wolff et al. [14] demonstrated that the effective tensions take place in the bone–implant interface under unidirectional axial load. Four types of implants showed bone loss resulting from pathological tensions >3000 $\mu\varepsilon$. The groups analyzed in the present work were in the rank of pathological overload; this favored the micro deformations and the displacements of the implant/abutment connections.

Villarinho et al. [41] inserted 46 single implants of 4.1 × 6 mm in the posterior areas of the maxilla and the mandible in 20 patients; after 45 ± 9 months the percentages of success were 65.2% and 95%, with more probabilities of implant loss in the jaw than in the maxilla. The crown–implant ratio and the time were significant predictive values for bone loss ($p < 0.001$). In this research that GA two splinted short implants were observed, which would have the best stress distribution and, therefore, more possibility of permanence in the mouth, and which would give the joint prosthesis-implant greater stability in the long-term.

5. Conclusions

Within the limitations of this FEA:

- PPFIVD on two extra-short dental implants could be used as a viable option;
- The tensions are distributed in the cervical third of the implants and to the implant/abutment interface in the form of micro deformations;
- PPFIVD over single extra short implants of 4.1 × 4 mm possess a high risk or mechanical failure; and
- The forces generated during the functional load in the posterior area of the maxilla would affect the prosthetic restoration with distal cantilever and would affect the peri-implant bone that surrounds the extra-short dental implants.

Author Contributions: Conceptualization, Enrique Fernández Bodereau.; methodology, Rafael Arcesio Delgado Ruiz, Viviana Yolanda Flores.; software, Viviana Yolanda Flores.; validation, Enrique Fernández Bodereau. and Viviana Yolanda Flores.; formal analysis, Juan Manuel Aragoneses, Viviana Yolanda Flores.; investigation, Viviana Yolanda Flores.; resources, José Luis Calvo Guirado.; data curation, Viviana Yolanda Flores.; writing—original draft preparation, Rafael Arcesio Delgado Ruiz, José Luis Calvo Guirado.; writing—review and editing, Enrique Fernández Bodereau and Viviana Yolanda Flores.; visualization, Juan Manuel AragonesesViviana Yolanda Flores and José Luis Calvo Guirado.; supervision, Enrique Fernández Bodereau.; project administration, Enrique Fernández Bodereau.; funding acquisition, Enrique Fernández Bodereau."

Acknowledgments: To the engineer Domínguez A., for his technical collaboration in obtaining the consigned data.

References

1. Brånemark, P.I. Osseointegration and its experimental background. *J. Prosthet. Dent.* **1983**, *50*, 399–410. [CrossRef]
2. Cervino, G.; Romeo, U.; Lauritano, F.; Bramanti, E.; Fiorillo, L.; D'Amico, C.; Milone, D.; Laino, L.; Campolongo, F.; Rapisarda, S.; et al. Fem and Von Mises Analysis of OSSTEM® Dental Implant Structural Components: Evaluation of Different Direction Dynamic Loads. *Open Dent. J.* **2018**, *12*, 219–229. [CrossRef] [PubMed]
3. Moraschini, V.; Poubel, L.; Ferreira, V.; Barboza Edos, S. Evaluation of survival and success rates of dental implants reported in longitudinal studies with a follow-up period of at least 10 years: A systematic review. *Int. J. Oral Maxillofac. Surg.* **2015**, *44*, 377–388. [CrossRef] [PubMed]
4. Ibáñez, J.C.; Tahhan, M.J.; Zamar, J.A. Performance of Double Acid-Etched Surface External Hex Titanium Implants in relation to One-and Two-Stage Surgical Procedures. *J. Periodontol.* **2003**, *74*, 1575–1581. [CrossRef] [PubMed]
5. Dawson, J.H.; Hyde, B.; Hurst, M.; Harris, B.T.; Lin, W.S. Polyetherketoneketone (PEKK), a framework material for complete fixed and removable dental prostheses: A clinical report. *J. Prosthet. Dent.* **2018**, *119*, 867–872. [CrossRef] [PubMed]
6. Najeeb, S.; Zafar, M.S.; Khurshid, Z.; Siddiqui, F. Applications of polyetheretherketone (PEEK) in oral implantology and prosthodontics. *J. Prosthodont. Res.* **2016**, *60*, 12–19. [CrossRef] [PubMed]
7. Thoma, S.D.; Cha, J.K.; Jung, U.W. Treatment concepts for the posterior maxilla and mandible: Short implants vs long implants in augmented bone. *J. Periodont. Implant Sci.* **2017**, *47*, 2–12. [CrossRef] [PubMed]
8. Raviv, E.; Turcotte, A.; Harel Raviv, M. Short dental implants in reduced alveolar bone height. *Quintessence Int.* **2010**, *41*, 505–509.
9. Felice, P.; Checchi, L.; Barausse, C.; Pistilli, R.; Sammartino, G.; Masi, I.; Ippolito, D.R.; Esposito, M. Posterior jaws rehabilitated with partial prostheses supported by 4.0 × 4.0 mm or by longer implants: One-year post-loading results from a multicenter randomized controlled trial. *Eur. J. Oral Implantol.* **2016**, *9*, 35–45.
10. Blanes, R.J.; Bernard, J.P.; Blanes, Z.M.; Belser, U.C. A 10-year prospective study of ITI dental implants placed in the posterior region. II: Influence of the crown-to-implant ratio and different prosthetic treatment modalities on crestal bone loss. *Clin. Oral Implants Res.* **2007**, *18*, 707–714. [CrossRef]
11. Urdaneta, R.A.; Rodriguez, S.; McNeil, D.C.; Weed, M.; Chuang, S.K. The effect of increased Crown-to-Implant Ratio on Single Tooth Locking Taper Implants. *Int. J. Oral Maxillofac. Implants* **2010**, *25*, 709–743.

12. Zurdo, J.; Romao, C.; Wennstrom, J.L. Survival and complication rates of implant-supported fixed partial dentures with cantilevers: A systematic review. *Clin. Oral Implants Res.* **2009**, *20*, 59–66. [CrossRef] [PubMed]
13. Salvi, G.E.; Brägger, U. Mechanical and technical risks in implant therapy. *Int. J. Oral Maxillofac. Implants* **2009**, *24*, 69–85. [PubMed]
14. Wolff, J.; Narra, N.; Antalainen, A.K.; Valášek, J.; Kaiser, J.; Sándor, G.K.; Marcián, P. Finite element analysis of bone loss around failing implants. *Mater. Des.* **2014**, *61*, 177–184. [CrossRef]
15. Cicciù, M.; Cervino, G.; Milone, D.; Risitano, G. FEM Investigation of the Stress Distribution over Mandibular Bone Due to Screwed Overdenture Positioned on Dental Implants. *Materials* **2018**, *11*, 1512.
16. Lauritano, F.; Runci, M.; Cervino, G.; Fiorillo, L.; Bramanti, E.; Cicciù, M. Three-dimensional evaluation of different prosthesis retention systems using finite element analysis and the Von Mises stress test. *Minerva Stomatol.* **2016**, *65*, 353–367. [PubMed]
17. Sahin, S.; Cehreli, M.C.; Yalcin, E. The influence of functional forces on the biomechanics of implant-supported prosthesis—A review. *J. Dent.* **2002**, *30*, 271–282. [CrossRef]
18. Mellal, A.; Wiskott, H.W.; Botsis, J.; Scherer, S.S.; Belser, U.C. Stimulating effect of implant loading on the surrounding bone. Comparison of three numerical models and validation by in vivo data. *Clin. Oral Implants Res.* **2004**, *15*, 239–248. [CrossRef] [PubMed]
19. Geng, J.P.; Tan, K.B.C.; Liu, G.R. Application of finite element analysis in implant dentistry: A review of the literature. *J. Prosthet. Dent.* **2001**, *85*, 585–598. [CrossRef]
20. Sohn, B.S.; Heo, S.J.; Koak, J.Y.; Kim, S.K.; Lee, S.Y. Strain of implants depending on occlusion types in mandibular implant-supported fixed prostheses. *J. Adv. Prosthodont.* **2011**, *3*, 1–9. [CrossRef] [PubMed]
21. Fernández Bodereau, E., Jr.; Fernández Bodereaum, E. Prótesis a Puente. Selección y valoración de places. In *Prótesis Fija e Implantes. Práctica Clínica*; Ed Avances Médico-Dentales SL: Madrid, Spain, 1996; pp. 295–320.
22. Fazi, G.; Tellini, S.; Vangi, D.; Branchi, R. Three-dimensional finite element analysis of different implant configuration for mandibular fixed prosthesis. *Int. J. Oral Maxillofac. Implants* **2011**, *26*, 752–759. [PubMed]
23. Turner, M.J. Stiffness and Deflection Analysis of Complex Structures. *J. Aeronaut. Sci.* **1956**, *23*, 805–823. [CrossRef]
24. Okumura, N.; Stegaroiu, R.; Kitamura, E.; Kurokawa, K.; Nomura, S. Influence of maxillary cortical bone thickness, implant design and implant diameter on stress around implants: A three-dimensional finite element analysis. *J. Prosthodont. Res.* **2010**, *54*, 133–142. [CrossRef] [PubMed]
25. De Almeida, E.O.; Rocha, E.P.; Freitas, A.C., Jr.; Freitas, M.M., Jr. Finite Element Stress Analysis of Edentulous Mandibles with Different Bone Types Supporting Multiple-Implant Superstructures. *Int. J. Oral Maxillofac. Implants* **2010**, *25*, 1108–1114. [PubMed]
26. Romeo, E.; Tomasi, C.; Finini, I.; Casentini, P.; Lops, D. Implant-supported fixed cantilever prosthesis in partially edentulous jaws: A cohort prospective study. *Clin. Oral Implants Res.* **2009**, *20*, 1278–1285. [CrossRef] [PubMed]
27. Céa, J. Approximation Variationnelle des Problèmes aux Limites. *Ann. Inst. Fourier.* **1964**, *14*, 345–444. [CrossRef]
28. Sotto Maior, B.S.; Senna, P.M.; da Silva, W.J.; Rocha, E.P.; Del Bel Cury, A.A. Influence of crown-to-implant ratio. Retention system, restorative material, and occlusal loading on stress concentrations in single short implants. *Int. J. Oral Maxillofac. Implants* **2012**, *27*, 13–18.
29. Bolle, C.; Felice, P.; Barausse, C.; Pistilli, V.; Trullenque-Eriksson, A.; Esposito, M. 4 mm long vs longer implants in augmented bone in posterior atrophic jaws: 1-Year post-loading results from a multicentre randomized controlled trial. *Eur. J. Oral Implantol.* **2018**, *11*, 31–47.
30. Toti, P.; Marchionni, S.; Menchini-Fabris, G.B.; Marconcini, S.; Covani, U.; Barone, A. Surgical techniques used in the rehabilitation of partially edentulous patients with atrophic posterior mandible: A systematic review and meta-analysis of randomized controlled clinical trials. *J. Craniomaxillofac. Surg.* **2017**, *45*, 1236–1245. [CrossRef]
31. Tabrizi, R.; Arabion, H.; Aliabadi, E.; Hasanzadeh, F. Does increasing the number of short implants reduce marginal bone loss in the posterior mandible? A prospective study. *Br. J. Oral Maxillofac. Surg.* **2016**, *54*, 731–735. [CrossRef]

32. Gastaldi, G.; Felice, P.; Pistilli, V.; Barausse, C.; Ippolito, D.R.; Esposito, M. Posterior atrophic jaws rehabilitated with prostheses supported by 5 × 5 mm implants with a nanostructured calcium-incorporated titanium surface o by longer implants in augmented bone. 3-Year results from a randomized controlled trial. *Eur. J. Oral Implantol.* **2018**, *11*, 49–61. [PubMed]
33. Chou, H.Y.; Müftü, S.; Bozkava, D. Combined effects of implants insertion depth and alveolar bone quality on peri-implant bone strain induced by a wide-diameter, short implant, and a narrow-diameter, long implant. *J. Prosthet. Dent.* **2010**, *104*, 293–300. [CrossRef]
34. Sahrmann, P.; Schoen, P.; Naenni, N.; Jung, R.; Attin, T.; Schmidlin, P.R. Peri-implant Bone Density around Implants of Different Length: A 3-year Follow-up of Randomized Clinical Trial. *J. Clin. Periodontol.* **2017**, *44*, 762–768. [CrossRef] [PubMed]
35. Peixoto, R.F.; Macedo, A.P.; Martinelli, J.; Faria, A.C.; Tiossi, R.; Ribeiro, R.F.; de Mattos, M.D. A Digital Image Correlation Analysis of Strain Generated by 3-Unit Implant-Supported Fixed Dental Prosthesis: An In Vitro Study. *Implant Dent.* **2017**, *26*, 567–573. [CrossRef] [PubMed]
36. Esfahrood, Z.R.; Ahmadi, L.; Karami, E.; Asghari, S. Short dental implants in the posterior maxilla: A review of the literature. *J. Korean Assoc. Oral Maxillofac. Surg.* **2017**, *43*, 70–76. [CrossRef] [PubMed]
37. Lemos, C.A.; Ferros-Alves, M.L.; Okamoto, R.; Mendonca, M.R.; Pellizzer, E.P. Short dental implants vs standard dental implants placed in the posterior jaw: A systematic review and meta-analysis. *J. Dent.* **2016**, *47*, 8–17. [CrossRef] [PubMed]
38. Block, J.; Matalon, S.; Tanase, G.; Ormianer, Z. Effect of Restorative Configurations and Occlusal Schemes on Strain Levels on Bone Surrounding Implants. *Implant Dent.* **2017**, *26*, 574–580. [CrossRef]
39. De Souza Batista, V.E.; Verri, F.R.; Almeida, D.A.; Santiago Junior, J.F.; Lemos, C.A.; Pellizzer, E.P. Finite element analysis of implant-supported prosthesis with pontic and cantilever in the posterior maxilla. *Comput. Methods Biomech. Biomed. Eng.* **2017**, *20*, 663–670. [CrossRef]
40. Ormianer, Z.; Matalon, S.; Block, J.; Kohen, J. Dental Implant Thread Design and the Consequences on Long-Term Marginal Bone Loss. *Implant Dent.* **2016**, *25*, 471–477. [CrossRef]
41. Villarinho, E.A.; Triches, D.F.; Alonso, F.R.; Mezzomo, L.A.M.; Teixeira, E.R.; Shinkai, R.S.A. Risk factors for single crowns supported by shorts (6-mm) implants in the posterior region: A prospective clinical and radiographic study. *Clin. Implant Dent. Relat. Res.* **2017**, *19*, 671–680. [CrossRef]

5

Influence of Mucosal Thickness, Implant Dimensions and Stability in Cone Morse Implant Installed at Subcrestal Bone Level on the Peri-Implant Bone: A Prospective Clinical and Radiographic Study

Sergio Alexandre Gehrke [1,2,*], Mauro Bercianos [3], Jorge Gonzalo Aguerrondo [3], José Luis Calvo-Guirado [4] and Juan Carlos Prados-Frutos [5]

1 Biotecnos Research Center, 11100 Montevideo, Uruguay
2 Master Postgraduate Program in Biotechnology of UCAM, 11100 Montevideo, Uruguay
3 Postgraduate Program in Biotechnology of UCAM, 11100 Montevideo, Uruguay
4 Oral and Implant Surgery, Faculty of Health Sciences, Universidad Católica San Antonio de Murcia (UCAM), 30107 Murcia, Spain
5 Department of Medicine and Surgery, Rey Juan Carlos University, Alcorcón, 28922 Madrid, Spain
* Correspondence: sergio.gehrke@hotmail.com

Abstract: The objective of this observational clinical study was to analyze the behavior of peri-implant tissues around cone Morse dental implants installed in the subcrestal bone position considering different clinical variables: Mucosal thickness, implant diameter, and implant length. Thirty patients were selected and included in the present study. Initially the thickness of the mucosa was measured by periapical radiographic and clinically (after the mucosal displaced). According to the planning for each treatment, implants with different dimensions (in length and diameter) were selected and used. Periapical radiographs were obtained at different times: Immediate postoperative (time t1) and 90 days after implantation (time t2). The initial stability of the implants (ISQ) was measured immediately of the implant insertion and 90 days after. The means and standard deviations of the ISQ values were in time t1 was 63.2 ± 6.99 (95% confidence interval (CI): 41 to 83) and in time t2 was 69.7 ± 7.09 (95% CI: 61 to 87). Overall mean of mesial and distal bone loss 90 days after the implantations were 1.11 ± 1.16 mm and 1.11 ± 1.15 mm, respectively. When the variables were considered, in all situations proposed, the bone loss showed differences statistically significant. In conclusion, the implant diameter and mucosal thickness variables showed an important effect on bone loss values. However, the implant length did not show an effect on the peri-implant behavior.

Keywords: crestal bone; cone Morse implants; mucosal thickness; implant dimensions; resonance frequency analysis

1. Introduction

Implantology as a surgical procedure implies the management of a wound involving the soft and hard tissues. After the implant osseointegration, the bone and the mucosa required by its new function of protection of underlying peri-implant structures, is transformed into the peri-implantar mucosa acquiring particular morphological characteristics. For this new sealing function, the epithelial and connective tissues require an appropriate dimension, and if it does not exist it will be created at the expense of bone resorption. Berglund and Lindhe [1] carried out a study with the purpose of confirming this concept, where thinning the tissues also proves that the conformation of the seal requires a minimal mucosal dimension, otherwise it would be created at the expense of bone resorption. In this way, the biology demands a dimension of minimal epithelial and connective tissue adequate for the protection of the underlying structures. In this sense, other authors begin to give importance to the mucosal thickness as a relevant factor independent of the aforementioned bone resorption, using in its clinical trials different types of technology in the area of the implant connection, noticing the inefficacy of these technologies in the control of crestal bone resorption when the mucosa shows little thickness [2–7].

In addition, other factors may affect the behavior of peri-implant tissues, such as: Microgap, micromovement, microtopography of the interface, repeated removal of the abutment, and the platform design (switching or no) [8–11]. Several studies carried out by our group demonstrated that Morse taper implants present a better condition and behavior when compared to implants of internal and external connection, referring to the factors previously described [12,13]. In this way, a recent important systematic review that was published about the performance of the Morse taper connection [14] showed evidence that this type of connection appeared to be superior in terms of bacterial sealing compared with the traditional ones emphasizing that no connection has a 100% bacterial sealing. Morse taper connection systems appear to be more resistant to abutment movement and increased under load space compared to internal and external hexagon implants [15]. Moreover, the Morse taper connection have greater resistance to torque loss than other connection models [16]. This system seems to have less tension on the abutment screw, the cone compensates for the high stresses and protects the screw from overload [17].

Marginal bone stability around dental implants has always been considered one of the main criteria for defining implant success [18]. Then, with the current advancements and new technologies in implant dentistry, we should strive both for bone loss close to zero and to seek out variables that cause higher or lower rates of resorption. Albrektsson et al. reported that the extensive bone resorption after the first year is generally due to an exacerbation of adverse body reactions caused by non-optimal implant components, adverse surgery or prosthodontics, and/or compromised patient factors [19]. In a recent review study of the evidence regarding marginal bone loss around dental implants, Sasada and Cochran concluded that there is a strong indication that contaminated implant-abutment connections may have an effect on peri-implantitis and failure over time [20].

Although the in vitro results show better results in implants of conical internal connection and in vivo results with lower marginal bone loss, all models show comparable rates in terms of implant success and survival. However, these Morse tapered implants need to be evaluated for their clinical behavior in relation to peri-implant tissues, as many manufacturers recommend their infra-osseous installation without explaining the need for this procedure. In this sense, the aim of the present study was to evaluate the clinical performance of an implant with Morse taper connection (submerged 2 mm infra-osseous) and comparing different clinical variables (mucosal thickness, implant dimensions, and implant stability) with the marginal bone behavior. It was hypothesized that mucosal thickness plays a fundamental role in the maintenance of peri-implant bone and soft tissues.

2. Material and Methods

2.1. Patient Population and Research Design

For the present study, patients aged between 20 to 63 years, that needed replacement of missing teeth in the posterior region of the mandible with adequate condition of remaining bone (height ≥10 mm and width ≥6 mm) and adequate prosthetic space to rehabilitation, were selected in a private clinic (Montevideo, Uruguay). A total of 30 patients, 18 women and 12 men, were consecutively included. All patients signed a written Helsinki informed consent for participation and permission to use the data obtained for research purposes prior to the procedures. The general health condition stability of the participants in the study was considered and their ability to withstand surgery to install the planned implants. Patients with systemic alterations (diabetes, hypertension, or osteoporosis) or local changes (oral pathology in soft or hard tissues, bruxism, and smoking) were excluded from this study.

In addition, patients with uncontrolled and/or untreated periodontal disease, lack of adequate bone tissue for implant insertion, and/or presence of inflammatory events were not included in the study.

Sixty dental implants of conical macro design with cone Morse connection manufactured in grade IV titanium (Implacil De Bortoli, São Paulo, Brazil) were used in the implantations. The implants dimensions used were 3.5 and 4 mm in diameter and 7, 9, and 11 mm in length. Moreover, five implants were used to the surface analysis. The Figure 1 show a representative image of the macro design and the connection characteristics of the implant used in the present study.

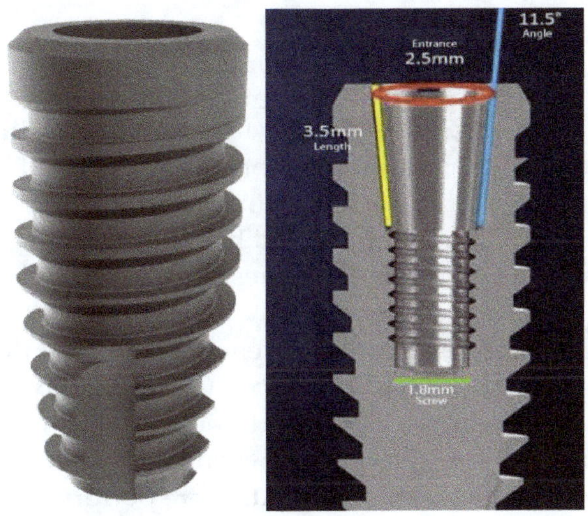

Figure 1. Representative image of the macro design and the connection characteristics of the implants used in the study, respectively.

2.2. *Dental Implant Surface Topography*

All implants are treated with sandblasted acid-etched surface technology as previously described by Gehrke et al. [21]. The implants were blasted with 50–100 μm TiO_2 microparticles and, following, the surface was ultrasonically cleaned with an alkaline solution, washed in distilled water, and pickled with maleic acid ($HO_2CCHCHCO_2H$). After these treatments, five implants were used to evaluate the surface characteristics by scanning electron microscopy (SEM, model JSM 5200, JEOL Ltd., Tokyo, Japan) and the roughness parameters, which was measured on the profilometer (Perthometer S2, Mahr GmbH, Göttingen, Germany), where Ra is the absolute value of all profile points, and Rz is the value of the absolute heights of the five highest peaks and the depths of the five deepest valleys.

2.3. *Surgical Procedure of Implant Placement*

All procedures (pre, trans, and postoperative) were performed by two specialists in implantology (MB and JGA). In all patients, mucosal thickness was measured at the local determined for implant installation through a periapical X-ray images. The measurement of the mesio-distal diameter of clinical crown of the tooth adjacent to the place where the implant will be installed was used to calibrate the program. The surgical procedures routinely used to install dental implants were applied. Surgical guides were prepared and used for the installation of all implants. All patients were given antibiotic premedication that was administered orally (2 g of Amoxicillin, 2 h before surgery) and continued in the postoperative for another five days (500 mg every 8 h). After the application of local anesthesia using Articaine 2% (DFL Ltd.a, Rio de Janeiro, Brazil), an incision was performed in the central area of the mucosal crest, and only the buccal flap was displaced, keeping the lingual mucosa in position for the proper measurement of its clinical thickness. The mucosa thickness was measured using a periodontal probe (Hu-Friedy, Chicago, IL, USA), from the crestal bone to the more apical area of the mucosa. Then, the lingual flap was raised, and the implant procedures were performed in accordance to the manufacturer's instructions.

The dimensions of the implants were previously determined during the planning of each case. For osteotomies, a Driller BLM600 motor and a counter angle with a 20:1 reduction (Driller, São Paulo, Brazil) was used under intense external irrigation with 0.9% saline solution. All implants were positioned 2 ± 0.2 mm subcrestally. All sutures were performed using simple point with Nylon 5-0 (Ethicon US, Bridgewater, NJ, USA). For the post-operative pain and inflammation control was administrated Cetoprofeno (200 mg/day) for four days plus paracetamol (750 mg, in case of pain). Ninety days after performing the surgery for the installation of the implants, the rehabilitation procedures were started.

2.4. Clinical Stability and Radiographic Evaluations

The stability of all implants was evaluated by resonance frequency immediately after the installation (t1) and 90 days (t2) in the reentry surgery to install the healing abutment. This evaluation was performed using the Ostell™ Mentor (Integration Diagnostics AB, Goteborg, Sweden) plus the Smartpeg™ (Integration Diagnostics AB) devices. Smartpeg sensors were installed in each implant using a controlled torque of 10 Ncm, as recommended by a recent study [22]. A mean was performed with the values obtained in the measurements in the vestibule-lingual direction (V-L) and mesio-distal direction (M-D).

Three periapical radiographies were made for each patient to measure the mucosa thickness (before implant placement) and the marginal bone loss (immediately after the surgery and 90 days later). Parallel profile radiography using a digital ring holder was used to standardize the analysis and decrease the image distortions. The relation between the implant platform and the crestal bone position was measured. All radiographic measurements were performed using the ImageJ software for Windows (developed at the U.S. National Institutes of Health and available at http://rsb.info.nih.gov/ij). In the first radiography the mucosa width was measured and compared with the clinical measurements. Then, the implants were grouped according to the measured thickness of the mucosa in each implant: Patients with mucosal thickness (MT) between 1.0 and 2.0 mm (MT1); mucosal thickness between 2.1 and 3.0 mm (MT2); and, mucosal thickness more 3.1 mm (MT3). In the radiographs post-implantation, the cortical bone level to the platform was measured and recorded at the mesial-marginal bone loss (m-MBL) and distal-marginal bone loss (d-MBL) side of each implant.

2.5. Statistical Analyses

The methodology and statistical data analyses were reviewed by an independent statistician. The outcomes were longitudinally analyzed among the two initial stability of the implants (ISQ) tests and the bone level between the variables using the one-way analysis of variance (ANOVA) test for repeated measures. The comparison between the clinical and radiographic measurements was performed using the z-test for unpaired samples. The Kolmogorov-Smirnov normality test and the Levene's homogeneity of variance test were used. For bivariate analysis, Mann-Whitney U, and Students-t tests were used. Repeated-measures ANOVA was used to analyze the reduction in marginal bone loss. All comparison analysis was performed using GraphPad Prism 5 software for Windows (GraphPad Software, San Diego, CA, USA). The level of significance was set at $\alpha = 0.05$.

3. Results

The mean and standard deviation of the absolute values of all profile points (Ra) was 0.87 ± 0.14 μm, the root-mean-square of the values of all points (Rq) was 1.12 ± 0.18 μm, and the average value of the absolute heights of the five highest peaks and the depths of the five deepest valleys (Rz) was 5.14 ± 0.69 μm. In the Figure 2 are showed the implant macro design and the surface images of the morphology.

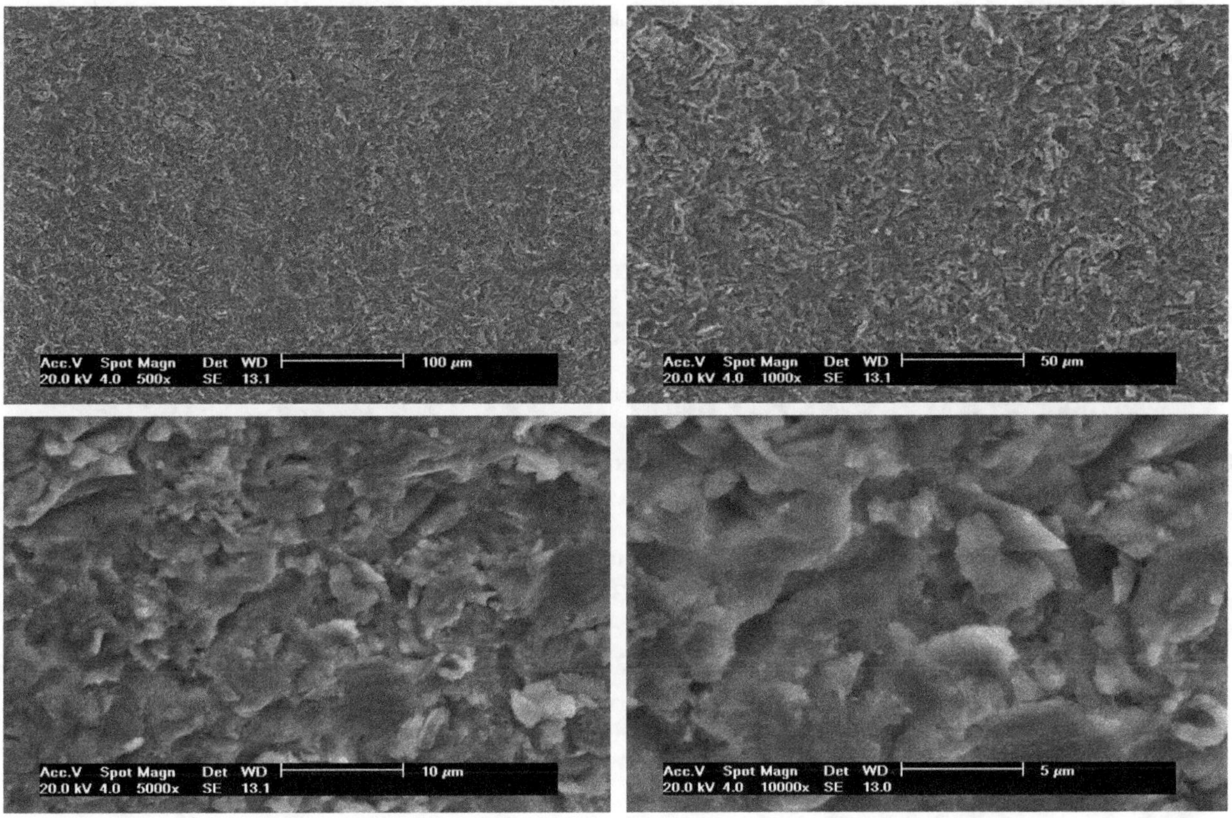

Figure 2. SEM images of the implant surface in different increases.

A total of 60 conical implants of Morse taper connections were installed and the evaluated variables were the diameter of 3.5 mm (n = 17) and 4 mm (n = 43), the different lengths that ranged from 7 mm (n = 21), 9 mm (n = 24), and 11 mm (n = 15) and the mucosa thickness MT1 (n = 19), MT2 (n = 24), and MT3 (n = 17). Thirty patients (18 women and 12 men; ages from 20 to 63 years) received dental implants. After the initial period of 90 days, only one implant was loose throughout the study period and re-implanted with success. Then, the analysis was performed with a total implant quantity (60 implants). No patient dropout was observed during the observation period.

The analyses between the radiographic and clinical measurements showed similar values for the mucosal thickness, no presenting statistical differences ($p = 0.634$), with a mean and standard deviation of 2.26 ± 0.72 and 2.34 ± 1.27, for clinical and radiographic measurements, respectively. The Figure 3 show a box plots graph to compare the measured values and the Figure 4 shows the clinical and radiographic representative image of these measurements.

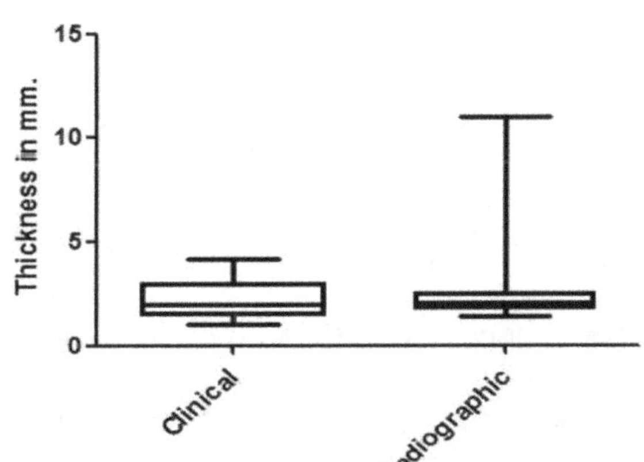

Figure 3. Box-plots graph of the values measured clinical and radiographically.

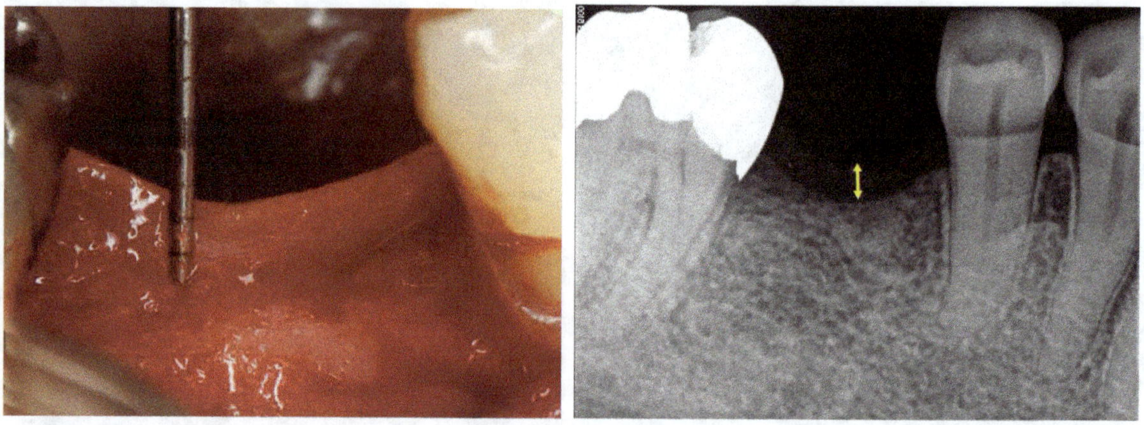

Figure 4. Representative clinical image of the mucosal thickness measurement after the mucosal flap and a periapical x-ray image of the mucosal measurement.

The measured ISQ values showed an overall mean and standard deviation in each proposed time as following: In time t1 was 63.6 ± 2.90 (95% CI: 53 to 70) and in t2 was 69.0 ± 4.14 (95% CI: 49 to 75). The values (mean, SD, and median) are summarized in the Table 1. Figure 5 showed a box-plots graph of the ISQ evolution in each time. No statistical difference of ISQ was observed regarding the implant diameter and length ($p > 0.05$). However, comparing the values of t1 versus t2, an expected statistical difference was found ($p < 0.0001$).

Table 1. Initial stability of the implants (ISQ) analysis and measurements at initial day (baseline) and 90 days after the implant installation. Results as mean and medians.

ISQ Value	Baseline		90 Days	
	Mean ± SD	**Median**	**Mean ± SD**	**Median**
Mesio-distal	63.4 ± 2.94	63.75	68.0 ± 3.85	69.53
Vestibule-lingual	63.7 ± 2.89	64.45	69.9 ± 4.14	70.80

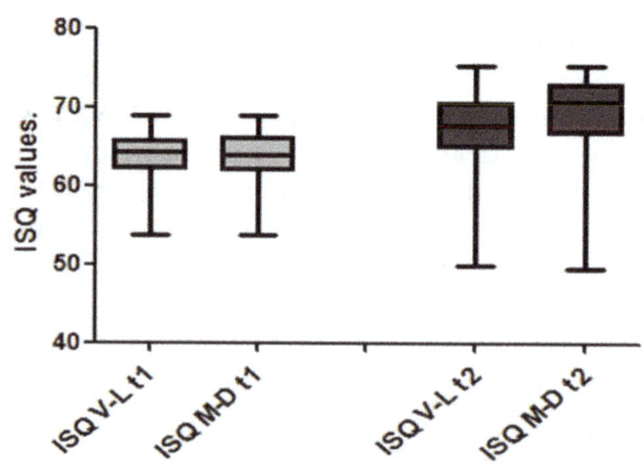

Figure 5. Box-plots graph of the ISQ measured values in the time 1 (t1) and time 2 (t2). V-L = vestibule-lingual direction and M-D = mesio-distal direction.

The comparative data measured between mesial and distal marginal bone loss with the observed variables. Overall mean of mesial and distal MBL were 1.11 ± 1.16 mm and 1.11 ± 1.15 mm, respectively, resulted in non-statistically significant differences ($p > 0.05$). The comparison of the bone loss between the patient's sex showed non-statistically significant differences ($p > 0.05$), where the woman patient's show an MBL mean value of 1.1 ± 1.25 mm and the man patient´s 1.0 ± 0.93 mm. The images of the Figure 6 show a sequence of measurements of the MBL.

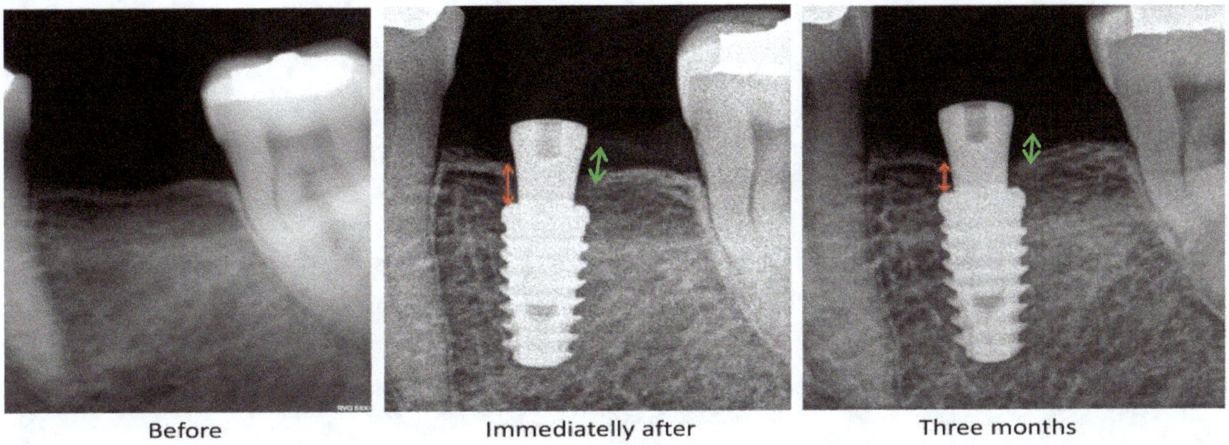

Figure 6. Radiograph sequence used to evaluate and measure the bone level. The measurements were performed from the implant platform to the crestal bone (red arrows = m-MBL and green arrows = d-MBL).

Regarding the implant dimensions, the diameter showed a mean value of MBL in 0.73 ± 0.8 mm for the implants of 3.5 mm and 1.05 ± 1.1 mm for the implant of 4.0 mm, with significant statistical difference ($p < 0.001$). The bar graph of the Figure 7 shows the values of mesial and distal MBL measurements.

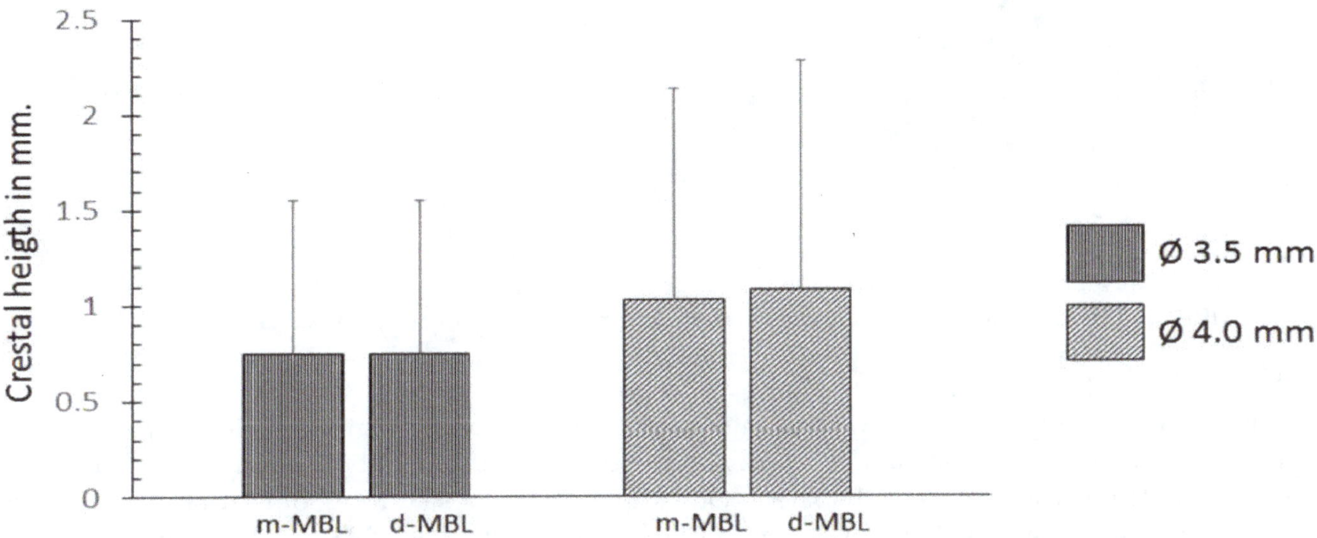

Figure 7. Bar graph showing the mean and standard deviation of the MBL values measured in mesial (m-MBL) and distal (d-MBL) position of each implant in the two implant diameters.

However, the MBL values measured at different implant lengths showed very similar values (Figure 8), without statistically significant differences ($p > 0.05$).

The mucosal thickness (MT1, MT2, and MT3) resulted in statistically significant differences ($p < 0.05$). The mean value of MBL in the MT1 was 1.5 ± 0.8 mm, in the MT2 was 0.75 ± 0.5 and in the MT3 was 0.9 ± 0.8 mm. The bar graph of the Figure 9 shows the values for mesial and distal measurements. In general, the better behavior was observed in the MT2 (mucosal thickness between 2.1 and 3.0 mm), with 0.7 ± 0.6 mm for m-MBL and 0.8 ± 0.5 mm for d-MBL.

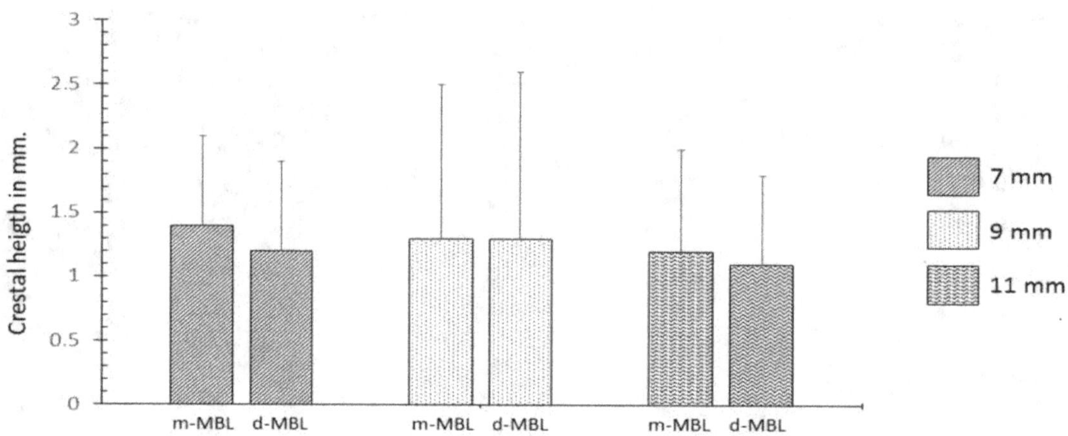

Figure 8. Bar graph showing the mean and standard deviation of the MBL values measured in mesial (m-MBL) and distal (d-MBL) position of each implant in the three implant lengths used.

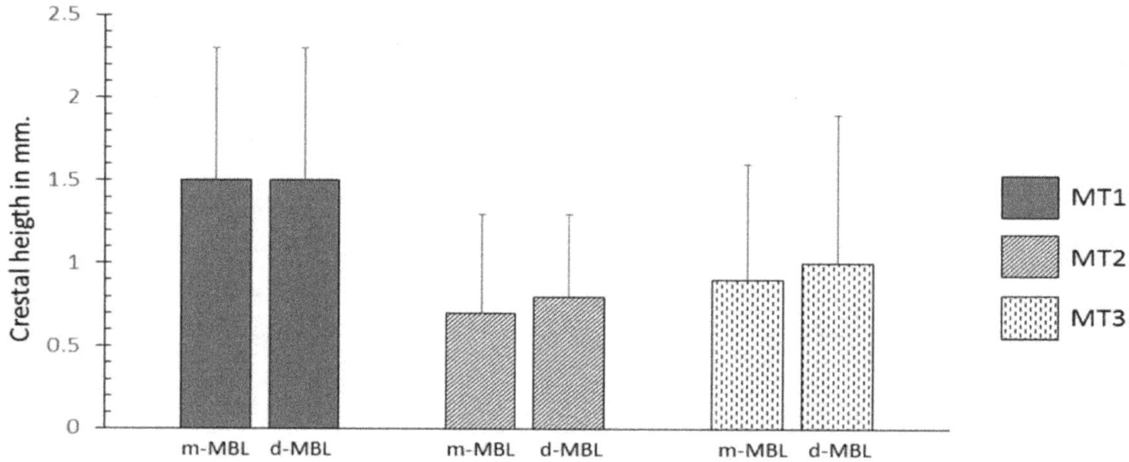

Figure 9. Bar graph showing the mean and standard deviation of the MBL values measured in mesial (m-MBL) and distal (d-MBL) position of each implant in the three mucosal thickness.

4. Discussion

This clinical study describes an analysis the marginal bone behavior considering of different variables after the implants installed in the posterior area of mandible: Patient sex, implant dimensions (diameter and length), and mucosa thickness. One implant was loose throughout the study period and re-implanted, and the survival rate of dental implants considered was of 98.3%. This study was made without patient selection, the only criterion was the posterior inferior region selection, this makes a random distribution of the ridges with the difficulty of achieving uniformity in the height and width of the ridge and the trouble of achieving the 2 mm of supracrestal bone in all cases, as well as having bone in around the 100% of the perimeter, simply because of the anatomy of the area. These could be factors that may affect the mucosal position and the behavior around the implant.

All implants measured the mucosa thickness on the radiographic images and compared with the clinical measurements, and the results confirmed no statistical differences among these collected data. Then, the measurement of the mucosa in radiographic images can be used for planification of the implant position (depth position). Therefore, the ISQ and the bone height in relation of the implant platform were measured immediately after the implant placement (baseline) and after 90 days. The relation of the marginal bone behavior and the variables with significant statistical differences are discussed separately follow.

Surface topography refers to the degree of surface roughness and the orientation of surface irregularities, which can directly stimulate osseointegration, increasing and/or accelerating the events involved in this process [8,21]. In this sense, we use implants with a surface roughness considered moderate, similar to that used by many other brands of implants. This data is important so that in future studies researchers can compare their results or reproduce in new investigations. In addition, since stability measurements were taken 90 days after implantation, the results are directly affected by the type of surface used in the implants.

4.1. Initial Implant Stability

The initial stability of the implants, a measure that can be represented by ISQ, is of fundamental importance for osseointegration. Several studies describe a direct relationship between bone density and measured ISQ values [23–27]. Both the thickness of the cortical bone and the pattern presented by the medullary portion (trabecular), which are in contact with the installed implant, are determinant factors for stability (bone and implant contact) [28]. The aim of this study was to observe the consequences of the placing Morse taper implants subcrestally and the relation between bone remodeling and soft tissue thickness. The initial results in these three months of studies show that the sectors in which the mucosal thickness was 1 to 2 mm suffered greater bone remodelation compared to the sectors where the width of the soft tissue was 2 mm or more.

The clinical methods that are commonly used to verify implant stability and osseointegration include percussion, mobility, and radiographic studies. However, these methods have an important limitation in their standardization, since they have a great dependence on the sensitivity and susceptibility with respect to the professional executor [29,30]. In this sense, more precise and non-invasive techniques were developed. These analyzes are called according to the method by which they are performed, i.e., resonance frequency analysis (RFA), and are used to verify and measure the stability of implants installed in bone tissue at different clinical periods [30,31]. The use of this technique is mainly based on being easy to perform, fast, and direct and, moreover, can be applied routinely in the clinic because it does not present discomfort to the patient.

The measured values of ISQ varied during the phases of osseointegration evaluated. At the trans-operative time, the mean and standard deviations of the ISQ values measured was 63.6 ± 2.90 varying of 53 to 70, indicating adequate primary stability, similar to the results reported in other studies that presented averages from 60.3 to 62.6 [31–34]. While, in the second time measured, 90 days after the implantations, the means and standard deviations of the ISQ values was 69.7 ± 7.09 varying of 49 to 75. Such overall result for the ISQ values for the time of 90 days are within the mean values shown in several similar studies, where the values varied from 67.0 to 72.1 [31,32,35,36].

4.2. Mucosal Thickness

Linkevicius and colleagues studied the main factors related with the bone remodeling [2,3], understanding and trying to make a relation between mechanic factors and mucosal thickness. Isolating the connection factor even when this was 2 mm supracrestal and the mucosa was thin, there was bone remodeling consequence of the biological width formation [2]. Using implants with platform switching concept did not prevent the bone remodeling also when the mucosal thickness shows little thickness [3,4]. The use of Morse-cone implants for this study is based on the minimal number of microorganisms penetrating the implant/abutment microgap as well as the absence of movement [37]. This rigid type of connection eliminates a potential remodeling bone factor and with the subcrestal position opens a new way in which the biologic width can be conformed [37–40]. Studies showed the possibility of having no bone remodeling reaction at the abutment-implant interface and making a new configuration of the biological space and the mucosa characteristics surrounding the implant [41–44].

The results are in agreement with the studies mentioned previously, although in our study the evaluation time was less than one year, the first case (MT1), where the mucosa was between 1 and 2 mm, suffered much more bone loss than de MT2 and MT3 where the mucosal width was two or more millimeters. The group MT2 and MT3 had very similar measures in respect of bone remodeling. However, the MT3 not show superior behavior in comparison with the MT1 and MT2, possibly because in this group the biological space exceeded the value considered ideal for the position of implant-abutment junction (IAJ). Conversely, controversial information is available regarding implants placed subcrestally. Some authors recommended placement of the implant platform 1 or 2 mm below the alveolar crest to better maintain marginal bone levels [45,46]. However, other studies reported an increased extension of inflammatory infiltrate due to deep positioning of the IAJ, resulting in greater MBL compared to implants placed equicrestally [47,48]. In the case of implants with mucosal thickness 3 mm (MT3), added to 2 mm positioning subcrestal implants, the final positioning distance of the AIJ was greater than 5 mm, which probably explains the behavior of the implants in this condition.

Clinically the time bone loss around implants can influence the planned aesthetic results, mainly because it alters the final positioning of the tissue because its final volume decreased.

4.3. *Implant Dimensions (Diameter and Length)*

Several studies showed that the implant dimensions have direct influence on the stress distribution to the bone [41–45] as the implant directly affects the area of possible bone retention [49]. Moreover, other authors have advocated the use of implants as long and wide as possible [50]. However, when bone loss around the implants was evaluated, there is a controversy regarding the influence of length in these alterations, and some studies present results of larger losses in the short implants, other authors report that the length of the implant has little influence on the quantity of vertical load stress, and may have a lower effect on the distribution of stresses to bone tissue when compared to the variation in implant diameter [49,51]. In this way, Koutouzis and collaborates not found statistical difference in the values of bone resorption in larger diameter implants, comparing small diameter (3.5 mm) with larger diameter (4.5 mm) [52]. Unlike most of the cited reports, an important fact that the research revealed was the better behavior of the 3.5 mm implants when compared to the 4.0 mm diameter implants in terms of bone remodeling, that is, the smaller implants diameters showed lower bone resorption. On the other hand, when the implants were compared in terms of length (7, 9, and 11 mm), the results obtained in the present study did not present statistical differences, with very similar values among the sizes used. However, in the present study the implants evaluated were not placed under masticatory loads, which may be the reason for the difference in results between the studies. Previous FEA studies have shown that a decrease in diameter increases the stress transferred to crestal bone [53].

5. Conclusions

Within the limitations of this prospective study, although in our study the evaluation time was short after the implantation, we concluded that cone Morse implants placed 2 mm subcrestal level showed different values of bone loss depending of the mucosal thickness and implant diameter. However, the initial stability and implant length not showed influence on the marginal bone loss.

Author Contributions: Conceptualization, J.C.P.-F.; Data curation, S.A.G., M.B. and J.A.; Formal analysis, S.A.G. and J.C.P.-F.; Investigation, M.B. and J.A.; Methodology, J.L.C.-G., S.A.G. and J.C.P.-F.; Project administration, M.B., J.L.C.-G.; Resources, J.A.; Software, M.B. and J.A.; Supervision, S.A.G. and J.C.P.-F.; Visualization, J.C.P.-F.; Writing—original draft, M.B. and J.A.; Writing—review and editing, J.L.C.-G. and S.A.G.

Acknowledgments: The authors are grateful to the Paulo Rossetti from the Dental School of the University of São Paulo, Bauru, Brazil, for their kind support as independent statistician. The authors are grateful to Implacil De Bortoli (São Paulo, Brazil) for the products support.

References

1. Berglundh, T.; Lindhe, J. Dimension of the periimplant mucosa. Biological width revisited. *J. Clin. Periodontol.* **1996**, *23*, 971–973. [CrossRef] [PubMed]
2. Linkevicius, T.; Apse, P.; Grybauskas, S.; Puisys, A. The influence of soft tissue thickness on crestal bone changes around implants: A 1-year prospective controlled clinical trial. *Int. J. Oral Maxillofac. Implant.* **2009**, *24*, 712–719.

3. Linkevicius, T.; Apse, P.; Grybauskas, S.; Puisys, A. Influence of thin mucosal tissues on crestal bone stability around implants with platform switching: A 1-year pilot study. *J. Oral Maxillofac. Surg.* **2010**, *68*, 2272–2277. [CrossRef] [PubMed]
4. van Eekeren, P.; Tahmaseb, A.; Wismeijer, D. Crestal bone changes in macrogeometrically similar implants with the implant-abutment connection at the crestal bone level or 2.5 mm above: A prospective randomized clinical trial. *Clin. Oral Implant. Res.* **2016**, *27*, 1479–1484. [CrossRef] [PubMed]
5. Linkevicius, T.; Puisys, A.; Svediene, O.; Linkevicius, R.; Linkeviciene, L. Radiological comparison of laser-microtextured and platform-switched implants in thin mucosal biotype. *Clin. Oral Implant. Res.* **2015**, *26*, 599–605. [CrossRef]
6. Puisys, A.; Linkevicius, T. The influence of mucosal tissue thickening on crestal bone stability around bone-level implants. A prospective controlled clinical trial. *Clin. Oral Implant. Res.* **2015**, *26*, 123–129. [CrossRef]
7. Linkevicius, T.; Puisys, A.; Steigmann, M.; Vindasiute, E.; Linkeviciene, L. Influence of Vertical Soft Tissue Thickness on Crestal Bone Changes Around Implants with Platform Switching: A Comparative Clinical Study. *Clin. Implant Dent. Relat. Res.* **2015**, *17*, 1228–1236. [CrossRef]
8. Gehrke, S.A.; da Silva Neto, U.T. Evaluation of the Surface Treatment on Bone Healing in a Transmucosal 1-mm Area of Implant Abutment: An Experimental Study in the Rabbit Tibia. *Clin. Implant Dent. Relat. Res.* **2016**, *18*, 489–497. [CrossRef]
9. van Eekeren, P.J.; Tahmaseb, A.; Wismeijer, D. Crestal Bone Changes Around Implants with Implant-Abutment Connections at Epicrestal Level or Above: Systematic Review and Meta-Analysis. *Int. J. Oral Maxillofac. Implant.* **2016**, *31*, 119–124. [CrossRef]
10. Schwarz, F.; Hegewald, A.; Becker, J. Impact of implant-abutment connection and positioning of the machined collar/microgap on crestal bone level changes: A systematic review. *Clin. Oral Implant. Res.* **2014**, *25*, 417–425. [CrossRef]
11. Hermann, J.S.; Schoolfield, J.D.; Schenk, R.K.; Buser, D.; Cochran, D.L. Influence of the size of the microgap on crestal bone changes around titanium implants. A histometric evaluation of unloaded non-submerged implants in the canine mandible. *J. Periodontol.* **2001**, *72*, 1372–1383. [CrossRef] [PubMed]
12. Zanatta, L.C.; Dib, L.L.; Gehrke, S.A. Photoelastic stress analysis surrounding different implant designs under simulated static loading. *J. Craniofacial Surg.* **2014**, *25*, 1068–1071. [CrossRef] [PubMed]
13. Stein, A.E.; McGlmphy, E.A.; Johnston, W.M.; Larsen, P.E. Effects of implant design and surface roughness on crestal bone and soft tissue levels in the esthetic zone. *Int. J. Oral Maxillofac. Implant.* **2009**, *24*, 910–919.
14. Schmitt, C.M.; Nogueira-Filho, G.; Tenenbaum, H.C.; Lai, J.Y.; Brito, C.; Döring, H.; Nonhoff, J. Performance of conical abutment (Morse Taper) connection implants: A systematic review. *J. Biomed. Mater. Res. Part A* **2014**, *102*, 552–574. [CrossRef] [PubMed]
15. Baj, A.; Bolzoni, A.; Russillo, A.; Lauritano, D.; Palmieri, A.; Cura, F.; Silvestre, F.J.; Giannì, A.B. Cone-morse implant connection system significantly reduces bacterial leakage between implant and abutment: An in vitro study. *J. Biol. Regul. Homeost. Agents* **2017**, *31*, 203–208. [PubMed]
16. Gehrke, S.A.; Delgado-Ruiz, R.A.; Prados Frutos, J.C.; Prados-Privado, M.; Dedavid, B.A.; Granero Marín, J.M.; Calvo Guirado, J.L. Misfit of Three Different Implant-Abutment Connections Before and After Cyclic Load Application: An in Vitro Study. *Int. J. Oral Maxillofac. Implant.* **2017**, *32*, 822–829. [CrossRef] [PubMed]
17. Hanaoka, M.; Gehrke, S.A.; Mardegan, F.; Gennari, C.R.; Taschieri, S.; Del Fabbro, M.; Corbella, S. Influence of implant/abutment connection on stress distribution to implant-surrounding bone: A finite element analysis. *J. Prosthodont.* **2014**, *23*, 565–571. [CrossRef] [PubMed]
18. Albrektsson, T.; Zarb, G.; Worthington, P.; Eriksson, A.R. The long-term efficacy of currently used dental implants: A review and proposed criteria of success. *Int. J. Oral Maxillofac. Implant.* **1986**, *1*, 11–25.
19. Albrektsson, T.; Chrcanovic, B.; Östman, P.O.; Sennerby, L. Initial and long-term crestal bone responses to modern dental implants. *Periodontology 2000* **2017**, *73*, 41–50. [CrossRef]
20. Sasada, Y.; Cochran, D.L. Implant-Abutment Connections: A Review of Biologic Consequences and Peri-implantitis Implications. *Int. J. Oral Maxillofac. Implant.* **2017**, *32*, 1296–1307. [CrossRef]
21. Gehrke, S.A.; Ramírez-Fernandez, M.P.; Granero Marín, J.M.; Barbosa Salles, M.; Del Fabbro, M.; Calvo Guirado, J.L. A comparative evaluation between aluminium and titanium dioxide microparticles for blasting the surface titanium dental implants: An experimental study in rabbits. *Clin. Oral Implant. Res.* **2018**, *29*, 802–807. [CrossRef] [PubMed]

22. Salatti, D.B.; Pelegrine, A.A.; Gehrke, S.; Teixeira, M.L.; Moshaverinia, A.; Moy, P.K. Is there a need for standardization of tightening force used to connect the transducer for resonance frequency analysis in determining implant stability? *Int. J. Oral Maxillofac. Implant.* **2019**, *34*, 886–890. [CrossRef] [PubMed]
23. Balleri, P.; Cozzolino, A.; Ghelli, L.; Momichioli, G.; Varriale, A. Stability measurements of osseointegrated implants using Osstell in partially edentulous jaws after one year of loading: A pilot study. *Clin. Implant. Dent. Relat. Res.* **2002**, *4*, 128–132. [CrossRef] [PubMed]
24. Barewal, R.M.; Oates, T.W.; Meredith, N.; Cochran, D.L. Resonance frequency measurement of implant stability in vivo on implants with a sandblasted and acid-etched surface. *Int. J. Oral Maxillofac. Implant.* **2003**, *18*, 641–651.
25. Bischof, M.; Nedir, R.; Szmukler-Moncler, S.; Bernard, J.P.; Samson, J. Implant stability measurement of delayed and immediately loaded implants during healing. *Clin. Oral Implant. Res.* **2004**, *15*, 529–539. [CrossRef] [PubMed]
26. Nedir, R.; Bischof, M.; Szmulzkler-Moncler, S.; Bernard, J.P.; Samson, J. Predicting osseointegration by means of implant primary stability: A resonance frequency analysis with delayed and immediately loaded ITI SLA implants. *Clin. Oral Implant. Res.* **2004**, *15*, 520–528. [CrossRef] [PubMed]
27. Oates, T.W.; Valderrama, P.; Bischof, M.; Nedir, R.; Jones, A.; Simpson, J.; Toutenburg, H.; Cochran, D.L. Enhanced implant stability with a chemically modified SLA surface: A randomized pilot study. *Int. Oral Maxillofac. Implant.* **2007**, *22*, 755–760.
28. Meredith, N. Assessment of implant stability as a prognostic determinant. *Int. J. Prosthodont.* **1998**, *11*, 491–501.
29. Fischer, K.; Bäckström, M.; Sennerby, L. Immediate and early loading of oxidized tapered implants in the partially edentulous maxilla: A 1-year prospective clinical, radiographic, and resonance frequency analysis study. *Clin. Implant. Dent. Relat. Res.* **2009**, *11*, 69–80. [CrossRef]
30. Meredith, N.; Book, K.; Friberg, B.; Jemt, T.; Sennerby, L. Resonance frequency measurements of implant stability in vivo. A crosssectional and longitudinal study of resonance frequency measurements on implants in the edentulous and partially dentate maxilla. *Clin. Oral Implant. Res.* **1997**, *8*, 226–233. [CrossRef]
31. Gehrke, S.A.; da Silva Neto, U.T.; Rossetti, P.H.; Watinaga, S.E.; Giro, G.; Shibli, J.A. Stability of implants placed in fresh sockets versus healed alveolar sites: Early findings. *Clin. Oral Implant. Res.* **2016**, *27*, 577–582. [CrossRef] [PubMed]
32. Gehrke, S.A.; Tavares da Silva Neto, U. Does the time of osseointegration in the maxilla and mandible differ? *J. Craniofacial Surg.* **2014**, *25*, 2117–2120. [CrossRef] [PubMed]
33. Friberg, B.; Sennerby, L.; Linden, B.; Gröndahl, K.; Lekholm, U. Stability measurements of one-stage Branemark implants during healing in mandibles. A clinical resonance frequency analysis study. *Int. J. Oral Maxillofac. Surg.* **1999**, *28*, 266–272. [CrossRef]
34. Zix, J.; Hug, S.; Kessler-Liechti, G.; Mericske-Stern, R. Measurement of dental implant stability by resonance frequency analysis and damping capacity assessment: Comparison of both techniques in a clinical trial. *Int. J. Oral Maxillofac. Implant.* **2008**, *23*, 525–530.
35. da Silva Neto, U.T.; Joly, J.C.; Gehrke, S.A. Clinical analysis of the stability of dental implants after preparation of the site by conventional drilling or piezosurgery. *Br. J. Oral Maxillofac. Surg.* **2014**, *52*, 149–153. [CrossRef] [PubMed]
36. Gehrke, S.A.; da Silva, U.T.; Del Fabbro, M. Does Implant Design Affect Implant Primary Stability? A Resonance Frequency Analysis-Based Randomized Split-Mouth Clinical Trial. *J. Oral Implantol.* **2015**, *41*, e281–e286. [CrossRef]
37. Koutouzis, T.; Neiva, R.; Nair, M.; Nonhoff, J.; Lundgren, T. Cone beam computed tomographic evaluation of implants with platform-switched Morse taper connection with the implant-abutment interface at different levels in relation to the alveolar crest. *Int. J. Oral Maxillofac. Implant.* **2014**, *29*, 1157–1163. [CrossRef] [PubMed]
38. Koutouzis, T.; Neiva, R.; Nonhoff, J.; Lundgren, T. Placement of implants with platform-switched Morse taper connections with the implant-abutment interface at different levels in relation to the alveolar crest: A short-term (1-year) randomized prospective controlled clinical trial. *Int. J. Oral Maxillofac. Implant.* **2013**, *28*, 1553–1563. [CrossRef]

39. Fetner, M.; Fetner, A.; Koutouzis, T.; Clozza, E.; Tovar, N.; Sarendranath, A.; Coelho, P.G.; Neiva, K.; Janal, M.N.; Neiva, R. The Effects of Subcrestal Implant Placement on Crestal Bone Levels and Bone-to-Abutment Contact: A Microcomputed Tomographic and Histologic Study in Dogs. *Int. J. Oral Maxillofac. Implant.* **2015**, *30*, 1068–1075. [CrossRef]
40. Tesmer, M.; Wallet, S.; Koutouzis, T.; Lundgren, T. Bacterial colonization of the dental implant fixture-abutment interface: An in vitro study. *J. Periodontol.* **2009**, *80*, 1991–1997. [CrossRef]
41. Welander, M.; Abrahamsson, I.; Berglundh, T. Subcrestal placement of two-part implants. *Clin. Oral Implant. Res.* **2009**, *20*, 226–231. [CrossRef] [PubMed]
42. Weng, D.; Nagata, M.J.H.; Bell, M.; Bosco, A.F.; de Melo, L.G.N.; Richter, E.-J. Influence of microgap location and configuration on the periimplant bone morphology in submerged implants. An experimental study in dogs. *Clin. Oral Implant. Res.* **2008**, *19*, 1141–1147. [CrossRef] [PubMed]
43. Weng, D.; Nagata, M.J.H.; Leite, C.M.; de Melo, L.G.N.; Bosco, A.F. Influence of microgap location and configuration on radiographic bone loss in nonsubmerged implants: An experimental study in dogs. *Int. J. Prosthodont.* **2010**, *24*, 445–452.
44. Pilliar, R.M.; Deporter, D.A.; Watson, P.A.; Valiquette, N. Dental implant design: Effect on bone remodeling. *J. Biomed. Mater. Res.* **1991**, *25*, 467–483. [CrossRef] [PubMed]
45. Brunski, J.B. Biomechanical considerations in dental implant design. *Int. J. Oral Maxillofac. Implant.* **1988**, *5*, 31–34.
46. Holmgren, E.P.; Seckinger, R.J.; Kilgren, L.M.; Mante, F. Evaluating parameters of osseointegrated dental implants using finite element analysis—A two-dimensional comparative study examining the effects of implant diameter, implant shape, and load direction. *J. Oral Maxillofac. Implant.* **1998**, *24*, 80–88. [CrossRef]
47. Meijer, H.J.; Kuiper, J.H.; Starmans, F.J.; Bosman, F. Stress distribution around dental implants: Influence of superstructure, length of implants, and height of mandible. *J. Prosthet. Dent.* **1992**, *68*, 96–102. [CrossRef]
48. Iplikcioglu, H.; Akca, K. Comparative evaluation of the effect of diameter, length and number of implants supporting three-unit fixed partial prostheses on stress distribution in the bone. *J. Dent.* **2002**, *30*, 41–46. [CrossRef]
49. Himmlova, L.; Dostalova, T.; Kacovsky, A.; Konvickova, S. Influence of implant length and diameter on stress distribution: A finite element analysis. *J. Prosthet. Dent.* **2004**, *91*, 20–25. [CrossRef]
50. Winkler, S.; Morris, H.F.; Ochi, S. Implant survival to 36 months as related to length and diameter. *Ann. Periodontol.* **2000**, *5*, 22–31. [CrossRef]
51. Misch, C.E. Divisions of available bone. In *Contemporary Implant Dentistry*, 2nd ed.; Mosby: St Louis, MO, USA, 1999; pp. 91–94.
52. Koutouzis, T.; Fetner, M.; Fetner, A.; Lundgren, T. Retrospective evaluation of crestal bone changes around implants with reduced abutment diameter placed non-submerged and at subcrestal positions: The effect of bone grafting at implant placement. *J. Periodontol.* **2011**, *82*, 234 242. [CrossRef] [PubMed]
53. Qian, L.; Todo, M.; Matsushita, Y.; Koyano, K. Effects of implant diameter, insertion depth, and loading angle on stress/strain fields in implant/ jawbone systems: Finite element analysis. *Int. J. Oral Maxillofac. Implant.* **2009**, *24*, 877–886.

6

A Hybrid Model for Predicting Bone Healing around Dental Implants

Pei-Ching Kung, Shih-Shun Chien and Nien-Ti Tsou *

Department of Materials Science and Engineering, National Chiao Tung University, Ta Hsueh Road, Hsinchu 300, Taiwan; gong1014.mse06g@nctu.edu.tw (P.-C.K.); play_58032.05g@g2.nctu.edu.tw (S.-S.C.)
* Correspondence: tsounienti@nctu.edu.tw

Abstract: Background: The effect of the short-term bone healing process is typically neglected in numerical models of bone remodeling for dental implants. In this study, a hybrid two-step algorithm was proposed to enable a more accurate prediction for the performance of dental implants. Methods: A mechano-regulation algorithm was firstly used to simulate the tissue differentiation around a dental implant during the short-term bone healing. Then, the result was used as the initial state of the bone remodeling model to simulate the long-term healing of the bones. The algorithm was implemented by a 3D finite element model. Results: The current hybrid model reproduced several features which were discovered in the experiments, such as stress shielding effect, high strength bone connective tissue bands, and marginal bone loss. A reasonable location of bone resorptions and the stability of the dental implant is predicted, compared with those predicted by the conventional bone remodeling model. Conclusions: The hybrid model developed here predicted bone healing processes around dental implants more accurately. It can be used to study bone healing before implantation surgery and assist in the customization of dental implants.

Keywords: dental implant; tissue differentiation; bone remodeling; mechano-regulation theory; short-term healing; long-term healing

---

1. Introduction

Implant stability is one of the important indexes to determine dental implant survival rates in the clinic [1]. It is dominated by the bone healing around the surgery site. Bone healing is a series of complex physiological processes that involved the regulation of several tissue phenotypes. At the beginning of bone healing, micro-vessels, and new connective tissue form on the surface of the wound, which is collectively referred to as granulation tissue [2–5]. After the formation of granulation tissue, further tissue differentiation initiates. Cells then transfer into fibrous connective tissues, cartilages, and new bones according to biophysical stimulus [6–8]. The final stage of bone healing is referred to as bone remodeling, which is a lifelong process, where the skeletal system maintains a dynamic equilibrium, related to the regulation of osteoclasts and osteoblasts [9–11]. When the balance is disrupted by external forces, a new equilibrium state can be achieved spontaneously. Thus, according to the healing process mentioned above, tissue differentiation and bone remodeling stages have a great impact on the short-term and long-term stability of implants, respectively [12,13].

To efficiently predict the short-term stability of implants in advance, we aim to simulate the tissue differentiation process by using the mechano-regulation algorithm. The origin of the method is based on Pauwels [14] who first specified that distortional stress and hydrostatic compression dominate tissue differentiation. Carter et al. [15] implemented the theory into a finite element model (FEM), revealing the evolution of connective tissues. Prendergast et al. [16] modified the methods by adopting octahedral shear strain and fluid flow as the solid and fluid stimuli. Lacroix further improved the model by using poroelastic finite elements, which can describe the biological mechanism in bones more accurately [5]. In recent years, many studies have revealed the effect of the mechanical environment and the geometric design of implants on the performance of tissue differentiation [17,18].

Bone adapts itself based on its mechanical environment and loading conditions, greatly affecting the morphology of bone and long-term stability of implants [11,13,19]. Many scientists have developed numerical methods to describe the behavior of bone remodeling [20–24]. Carter et al. [15,25,26] proposed that bone apparent density is dominated by strain energy density and studied the energy transfer in hip stems. The internal changes in bone morphology and the aging of connective tissues affected by the external loads were also predicted by FEM. Huiskes et al. [27] adopted a similar approach and simulated the femoral cortex around intramedullary prostheses to reveal the relationship between stress shielding effect and bone resorption. The bone remodeling algorithm was then extended to predict the variation of bone apparent density after implantation treatment [28–31]. The algorithm was verified by computed tomographic (CT) images, showing a high degree of similarity [32]. Most of the studies assumed a simple initial state of the models, where uniform material properties were assigned around the implants [29,31,33,34], i.e., the short-term bone healing has no effect on bone remodeling results. However, short-term healing is crucial since bone remodeling is an iterative process, where different initial conditions may lead to different bone density distribution around dental implants.

In order to test the null hypothesis of the bone healing process in the conventional model, we proposed a hybrid algorithm that regards the procedure of bone healing as two stages: (1) the short-term stage which was simulated by a tissue differentiation model and (2) the long-term stage which simulated by a bone remodeling model. At the beginning of the tissue differentiation model, it was assumed that the wound was filled with granulation tissue. The mechano-regulation algorithm was then applied to determine the tissue phenotypes for the following time steps. Once a stable tissue differentiation has been reached, the current tissue distribution with the material properties, such as Young's modulus, apparent bone density, and Poisson's ratio, in callus around the implant then served as the initial condition for the bone remodeling model. Then, the resulting long-term distribution of Young's modulus and the remodeling stimulus will be discussed. and compared with the results which were similar to those done by Chou et al. [29], where the effect of short-term tissue differentiation was not considered.

The objective of this study is to develop a hybrid model that can predict the stability of dental implants and the strength of the surrounding bones with consideration of both the short-term and long-term bone healing process. The results of the current work can reveal the effect of bone with different material properties on bone healing, providing useful information for dental clinics. Furthermore, the proposed model can be used to rapidly examine the morphology design of dental implants (such as implant radius, length, thread geometry) and the placement protocol (such as insertion angle and depth) to improve the osseointegration between implants and bones.

2. Materials and Methods

Figure 1 shows the flowchart of the current hybrid algorithm, including short-term and long-term bone healing models. The distribution of strain, fluid velocity, and stem cell diffusion in the initial model ($t = 0$) was firstly calculated by FEM. Granulation tissues then differentiated into various tissue phenotypes based on the mechano-regulation algorithm. Next, the rule of mixture and smoothing procedure [35] was applied to determine the updated material properties and the detail will be discussed in Section 2.2. After the short-term healing process finished, the distribution of tissue phenotypes and the corresponding material properties around the implants was obtained and assigned to the bone remodeling model at the initial state for simulating the long-term healing process. Where bone remodeling algorithm adjusted the bone apparent density of each element iteratively until the equilibrium state of the remodeling stimulus under the given loading condition was achieved. The procedures will be discussed in more detail in Sections 2.2 and 2.3.

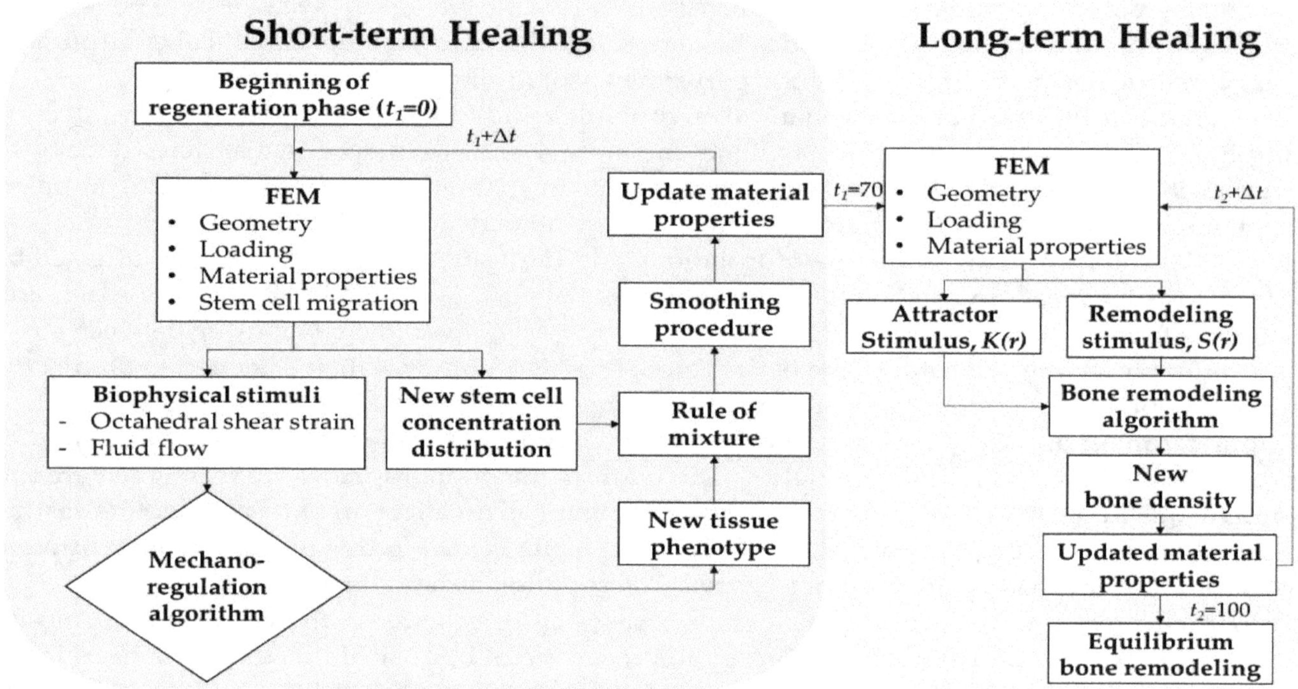

Figure 1. Flow chart of bone healing preoperative evaluation.

2.1. Three-Dimensional FEM Model

The current hybrid algorithm was applied to study the bone healing of the mandibular second molar (back teeth in the upper jaw), where the bone geometry, density, and other material properties were adopted based on Chou et al. [29]. The geometry of the bone structure was obtained by extruding a planar CT image with a thickness of 80 mm, as shown in Figure 2a. It was referred to as the bone-tooth system, consisting of a layer of cortical bone overlying on cancellous bone, and a natural tooth. The physiological stimulus of the healthy state, i.e., bone-tooth system, was served as the objective function (i.e., attractor stimulus) for the calculation of bone remodeling in the bone-implant-prosthesis system, details of the calculation will be introduced in the next section. Next, the bone-implant-prosthesis system replaced the tooth in the bone-tooth system by a prosthesis and a short implant with a size of 5.0 × 5.1 mm; the remaining region, i.e., the extraction socket, was filled with callus, as shown in Figure 2b.

The models of the two systems were built by a commercial finite element package ANSYS 18.0 (ANSYS, Inc., Canonsburg, PA, USA). The implant, tooth, and prosthesis were meshed by the built-in element type, SOLID185; the remaining parts of the tissues were meshed by CPT215, which allows the calculation of poroelastic material properties, such as the fluid velocity and pressure in the pores of the bones. There were approximately 138,000 elements and 94,500 nodes for both systems. To maintain the balance between computation time and accuracy, finer meshes were applied around the interfaces between bone and the tooth/implant, as shown in Figure 2. The interfaces were set to allow sliding with a friction coefficient of 0.3. A symmetry boundary condition was applied to the mesial side of the model. All of the nodes in the distal side were constrained in all degrees of freedom. A displacement of 10.5 μm was applied at nodes on the top of the tooth/prosthesis. This value was equivalent to a biting force of 100 N [36–38]; the angle of the displacement was set according to it used in Chou et al. [29]. Note that loading, setting, and properties of all materials, including bones, prosthesis, tooth, implant, and bone graft, used in the current work were based on Chou et al. [29] for comparison, as shown in Table 1. It is worth mentioning that, in the tissue differentiation process, the material properties of elements in the callus region transformed with iterations, i.e., they evolved according to the corresponding tissue phenotypes during the iteration process. Details of the mechanism of the mechano-regulation algorithm will be explained in the next section.

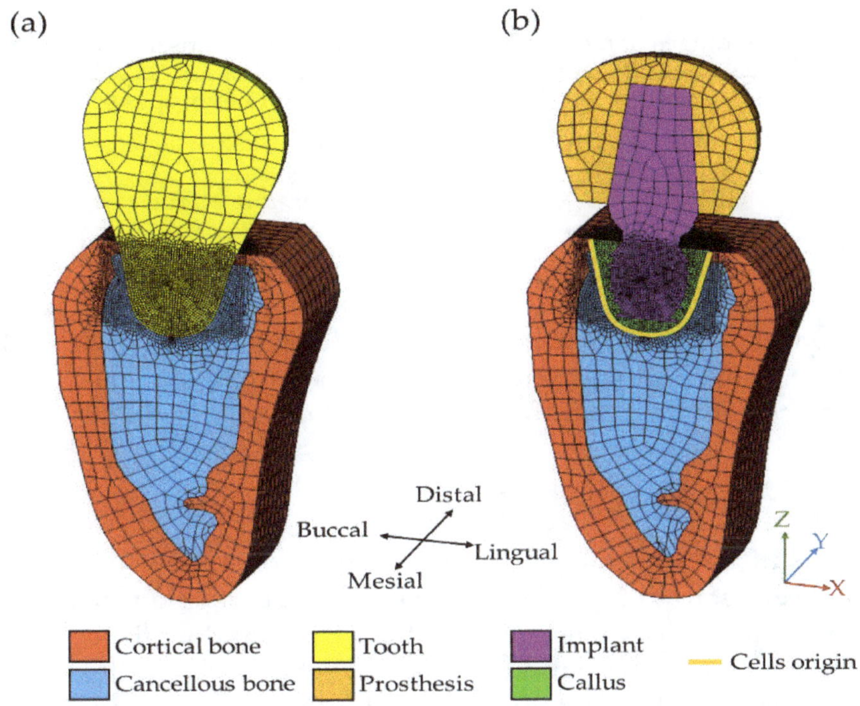

Figure 2. FEM model of (**a**) bone-tooth and (**b**) bone-implant-prosthesis systems.

Table 1. The material properties used in the current work [29].

Materials	Young's Modulus (GPa)	Poisson's Ratio	Permeability (m^4/Ns)
Ti6Al4V	113.8	0.34	N/A
Tooth	20	0.3	N/A
Prosthesis	80	0.3	N/A
Bone graft	2	0.3	N/A
Cortical bone	13.7	0.3	10^{-17}
Cancellous bone	2	0.3	3.7×10^{-13}
Granulation tissue	0.001	0.17	10^{-14}
Fibrous tissue	0.002	0.17	10^{-14}
Cartilage	0.01	0.17	5×10^{-15}
Immature bone	1	0.3	10^{-13}
Mature bone	6	0.3	3.7×10^{-13}

N/A: not applicable.

2.2. Mechano-Regulation Algorithm

The mechano-regulation algorithm proposed by Lacroix and Prendergast [5,35] was adopted in the current work to predict the distribution of tissue phenotypes. The procedures of the algorithm, including the calculation in each iteration, updates of material properties, and post-processing to the results, were implemented by MATLAB 2019 (The MathWorks, Inc., Natick, MA, USA). At the beginning of the calculation, elements in the callus region were set with the material properties of granulation tissues. According to the theory, tissue differentiation (TD) is induced by the combination of octahedral shear strain (γ) and fluid flow (ν) caused by external loads. It is referred to as biophysical stimulus S_{TD} such that:

$$S_{TD} = \frac{\gamma}{a} + \frac{\nu}{b} \quad (1)$$

where a = 0.0375 and b = 3 μm/s are empirical constants. Then, the tissue phenotype for the next iteration can be determined based on the value of S_{TD} as shown in Table 2. The material properties of the tissue phenotype were updated accordingly.

Table 2. The ranges of biophysical stimulus for different tissue phenotypes.

	S_{TD}		Tissue Phenotypes
3<	S_{TD}		Fibrous tissue
1<	S_{TD}	≤3	Cartilage
0.266<	S_{TD}	≤1	Immature bone
0.010<	S_{TD}	≤0.266	Mature bone
	S_{TD}	≤0.010	Initial resorption

The concentration of mesenchymal stem cells determined the level of the transition from granulation tissue to the other tissue phenotypes. The migration [39] and proliferate [40] of mesenchymal stem cell can be simplified as a classical isotropic diffusion, such that:

$$\frac{dn}{dt} = D\nabla^2 n \tag{2}$$

where t is time; D is the diffusion coefficient; n is the current concentration of mesenchymal stem cell. The migration of stem cells started from the boundary of the extraction socket, which is called cells origin and marked by yellow lines in Figure 2b. At the last iteration, the concentration of the stem cell reached the maximal value. In the current work, D is set as 8.85×10^{-14} m^2/s. Then, the effective material properties of tissues for the next iteration, including Young's modulus, Poisson's ratio, and permeability, can be obtained by a linear combination between the granulation tissue (X_g) and the differentiated tissue (X_d) as follows:

$$X_{mix} = \frac{n_{max} - n}{n_{max}} X_g + \frac{n}{n_{max}} X_d \tag{3}$$

where n^{max} is the maximum concentration; n is the current concentration of stem cells determined by Equation (2); X_d is material properties of the differentiated tissue phenotype shown in Table 1.

To avoid the instability and dramatic change of material properties between iterations, Lacroix and Prendergast [35] suggested a smooth procedure to average the material properties from the previous nine iterations, which can be written as:

$$X_i = \frac{1}{N}\left(X_{mix} + X_{i-1} + X_{i-2} + \ldots + X_{i-(N-1)}\right) \tag{4}$$

where $N = 10$; i is the current iteration number; X_{mix} is the effective material properties calculated from Equation (3). Note that when the iteration number is $i < 9$, smoothing operation is applied to the iteration i to the first [35]. The short-term healing time was set as 70 days, which is the average healing period for implantation surgeries [41–43]. The short-term healing process and the differentiated tissue phenotypes can then be predicted.

2.3. *Bone Remodeling Algorithm*

After the numerical calculation for the short-term healing, long-term healing, i.e., bone remodeling (BR), occurred to alter the internal structure of bones and reach a new equilibrium state based on the mechanical environment. Huskies et al. [27] proposed a bone remodeling theory assuming the driving force of self-adaptive activity is determined by remodeling stimulus (S_{BR}, unit: J/kg), such that:

$$S_{BR}\left(\vec{r},t\right) = \frac{u\left(\vec{r},t\right)}{\rho\left(\vec{r},t\right)} \tag{5}$$

where u is strain energy density (unit: J/m^3); ρ is the apparent bone density (kg/m^3), t is time; and $\vec{r}$ is the position vector [27]. When the value of remodeling stimulus S_{BR} is greater than the given threshold, bone formation occurred and Young's modulus and bone density increase accordingly. On the contrary, when the remodeling stimulus S_{BR} is less than the threshold, bone resorption occurred, and Young's modulus and bone density decrease. In addition, Carter [25] stated that bones maintain a state of homeostasis when the remodeling stimulus is in a certain range, which is referred to as a "lazy zone." Thus, the bone remodeling process can be expressed by nonlinear functions of the remodeling stimulus [27]:

$$\frac{d\rho}{dt} = \begin{cases} A_f\left[S_{BR} - (1+s)K\left(\vec{r}\right)\right]^2, & S_{BR} \geq (1+s)K\left(\vec{r}\right) & \text{(Formation)} \\ 0, & (1-s)K\left(\vec{r}\right) < S_{BR} \leq (1+s)K\left(\vec{r}\right) & \text{(Lazy zone)} \\ A_r\left[S_{BR} - (1-s)K\left(\vec{r}\right)\right]^3, & S_{BR} \leq (1-s)K\left(\vec{r}\right) & \text{(Resorption)} \end{cases} \tag{6}$$

where A_f and A_r are formation and resorption coefficients; s is the threshold of the lazy zone, which is set as 0.75 [44]; $K\left(\vec{r}\right)$ is the attractor stimulus induced by the biting force in the bone-tooth system, which is determined by Equation (5). The value of $K\left(\vec{r}\right)$ in the region of callus was set to 5, which is the average of the overall remodeling stimulus in bone element. It is worth noting that the rate of bone resorption is greater than that of bone formation based on clinical observations, resulting in a greater exponential term of resorption in Equation (6). The apparent density of a bone element m at the jth iteration can be derived by integrating Equation (6) with a forward Euler method [27,45–47], such that:

$$\rho_m^j = \begin{cases} \rho_m^{j-1} + A_f\Delta t\left[S_{BR}^{j-1} - (1+s)K\left(\vec{r}\right)\right]^2, & S_{BR}^{j-1} \geq (1+s)K(r) & \text{(Formation)} \\ 0, & (1-s)K(r) < S_{BR}^{j-1} \leq (1+s)K(r) & \text{(Lazy zone)} \\ \rho_m^{j-1} + A_r\Delta t\left[S_{BR}^{j-1} - (1-s)K\left(\vec{r}\right)\right]^3, & S_{BR}^{j-1} \leq (1-s)K(r) & \text{(Resorption)} \end{cases} \tag{7}$$

where Δt is the time increment [21,48]. Young's modulus (E, unit: GPa) of bone elements was associated with the corresponding apparent density based on the finding of Carter and Hayes [26], such that:

$$E = C\rho^3 \tag{8}$$

where C is constant. Note that the integration coefficients $A_f\Delta t$ and $A_r\Delta t$ in Equation (7) were set as 1×10^{-11} and the constant was set as 3.79, based on the setting used in Chou et al. [29]. The value of Young's modulus indicated the strength of the internal structure of bone, which affected the calculation at the next iteration. The average remodeling stimulus (S_{ave}) in each iteration was recorded and served as a measure of convergence of the model, such that:

$$S_{ave} = \frac{1}{N_{total}} \sum_{k=1}^{N_{total}} S_k \tag{9}$$

where N_{total} is the total number of bone elements; S_k is remodeling stimulus of the local bone element k. It is worth noting that long-term bone healing, i.e., bone remodeling, is a lifelong process and the bone system evolves to reach an equilibrium state according to its current mechanical environment. Thus, the time step used here is, in fact, a computational increment and is not associated with a real-life time scale. The end of the calculation depends on the convergence of S_{ave} as mentioned above.

3. Results

3.1. Short-Term Healing and Tissue Differentiation

Tissue differentiation and the evolution of bone ingrowth around the implant were evaluated by the mechano-regulation model. Figure 3 shows the percentage of tissue phenotypes in each day during the short-term healing process. In the early stage of tissue differentiation, granulation tissues still existed in the callus region. This is because tissue differentiation was initiated when the concentration of stem cells above certain levels. At this stage, the inner callus region has relatively low concentration as the stem cells diffused from the boundary of the callus region. Moreover, it was found that the soft tissue with a higher biophysical stimulus ($S_{TD} > 1$) such as cartilage and fibrous tissue decrease with time while the bone tissue increased continuously until the middle of the differentiation process (i.e., around the 35th day). After the 35th day, bones possessed a certain degree of strength, i.e., higher Young's modulus. This resulted in the decreasing values of bone stimuli, and thus, maturate and immature bones gradually became the dominant tissue phenotype in the entire callus region. Then, most of the immature bones transformed into maturate bones as the healing process was closed to the 70th day.

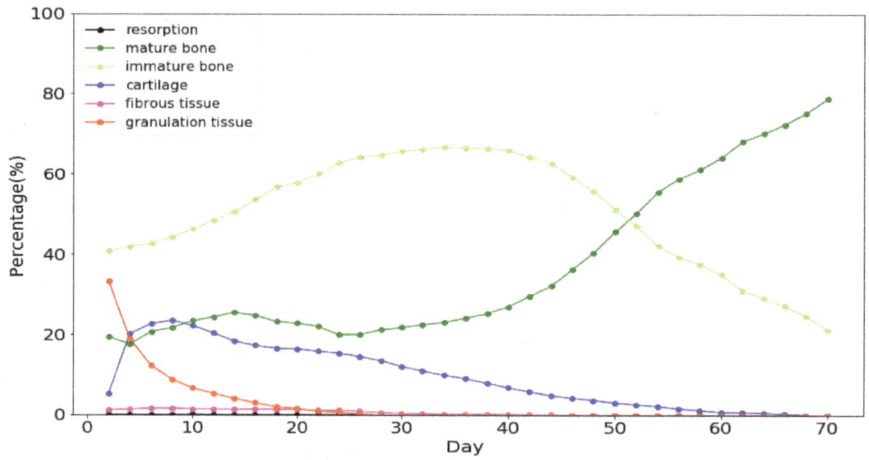

Figure 3. Percentage of various tissue phenotype in each day during the short-term bone healing process.

Details of the tissue phenotype at the specific days are shown in Figure 4. On the 4th day, more than half of the callus region remained as granulation tissue, as shown in Figure 4. It is observed that cartilages and fibrous tissues occurred around the threads in the middle part and the bottom of the implant, respectively. It is because the applied load caused the stress concentration around the threads and the bottom, giving higher biophysical stimulus to the elements in that region. Note that, although there were mature and immature bones, the effective material properties, such as Young's modulus, were still close to that of granulation tissue based on Equation (3), due to the low concentration of stem cell on the 4th day. Then, it can be observed that, on the 10th day, granulation tissues gradually transformed into mature and immature bones as the concentration of stem cells increased with time. It is worth noting that cartilages accumulated at tips of the threads since stress concentration was partially released with the increasing maturity of the surrounding bones. On the 30th day, granulation tissues were disappeared entirely. Cartilages were mainly located at the lingual side because of the oblique biting force. Then, maturate and immature bones gradually dominated the entire system around the implant on the 50th to 70th days. It is worth noting that there were very few elements of bone resorption on the 10th day and were not shown in the current cross-section in Figure 4. In this way, the short-term healing pattern around the implant was obtained.

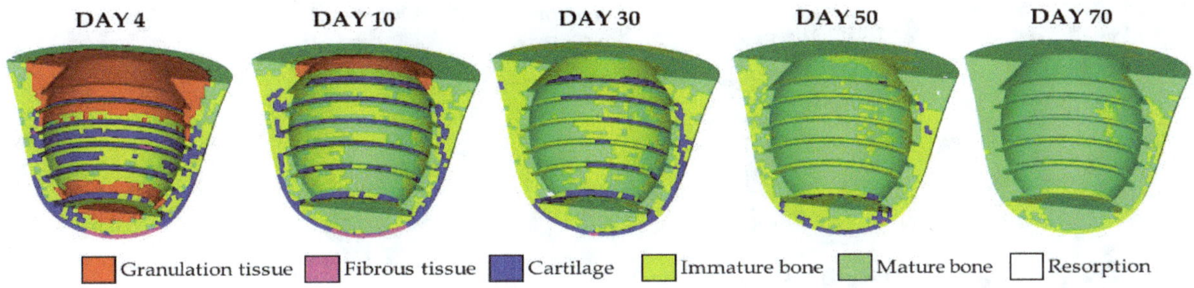

Figure 4. The tissue differentiation history predicted by the mechano-regulation algorithm.

3.2. Bone Remodeling

Now consider two bone remodeling models. The first, i.e., the current model, adopted the result at the end of short-term healing predicted by the mechano-regulation algorithm as the initial state; the second was the conventional model based on bone remodeling algorithm with the assumption that the extraction socket was filled with bone graft and regarded as the initial state where the material properties were set as uniform. The setting of the second model followed the work done by the literature [29]. Both models shared the same distribution of the objective attractor stimulus $K(\vec{r})$ based on the natural tooth, as shown in Figures 5a and 6a. Then, the bone remodeling models altered the bone apparent density of all the bone elements in the following iterations to achieve that objective distribution.

In the current model, the distribution of Young's modulus of the initial state is shown in Figure 5d. It can be observed that certain regions in the callus in Figure 5d were in dark and light blue colors giving low and high Young's modulus, ranging from 0.001 to 6 GPa based on Table 1, due to the non-uniform stem cell concentration and the presence of different tissue phenotypes. It is worth noting that the average value of Young's modulus in that region was around 2 GPa, having a good agreement with the value used in the conventional model where uniform Young's modulus was assumed, as shown in Figure 6d. The corresponding bone apparent density of each element in the callus region can then be obtained by Equation (8). The resulting model with the updated bone apparent density was then subjected to the biting force, giving the distribution of the remodeling stimulus (S_{BR}) for the 1st iteration, as shown in Figure 5b. The values are shown in Figure 5a,b were substituted into Equation (7) to obtain the updated bone apparent density for the next iteration. The corresponding distribution of Young's modulus in the 1st iteration was shown in Figure 5e. It can be observed that bone regions with high Young's modulus (above 12.18 GPa, colored in red) fully covered around the implant; most of the bones attached to the surface of the implant were also with non-uniform Young's modulus (ranging from 3.04 to 6.08 GPa). The calculation continued until the 100th iteration was achieved. It is worth noting that the average remodeling stimulus (S_{ave}) of the current model quickly converged around the 10th iteration, showing great stability. The converged values S_{ave} for both the current and conventional models were identical. The distribution of S_{BR} of the 100th iteration is shown in Figure 5c. It can be observed that most of the regions had the value of S_{BR} closed to those of the target, i.e., the objective attractor stimulus $K(\vec{r})$. The final state of bone remodeling gave the distribution of Young's modulus, shown in Figure 5f.

The average Young's modulus of the entire system predicted by the current model was around 4.77 GPa. It is worth noting that bone resorptions (colored in gray) occurred around the threads toward the lingual side and around the neck of the implant. The total volume fraction of bone resorption was 0.042%. Similar to the 1st iteration, bone regions with high Young's modulus were still fully covered around the implant. Two additional high strength bone tissue bands connected to cortical bones were formed in the bottom right (the lingual side) and top left (the buccal side) of the implant, which provided extra supports and enhanced the stability of the implant.

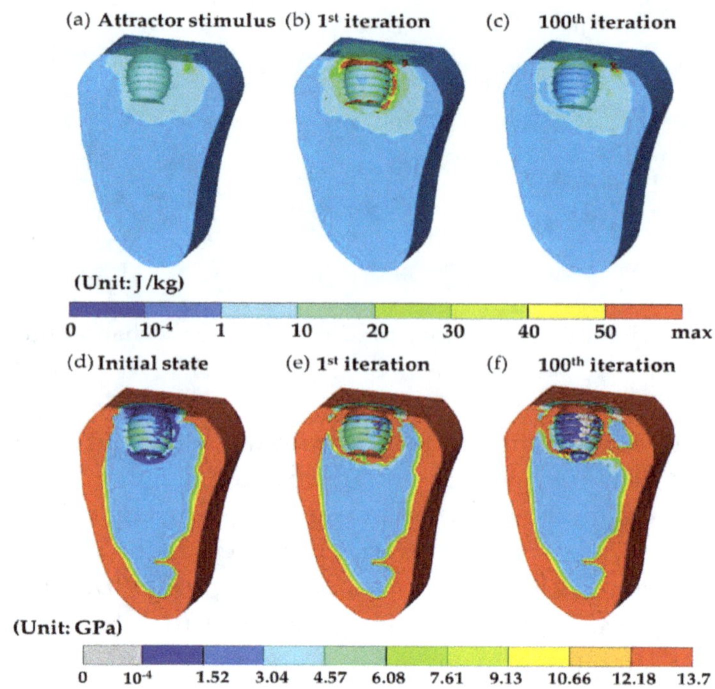

Figure 5. The results generated by the current model. (**a**) The target distribution of the attractor stimulus $K(\vec{r})$ based on the natural tooth. (**b**,**c**) are bone remodeling stimulus (S_{BR}) at the 1st and 100th iterations. (**d**–**f**) are the corresponding distribution of Young's modulus during the bone remodeling process at the initial state, 1st, and 100th iteration.

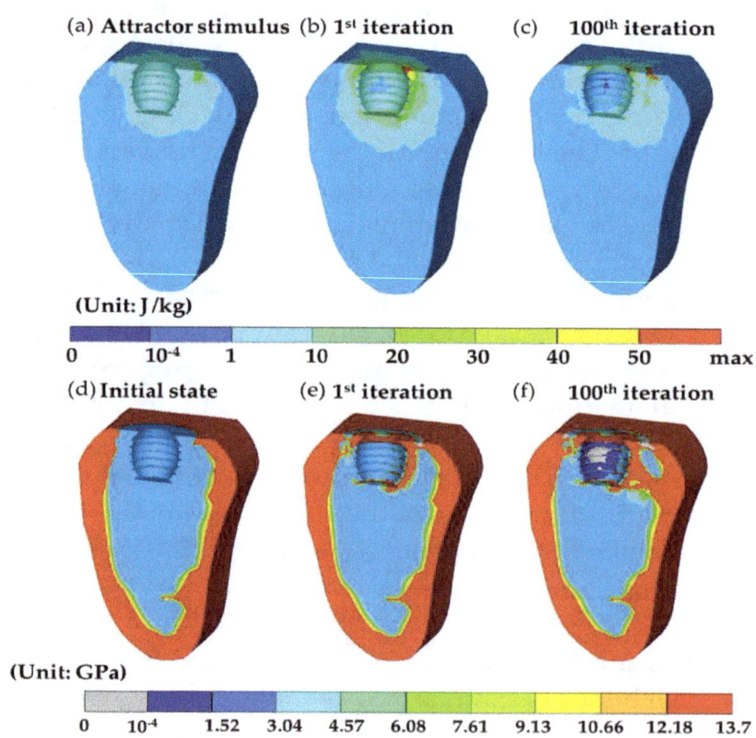

Figure 6. The results generated by the conventional model. (**a**) The target distribution of the attractor stimulus $K(\vec{r})$ based on the natural tooth. (**b**,**c**) are bone remodeling stimulus (S_{BR}) at the 1st and 100th iterations. (**d**–**f**) are the corresponding distribution of Young's modulus during the bone remodeling process at the initial state, 1st, and 100th iteration.

Next, Figure 6d shows the distribution of Young's modulus of the initial state adopted in the conventional model. It can be observed that constant Young's modulus of 2 GPa in the callus in Figure 6d was assumed without considering the result of differentiating tissue phenotypes during the short-term healing. Then, the distribution of the remodeling stimulus (S_{BR}) for the 1st iteration can be determined as shown in Figure 6b. In the 1st iteration, the distribution of S_{BR} was similar to that generated by the current model, apart from there was no high stimulus bands around the implant. However, such a small difference resulted in a very different distribution of Young's modulus shown in Figure 6e compared with that in Figure 5e, wherein, the high strength bones partially covered around the implant; most of the bones attached to the surface of the implant remained a constant Young's modulus of 2 GPa. Then, similar to the current model, the average remodeling stimulus (S_{ave}) quickly converged. Finally, the 100th iteration was achieved, giving the distribution of S_{BR} as shown in Figure 6c. The resulting Young's modulus distribution is shown in Figure 6f. The volume fraction of bone resorption was at the value of 0.044%, which was very similar to the current model. A significant difference between the results of the two models was the location of bone resorption. It was found that bone resorption (colored in grey) occurred in the buccal side in the conventional model while it appeared on the lingual side in the current model. This will be discussed in more detail in the next section. Another obvious difference between the two models was the distribution of high Young's modulus bands. The high Young's modulus band was absent in the buccal side, and thus, no supporting connection between the surface of the implant and cortical bone. The average Young's modulus at the 100th iteration was around 3.65 GPa which was relatively lower than that generated by the current model.

4. Discussion

The results mentioned above show that the initial state of bone remodeling can greatly affect the distribution of Young's modulus at the final state. In the current model, the initial state of bone remodeling was the result of the mechano-regulation model (short-term healing process), giving the top and bottom regions in the callus with lower Young's modulus. This leads to a higher strain energy density and a low corresponding bone apparent density base on Equation (8). Then, these regions had higher remodeling stimulus based on Equation (5), promoting the formation of bones, i.e., Young's modulus and apparent density increased. This non-uniform Young's modulus at the initial state leads to a dramatic change of Young's modulus in the entire callus region in the 1st iteration. On the contrary, in the conventional model, Young's modulus was assumed uniform, resulting in the change of Young's modulus around the implant only in the 1st iteration.

In the 100th iteration, it can be observed that the stability of the implants was greatly influenced by the initial states. In the current model, there were two high strength bone tissue bands connected to cortical bones, while there was only one connected bone tissue band in the result generated in the conventional model. In addition, the average Young's modulus in the current model was higher than it predicted by the current model. Thus, the stability of the implant was underestimated in the conventional model where uniform Young's modulus in the callus region at the initial state was assumed. This indicated that short-term healing can greatly affect the results of bone remodeling and cannot be neglected.

In the results of short-term healing generated by the mechano-regulation model, soft tissues occurred in the early stage and then replaced by bone tissues due to the decrease of biophysical stimulus in the later stage. This was in accordance with both the experimental [14] and computational [5] works in the literature. Where the literature reported that bone tissue forms after the formation of soft tissues (i.e., fibrous tissue and cartilage), and then bone began to differentiate, giving the increase of fluid flow since woven bone is more permeable. Furthermore, three additional features can be found in the remodeling result in the 100th iteration predicted by both the current and conventional models, which were in accordance with the clinical observations. Firstly, both models predicted a region of bone resorption at the top surface in the lingual (right) side. This phenomenon was known as marginal bone loss [49,50], which was an important factor for implant stability. Secondly, both models generated a bone resorption region in the middle of the bone-implant interface. This is the so-called stress shielding effect [27,47], which was the result of the occurrence of high strength bone tissue (colored in red) at the region around the first thread. However, the locations of the bone resorption region predicted by the two models were different, where the region predicted by the current model was in the lingual (right) side and that predicted by the conventional model was in the buccal (left) side. According to the literature [51], bone resorption occurred on the right-hand side when the loading direction was similar to that in the current work, i.e., the load was applied from the top right to the bottom left. The current model successfully captured this feature, reproduce the bone resorption region at the right-hand side at the bone-implant interface, while the conventional model predicted the location of bone resorption at the opposite side. This shows that the current model can give a more accurate result of bone remodeling procedure in the bone-implant-prosthesis system. Third, the result in the 100th iteration predicted by the current model shows that around 70% of the surface of the implant was covered by bone tissues (i.e., the elements with Young's modulus greater than that of immature bone, 2 GPa). This value was similar to that reported by Lian et al. [31], where they suggested around 60% contact between bone and implant when an equilibrium of bone remodeling is reached. Based on the features mentioned above, we conclude the rejection of the null hypothesis that short-term bone healing has no effect on bone remodeling results.

Since the current hybrid model was implemented by the finite element method, which can perform virtual tests on a wide variety of people characteristics and dental materials by simply changing the geometry of the model, boundary conditions, and material properties of bones. Thus, the current model can potentially provide estimated information and may even provide optimized dental implants for dentist clinics. Next, to demonstrate the applicability of the current model and reveal the effect of individual differences of the patients, we adopted the case of middle-aged male adults with higher strength material property of bone, referred to as to higher bone strength case. Where Young's modulus of cortical, cancellous, immature, and mature bone was 1.4 times [52] than it in Table 1, while the properties of the remaining tissues, such as fibrous tissue and cartilage, stayed unchanged. Then, the short- and long-term bone healing processes were evaluated by the current model. The corresponding results are shown in Figures 7 and 8, respectively. It was found that the trend of tissue differentiation in the short-term healing process was almost identical to it the standard case as shown in Figure 4. The only difference between the two cases was the averaged Young's modulus in the high strength case was about two times higher than it was in the standard case, which can be seen in Figure 8a, where the material properties in the callus region were assigned according to the tissue differentiation result. In the 100th iteration, there were several significant differences between the two cases. Firstly, there was merely no bone resorption in the higher bone strength case. The volume fraction of bone resorption was at a value of 0.0068%. Secondly, the connective tissue bands in the higher bone strength case were thicker than in the standard case. The two features indicate that the bone system in the higher bone strength case can provide excellent supports and enhance the stability of the implant. This result also has good agreement with the clinical observation, where the dental implant failure rate for the middle-aged male adults was relatively low [53].

Although the current model considered both the short-term and long-term healing process and reproduced many features that were discovered in the experiments, the model can be further improved by considering the physiological mechanism listed as follows. For example, a more complex diffusion mechanism of stem cell migration in the short-term healing process, such as the growth of vessels which can be implemented by the random-walk model [54]; periodontal ligaments (PDL), which play a crucial role in bone remodeling, can be simulated by taken the anisotropic and nonlinear elastic stress-strain behavior into account [55–57]. It is expected a more accurate prediction can be achieved if these factors were considered.

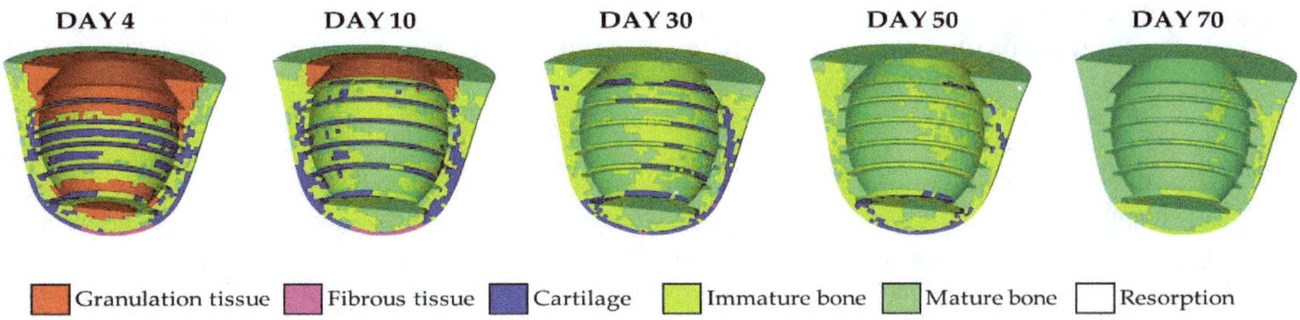

Figure 7. The tissue differentiation history predicted by the mechano-regulation algorithm in higher bone strength case.

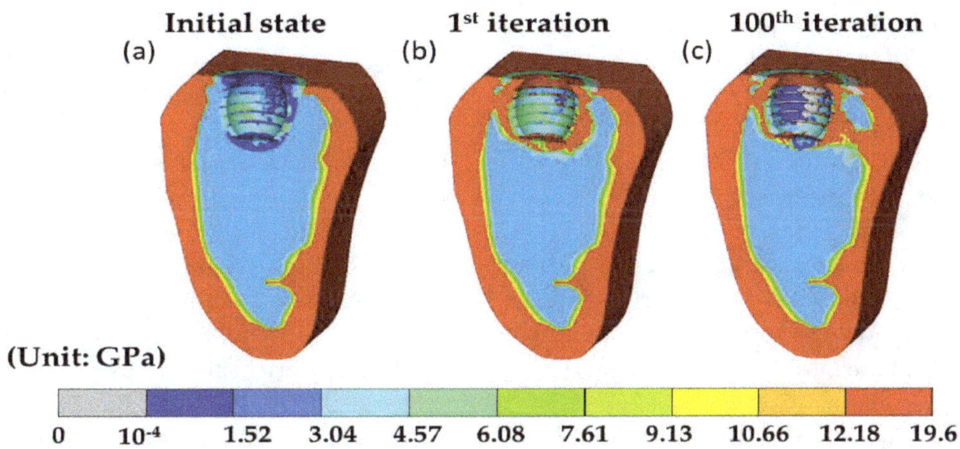

Figure 8. The results generated by the current model in higher bone strength case. (**a–c**) are the corresponding distribution of Young's modulus during the bone remodeling process at the initial state, 1st, and 100th iteration.

5. Conclusions

In this study, a hybrid numerical bone healing algorithm was developed to predict the morphology of bone around dental implants with the consideration of both short-term and long-term bone healing. The results showed that the effect of short-term bone healing should not be ignored, and the assumption of uniform material properties for the initial state in the bone remodeling model is inappropriate. The current hybrid model can reveal many bone healing features having a very good agreement with the literature. It can be extended to simulate different implant geometries, applied loads, and bone properties of patients, enabling an early prediction of the performance of clinical treatments.

Author Contributions: Conceptualization, S.-S.C. and N.-T.T.; methodology, P.-C.K. and S.-S.C.; software, P.-C.K. and S.-S.C.; validation, P.-C.K. and N.-T.T.; writing—original draft preparation, P.-C.K.; writing—review and editing, N.-T.T.; visualization, P.-C.K.; supervision, N.-T.T.; project administration, N.-T.T. All authors have read and agreed to the published version of the manuscript.

Acknowledgments: The authors would like to thank Ming-Jun Li for his comments and assistance to this work. The authors wish to acknowledge the National Center for High-Performance Computing, Taiwan, for providing the computational platform.

References

1. Meredith, N. Assessment of implant stability as a prognostic determinant. *Int. J. Prosthodont.* **1998**, *11*, 491–501. [PubMed]
2. Ammon, C.; Kreutz, M.; Rehli, M.; Krause, S.W.; Andreesen, R. Platelets induce monocyte differentiation in serum-free coculture. *J. Leukoc. Biol.* **1998**, *63*, 469–476. [CrossRef] [PubMed]

3. Spisani, S.; Giuliani, A.L.; Cavalletti, T.; Zaccarini, M.; Milani, L.; Gavioli, R.; Traniello, S. Modulation of neutrophil functions by activated platelet release factors. *Inflammation* **1992**, *16*, 147–158. [CrossRef] [PubMed]
4. Tang, Y.; Wu, X.; Lei, W.; Pang, L.; Wan, C.; Shi, Z.; Zhao, L.; Nagy, T.R.; Peng, X.; Hu, J.; et al. TGF-β1-induced migration of bone mesenchymal stem cells couples bone resorption with formation. *Nat. Med.* **2009**, *15*, 757. [CrossRef] [PubMed]
5. Lacroix, D.; Prendergast, P.J. A mechano-regulation model for tissue differentiation during fracture healing: Analysis of gap size and loading. *J. Biomech.* **2002**, *35*, 1163–1171. [CrossRef]
6. Crisan, M.; Yap, S.; Casteilla, L.; Chen, C.W.; Corselli, M.; Park, T.S.; Andriolo, G.; Sun, B.; Zheng, B.; Zhang, L.; et al. A perivascular origin for mesenchymal stem cells in multiple human organs. *Cell Stem Cell* **2008**, *3*, 301–313. [CrossRef] [PubMed]
7. Wollert, K.C.; Meyer, G.P.; Lotz, J.; Lichtenberg, S.R.; Lippolt, P.; Breidenbach, C.; Fichtner, S.; Korte, T.; Hornig, B.; Messinger, D.; et al. Intracoronary autologous bone-marrow cell transfer after myocardial infarction: The BOOST randomised controlled clinical trial. *Lancet* **2004**, *364*, 141–148. [CrossRef]
8. Ashton, B.A.; Allen, T.D.; Howlett, C.R.; Eaglesom, C.C.; Hattori, A.; Owen, M. Formation of bone and cartilage by marrow stromal cells in diffusion chambers in vivo. *Clin. Orthop. Relat. Res.* **1980**, *151*, 294–307. [CrossRef]
9. Hadjidakis, D.J.; Androulakis, I.I. Bone remodeling. *Ann. N. Y. Acad. Sci.* **2006**, *1092*, 385–396. [CrossRef]
10. Frost, H.M. Tetracycline-based histological analysis of bone remodeling. *Calcif. Tissue Int.* **1969**, *3*, 211–237. [CrossRef]
11. Wolff, J. *The Law of Bone Remodelling*, 1st ed.; Springer: Berlin/Heidelberg, Germany, 1986; ISBN 978-3-642-71031-5.
12. Ghiasi, M.S.; Chen, J.; Vaziri, A.; Rodriguez, E.K.; Nazarian, A. Bone fracture healing in mechanobiological modeling: A review of principles and methods. *Bone Rep.* **2017**, *6*, 87–100. [CrossRef] [PubMed]
13. Mohaghegh, K.; Pérez, M.A.; García-Aznar, J.M. Accelerating numerical simulations of strain-adaptive bone remodeling predictions. *Comput. Methods Appl. Mech. Eng.* **2014**, *273*, 255–272. [CrossRef]
14. Pauwels, F. A new theory on the influence of mechanical stimuli on the differentiation of supporting tissue. The tenth contribution to the functional anatomy and causal morphology of the supporting structure. *Z. Anat. Entwicklungsgesch.* **1960**, *121*, 478–515. [CrossRef] [PubMed]
15. Carter, D.R.; Fyhrie, D.P.; Whalen, R.T. Trabecular bone density and loading history: Regulation of connective tissue biology by mechanical energy. *J. Biomech.* **1987**, *20*, 785–794. [CrossRef]
16. Prendergast, P.J.; Huiskes, R.; Søballe, K. Biophysical stimuli on cells during tissue differentiation at implant interfaces. *J. Biomech.* **1997**, *30*, 539–548. [CrossRef]
17. Chou, H.Y.; Müftü, S. Simulation of peri-implant bone healing due to immediate loading in dental implant treatments. *J. Biomech.* **2013**, *46*, 871–878. [CrossRef]
18. Sotto-maior, B.S.; Graciliano, E.; Mercuri, F.; Mendes, P.; Maria, N.; Picorelli, S.; Francischone, C.E.; Maria, N.; Picorelli, S.; Francischone, C.E.; et al. Computer Methods in Biomechanics and Biomedical Engineering Evaluation of bone remodeling around single dental implants of different lengths: A mechanobiological numerical simulation and validation using clinical data. *Comput. Methods Biomech. Biomed. Engin.* **2016**, *19*, 699–706. [CrossRef]
19. Fernández, J.R.; García-Aznar, J.M.; Martínez, R.; Viaño, J.M. Numerical analysis of a strain-adaptive bone remodelling problem. *Comput. Methods Appl. Mech. Eng.* **2010**, *199*, 1549–1557. [CrossRef]
20. Cowin, S.C.; Hegedus, D.H. Bone remodeling I: Theory of adaptive elasticity. *J. Elast.* **1976**, *6*, 313–326. [CrossRef]
21. Frost, H.M. Bone "mass" and the "mechanostat": A proposal. *Anat. Rec.* **1987**, *219*, 1–9. [CrossRef] [PubMed]
22. Kim, Y.; Park, S.; Shin, K. Effect of cycloid movement on plate-to-roll gravure offset printing. *Microsyst. Technol.* **2016**, *22*, 357–365. [CrossRef]
23. Hegedus, D.H.; Cowin, S.C. Bone remodeling II: Small strain adaptive elasticity. *J. Elast.* **1976**, *6*, 337–352. [CrossRef]
24. Hart, R.T.; Davy, D.T.; Heiple, K.G. A computational method for stress analysis of adaptive elastic materials with a view toward applications in strain-induced bone remodeling. *J. Biomech. Eng.* **1984**, *106*, 342–350. [CrossRef] [PubMed]

25. Carter, D.R. Mechanical loading histories and cortical bone remodeling. *Calcif. Tissue Int.* **1984**, *36*, S19–S24. [CrossRef] [PubMed]
26. Carter, D.R.; Hayes, W.C. The compressive behavior of bone as a two-phase porous structure. *J. Bone Jt. Surg. Am.* **1977**, *59*, 954–962. [CrossRef]
27. Huiskes, R.; Weinans, H.; Grootenboer, H.J.; Dalstra, M.; Fudala, B.; Slooff, T.J. Adaptive bone-remodeling theory applied to prosthetic-design analysis. *J. Biomech.* **1987**, *20*, 1135–1150. [CrossRef]
28. Lin, D.; Li, Q.; Li, W.; Zhou, S.; Swain, M.V. Design optimization of functionally graded dental implant for bone remodeling. *Compos. Part B Eng.* **2009**, *40*, 668–675. [CrossRef]
29. Chou, H.-Y.; Romanos, G.; Müftü, A.; Müftü, S. Peri-implant bone remodeling around an extraction socket: Predictions of bone maintenance by finite element method. *Int. J. Oral Maxillofac. Implants* **2012**, *27*, 39–48.
30. Crupi, V.; Guglielmino, E.; LaRosa, G.; VanderSloten, J.; VanOosterwyck, H. Numerical analysis of bone adaptation around an oral implant due to overload stress. *Proc. Inst. Mech. Eng. Part H J. Eng. Med.* **2004**, *218*, 407–415. [CrossRef]
31. Lian, Z.; Guan, H.; Ivanovski, S.; Loo, Y.-C.; Johnson, N.W.; Zhang, H. Effect of bone to implant contact percentage on bone remodelling surrounding a dental implant. *Int. J. Oral Maxillofac. Surg.* **2010**, *39*, 690–698. [CrossRef]
32. Reina, J.M.; García-Aznar, J.M.; Domínguez, J.; Doblaré, M. Numerical estimation of bone density and elastic constants distribution in a human mandible. *J. Biomech.* **2007**, *40*, 828–836. [CrossRef] [PubMed]
33. Lin, D.; Li, Q.; Li, W.; Swain, M. Bone remodeling induced by dental implants of functionally graded materials. *J. Biomed. Mater. Res. Part B Appl. Biomater.* **2010**, *92*, 430–438. [CrossRef] [PubMed]
34. Li, J.; Li, H.; Shi, L.; Fok, A.S.L.; Ucer, C.; Devlin, H.; Horner, K.; Silikas, N. A mathematical model for simulating the bone remodeling process under mechanical stimulus. *Dent. Mater.* **2007**, *23*, 1073–1078. [CrossRef]
35. Lacroix, D.; Prendergast, P.J. A homogenization procedure to prevent numerical instabilities in poroelastic tissue differentiation models. In Proceedings of the Eighth Annual Symposium: Computational Methods in Orthopaedic Biomechanics, Orlando, FL, USA, 11 March 2000.
36. Barbier, L.; VanderSloten, J.; Krzesinski, G.; Schepers, E.; Van DerPerre, G. Finite element analysis of non-axial versus axial loading of oral implants in the mandible of the dog. *J. Oral Rehabil.* **1998**, *25*, 847–858. [CrossRef] [PubMed]
37. Jansen, V.K.; Conrads, G.; Richter, E.J. Microbial leakage and marginal fit of the implant-abutment interface. *Int. J. Oral Maxillofac. Implants* **1997**, *12*, 23.
38. Streckbein, P.; Streckbein, R.G.; Wilbrand, J.F.; Malik, C.Y.; Schaaf, H.; Howaldt, H.P.; Flach, M. Non-linear 3D evaluation of different oral implant-abutment connections. *J. Dent. Res.* **2012**, *91*, 1184–1189. [CrossRef]
39. Zohar, R.; Cheifetz, S.; McCulloch, C.A.G.; Sodek, J. Analysis of intracellular osteopontin as a marker of osteoblastic cell differentiation and mesenchymal cell migration. *Eur. J. Oral Sci.* **1998**, *106*, 401–407. [CrossRef]
40. Iwaki, A.; Jingushi, S.; Oda, Y.; Izumi, T.; Shida, J.I.; Tsuneyoshi, M.; Sugioka, Y. Localization and quantification of proliferating cells during rat fracture repair: Detection of proliferating cell nuclear antigen by immunohistochemistry. *J. Bone Miner. Res.* **1997**, *12*, 96–102. [CrossRef]
41. Monjo, M.; Lamolle, S.F.; Lyngstadaas, S.P.; Rønold, H.J.; Ellingsen, J.E. In vivo expression of osteogenic markers and bone mineral density at the surface of fluoride-modified titanium implants. *Biomaterials* **2008**, *29*, 3771–3780. [CrossRef]
42. Papalexiou, V.; Novaes, A.B., Jr.; Grisi, M.F.M.; Souza, S.S.L.S.; Taba, M., Jr.; Kajiwara, J.K. Influence of implant microstructure on the dynamics of bone healing around immediate implants placed into periodontally infected sites: A confocal laser scanning microscopic study. *Clin. Oral Implants Res.* **2004**, *15*, 44–53. [CrossRef]
43. JR, S.A.; Allegrini, M.R.F.; Yoshimoto, M.; JR, B.K.; Mai, R.; Fanghanel, J.; Gedrange, T. Soft tissue integration in the neck area of titanium implants–an animal trial. *J. Physiol. Pharmacol.* **2008**, *59*, 117–132.
44. Huiskes, R.; Weinans, H.; VanRietbergen, B. The relationship between stress shielding and bone resorption around total hip stems and the effects of flexible materials. *Clin. Orthop. Relat. Res.* **1992**, 124–134. [CrossRef]
45. Turner, C.H.; Anne, V.; Pidaparti, R.M. VA uniform strain criterion for trabecular bone adaptation: Do continuum-level strain gradients drive adaptation? *J. Biomech.* **1997**, *30*, 555–563. [CrossRef]

46. Turner, C.H. Three rules for bone adaptation to mechanical stimuli. *Bone* **1998**, *23*, 399–407. [CrossRef]
47. Weinans, H.; Huiskes, R.; Grootenboer, H.J. The behavior of adaptive bone-remodeling simulation models. *J. Biomech.* **1992**, *25*, 1425–1441. [CrossRef]
48. Frost, H.M. Bone's mechanostat: A 2003 update. *Anat. Rec. Part A Discov. Mol. Cell. Evol. Biol.* **2003**, *275*, 1081–1101. [CrossRef]
49. Akca, K.; Cehreli, M.C. Biomechanical consequences of progressive marginal bone loss around oral implants: A finite element stress analysis. *Med. Biol. Eng. Comput.* **2006**, *44*, 527–535. [CrossRef]
50. Esposito, M.; Ekestubbe, A.; Gröndahl, K. Radiological evaluation of marginal bone loss at tooth surfaces facing single Brånemark implants. *Clin. Oral Implants Res.* **1993**, *4*, 151–157. [CrossRef]
51. Arifin, A.; Sulong, A.B.; Muhamad, N.; Syarif, J.; Ramli, M.I. Material processing of hydroxyapatite and titanium alloy (HA/Ti) composite as implant materials using powder metallurgy: A review. *Mater. Des.* **2014**, *55*, 165–175. [CrossRef]
52. Miyaura, K.; Matsuka, Y.; Morita, M.; Yamashita, A.; Watanabe, T. Comparison of biting forces in different age and sex groups: A study of biting efficiency with mobile and non-mobile teeth. *J. Oral Rehabil.* **1999**, *26*, 223–227. [CrossRef]
53. Moy, P.K.; Medina, D.; Shetty, V.; Aghaloo, T.L. Dental implant failure rates and associated risk factors. *Int. J. Oral. Maxillofac. Implant.* **2005**, *20*, 569–577.
54. Pérez, M.A.; Prendergast, P.J. Random-walk models of cell dispersal included in mechanobiological simulations of tissue differentiation. *J. Biomech.* **2007**, *40*, 2244–2253. [CrossRef]
55. Toms, S.R.; Lemons, J.E.; Bartolucci, A.A.; Eberhardt, A.W. Nonlinear stress-strain behavior of periodontal ligament under orthodontic loading. *Am. J. Orthod. Dentofac. Orthop.* **2002**, *122*, 174–179. [CrossRef]
56. Vollmer, D.; Bourauel, C.; Maier, K.; Jäger, A. Determination of the centre of resistance in an upper human canine and idealized tooth model. *Eur. J. Orthod.* **1999**, *21*, 633–648. [CrossRef]
57. Provatidis, C.G. A comparative FEM-study of tooth mobility using isotropic and anisotropic models of the periodontal ligament. *Med. Eng. Phys.* **2000**, *22*, 359–370. [CrossRef]

7

Biological Responses to the Transitional Area of Dental Implants: Material- and Structure-Dependent Responses of Peri-Implant Tissue to Abutments

Jung-Ju Kim [1,†], Jae-Hyun Lee [2,†], Jeong Chan Kim [1], Jun-Beom Lee [1] and In-Sung Luke Yeo [3,*]

1 Department of Periodontology, Seoul National University School of Dentistry, Seoul 03080, Korea; freetist@gmail.com (J.-J.K.); perio_kjc@naver.com (J.C.K.); dent.jblee@gmail.com (J.-B.L.)
2 Department of Prosthodontics, One-Stop Specialty Center, Seoul National University Dental Hospital, Seoul 03080, Korea; jhlee.snudh@gmail.com
3 Department of Prosthodontics, School of Dentistry and Dental Research Institute, Seoul National University, Seoul 03080, Korea
* Correspondence: pros53@snu.ac.kr
† Jung-Ju Kim and Jae-Hyun Lee contributed equally to this work.

Abstract: The stability of peri-implant tissue is essential for the long-term success of dental implants. Although various types of implant connections are used, little is known about the effects of the physical mechanisms of dental implants on the stability of peri-implant tissue. This review summarizes the relevant literature to establish guidelines regarding the effects of connection type between abutments and implants in soft and hard tissues. Soft tissue seals can affect soft tissue around implants. In external connections, micromobility between the abutment and the hex component of the implant, resulting from machining tolerance, can destroy the soft tissue seal, potentially leading to microbial invasion. Internal friction connection implants induce strain on the surrounding bone via implant wall expansion that translates into masticatory force. This strain is advantageous because it increases the amount and quality of peri-implant bone. The comparison of internal and external connections, the two most commonly used connection types, reveals that internal friction has a positive influence on both soft and hard tissues.

Keywords: abutment; dental implant; implant connection; marginal bone; peri-implantitis

1. Introduction

A dental implant is an artificial organ that replaces a missing natural tooth. Implants should be able to function properly in the human body [1]. Long-term stability should be predictable and in line with current trends toward increased life expectancy [2–6]. For dental implants to function properly for a long time in the oral cavity, they should experience neither mechanical nor biological complications, including those related to soft and hard tissues surrounding the implant [7–11].

The stability of the implant–abutment connection is an important factor affecting the long-term success of dental implants in clinical practice [12,13]. To prevent complications resulting from unstable implant–abutment connections, implant–abutment biomechanics are investigated theoretically and experimentally. In this review, internal friction connection and external hex-type connection implant–abutment joints are explored. Dental implants belonging to these two systems are currently the most widely used in clinical practice [13–15]. The nature of these connections is summarized, and their effects on tissues surrounding implants are analyzed for both soft and hard tissues.

2. Typical Dental Implant Connection Types

2.1. External Hex Connection: Butt-Jointed Interface

In external hex-type connections, the abutment is connected to the implant by an abutment screw. This connection is also called a butt joint interface because the flat surfaces on the top of the implant and the bottom of the abutment are in direct contact with each other. This external connection is stabilized entirely by fastening of the abutment screw. When torque is applied to the abutment screw connecting the implant and the abutment, the abutment screw is elongated, generating a preload. Screw dynamics play an important role in this interaction because the mechanism linking this connection is fundamentally dependent on the preload of the screw [16]. The preload acts as a clamping force on the implant–abutment complex, and provides stability to the connection [17].

The Brånemark implant (NobelBiocare, Zurich, Switzerland), the first commercially available screw-shaped implant, is a representative external connection-type implant. When masticatory force is applied to this type of implant, the vertical component of the masticatory force is supported by the top platform of the implant. The lateral component of the masticatory force is placed on the hex structure of the top of the implant and the abutment screw, and the rotational component of this force is resisted by the hex structure.

Previous biomechanical analyses indicate that the manufacturer's recommended torque of 30–35 Ncm is not sufficient to prevent screw loosening [17,18]. Repeated tightening of the abutment screw is considered essential because of the preload loss in screw mechanics, which is the cause of screw loosening [17]. It is also helpful to use other methods in addition to screw tightening to maintain the stability of the implant–abutment connection. One option that makes this possible is the use of the frictional force generated between the interfaces.

2.2. Internal Friction Connection: Frictional Interface

In internal friction connections, stability is maintained by close contact between the inner surface of the implant and the outer surface of the abutment, in addition to the preload applied to the abutment screw. The tight contact between the abutment and implant creates frictional force, and this plays a major role in supporting the stability of the connection. Therefore, this type of connection is also called a friction-screw-retained connection.

The degree of tapering at the interface between the implant and the abutment is an important factor to consider when determining the abutment mobility of the internal conical connection. A wider tapering angle will result in a more unstable connection in this type of internal connection, although the possibility of implant fracture decreases [16,19]. In addition, the role of frictional forces in maintaining the stability of the connection is decreased, while the burden on the abutment screws is increased (Figure 1).

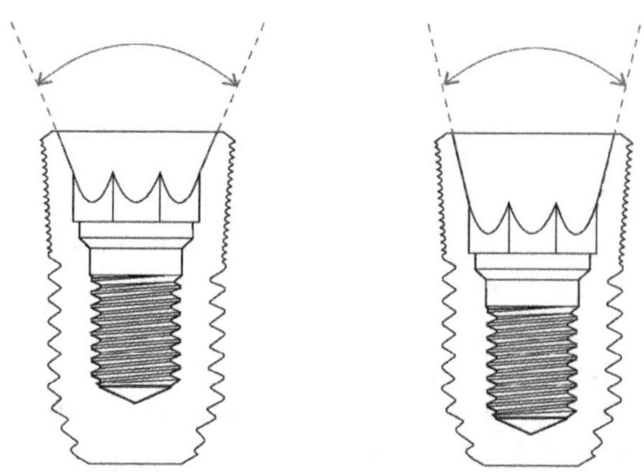

Figure 1. The degree of conical connection. A wider tapering angle (left) results in a more unstable connection for abutment mobility in internal connection-type implants.

A systematic review reported that internal friction connection provides less microleakage at the implant–abutment interface than external hex connection type in both static and dynamic loading tests [20]. The presence of gap could lead to accumulation of bacteria and the phenomenon might affect the success rate of implants.

When an abutment is connected to an internal conical connection-type implant, the abutment is first brought into contact with the upper part of the implant inner wall [19,21]. As the implant at the top is slightly flared, it comes into greater contact with the abutment as the implant is combined. The abutment screw becomes slightly loosened when the abutment is completely combined with the implant by opening the implant wall. Because of the preload loss from such an abutment sinking and settling effect, repeated screw tightening is essential [18,22].

3. Soft Tissue Responses to Different Implant System Materials and Structures

3.1. The Soft Tissue Seal Theory

Humans are exposed to a variety of external environments involving external forces, ultraviolet rays, and microorganisms. Human skin is the first line of defense that protects the human body against these external stresses. When human skin is pierced, the resulting hole must be closed by the immune system and healing mechanisms.

Teeth are one of the few organs in the human body that are located across the skin. The root of the tooth is surrounded by alveolar bone, while the part that penetrates through the soft tissue is in contact with epithelial tissue and/or the connective tissue of the mucosa [23]. Holes in the mucosa created by teeth are sealed by a special structure composed of epithelium and connective tissue [23]. An internal basal lamina and the hemi-desmosomes of epithelial tissue are attached to teeth, and a combination of dento-gingival fiber and cementum links teeth to the surrounding connective tissue. The holes connecting the inside and outside of the human body that contain teeth are secured by soft tissue attachments [23].

Like natural teeth, dental implants are an artificial organ located in a hole on the surface of the body, and the hole is sealed via a mechanism similar to the one that seals the holes around natural teeth using soft tissues. However, these sealing mechanisms are not identical to each other. Dental implants are in contact with the alveolar bone or soft tissue (epithelial and connective tissue) of the transition area (Figure 2) [24]. Fibers in the connective tissue attached to the abutment mainly run parallel to the surface and are circular in shape, whereas dento-gingival fibers, such as Sharpey's fibers, are attached vertically to the cementum in natural teeth (Figure 1) [24].

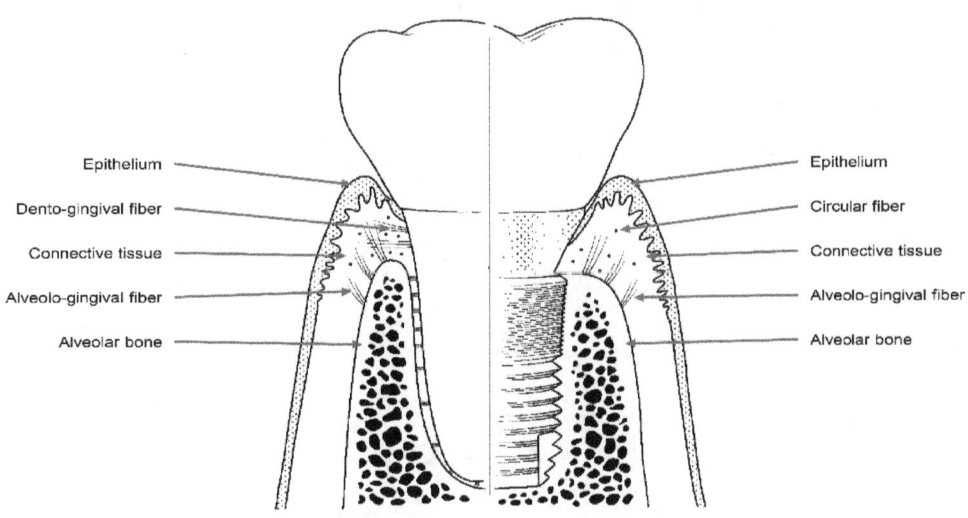

Figure 2. Soft and hard tissues with collagen fibers surrounding a natural tooth (**left**) and a dental implant (**right**).

A scanning electron microscopy study showed that there are two distinct layers in the area within 200 μm of where the implant abutment comes into contact with the connective tissue. The inner 40 μm of this layer contains multiple fibroblasts that are attached directly to the surface of the abutment, while the outer 160 μm of this layer contains numerous collagen fibers [25]. Hence, the attachment of connective tissue to the abutment is maintained by fibroblasts attached to the titanium surface of the implant, and the elasticity of circular collagen fibers. For this reason, compared with the attachments of natural teeth, which involve direct attachment to connective tissue, attachments formed by connective tissue around an implant abutment are weaker.

Epithelial tissue is attached to the implant abutment via an internal basal lamina and hemi-desmosomes in a manner similar to the attachment of natural teeth [26–29]. However, epithelium attachment includes the internal basal lamina and hemi-desmosomes formed only in the lower part of the peri-implant epithelium around the implant abutment, whereas in natural teeth, these attachments are widely distributed throughout the junctional epithelium–tooth interface [30–32]. Thus, epithelial adhesions that form around the implant abutment are more vulnerable than those that form around natural teeth owing to their limited area of distribution.

In summary, both epithelial and connective tissues are more weakly attached to implant abutments than to natural teeth. Hence, holes on the surface of the human body that contain implants are more vulnerable to containment failure. This mechanism of blockade by soft tissue is called a 'soft tissue seal' [30,33].

3.2. *Attachment of Soft Tissue*

The stability and immobility of soft tissue attachments in contact with the implant abutment are important factors that affect the long-term prognosis of the implant [30,33]. If the soft tissues around the implant are deformed owing to the movement of the lip, cheek, tongue, or jaw, the weak soft tissue seal surrounding the implant may be destroyed. This allows microbes to penetrate through the damaged mucosal seal, increasing the likelihood of disease around the implant [30,33]. Therefore, a stable soft tissue seal is essential to prevent microbial invasion and peri-implant disease [33–35].

The soft tissues around natural teeth are separated into the lining mucosa and masticatory mucosa, of which the masticatory mucosa is composed of the free and attached gingiva (Figure 3). The attached gingiva is in permanent and intimate contact with the surface of the enamel, the cementum, and the alveolar bone, thereby immobilizing the soft tissue [23]. It is, therefore, possible to retain the firmness and health of the mucosal seal by preventing it from detaching.

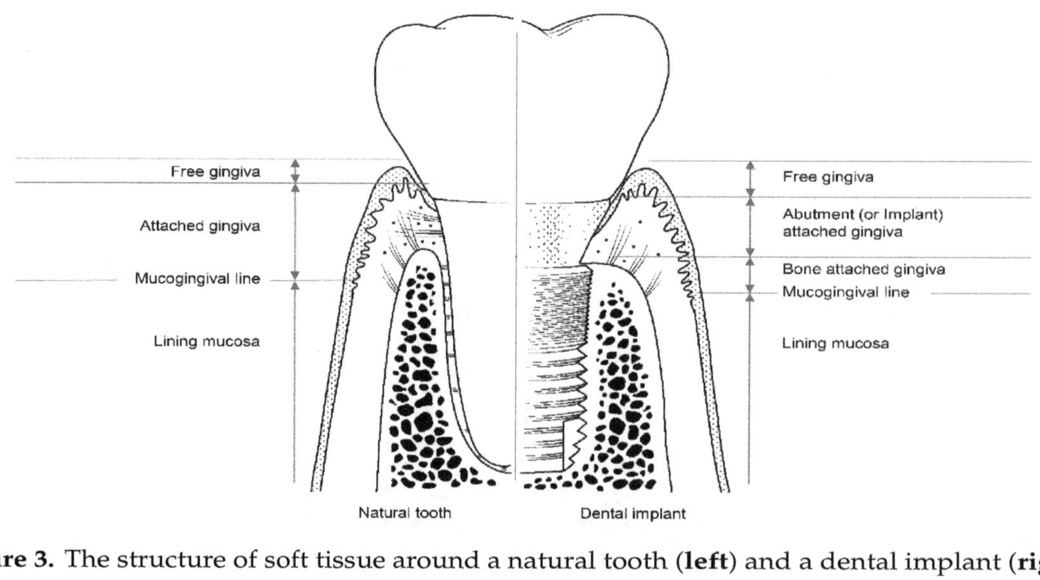

Figure 3. The structure of soft tissue around a natural tooth (**left**) and a dental implant (**right**).

Among the soft tissues surrounding an implant, the attached gingiva differs from those surrounding natural teeth [24]. The gingiva attached to the peri-implant can be divided into two parts: bone-attached and abutment (or implant)-attached gingiva (Figure 3). The bone-attached gingiva is identical to the corresponding tissue in natural gums, and rigidly immobilizes the soft tissue. However, as mentioned above, the abutment- (or implant)-attached gingiva more weakly adheres than the attachment gingiva that surrounds natural teeth [24]. Owing to the weak structure of the abutment- (or implant)-attached gingiva, the width of the bone-attached gingiva around the implant should be wide enough to prevent mucosal mobility, and thereby prevent the occurrence of peri-implant disease due to the collapse of the mucosal seal [24,33].

3.3. Disruption of the Soft Tissue Seal

The soft tissue seal is mainly destroyed via two mechanisms; instability of the peri-implant mucosa or the implant-abutment assembly. If there is no bone-attached gingiva around the implant, the soft tissue can become mobile, and the mucosal seal will inevitably rupture. When the mucosal seal is destroyed, bacteria can penetrate the internal environment through the transmucosal rupture site, potentially leading to peri-implant disease [36]. Therefore, because of the weakness of the soft tissue attachment, it is important to ensure there is sufficient bone-attached gingiva around the implant. Thus, a plan for implant surgery should be established to maintain the bone-attached gingiva following implant placement.

Instability in the connection between the implant and the abutment can also lead to the disruption of the soft tissue seal, which may present as mobility of the abutment or the implant. Mobility of the implant occurs only when osseointegration fails, but mobility of the abutment can occur as a result of various causes, including fractures of the abutment or implant, even following successful osseointegration. The most common cause of abutment mobility is the loosening of the abutment screw that connects it to the implant. Elongation and loosening of the screw caused by the lateral force of the masticatory load are more frequently observed in external connection-type implants than in internal connection-type implants [15].

In external-type implants, there is slight machining tolerance around the hex component, resulting in micromobility in the abutment. This external hex connection is, therefore, a mobile structure. Thus, most occlusal forces are concentrated on the abutment screw. This micromobility is likely to cause disruption of the soft tissue seal, bacterial infiltration, and peri-implant disease [37] (Figure 4). Implant systems with an external hex connection were originally developed for the mandibular restoration of a completely edentulous patient wearing a maxillary complete denture. The occlusal force in such patients is weak, and this mobile connection is able to bear this weak masticatory force with few screw loosening events or breakdown of the soft tissue seal. However, such unstable implant–abutment connections can provoke severe peri-implant problems for a partially edentulous patient with antagonistic natural teeth and a strong occlusal force. To reduce the micromobility of the abutment, the external hex must be lengthened, and the machining tolerance between the male and female components must be minimized. Furthermore, it may be possible to fabricate an abutment screw using a stronger material, or by widening the platform size of the top of the implant to minimize the force concentrated on the abutment screw. In addition, when the abutment is fastened to the implant, applying higher torque may also be employed to increase the stability of the connection. However, none of these methods can completely eliminate the micromobility of the abutment in external connection-type implants.

In internal connection-type implants, the abutment–implant connection is firm owing to a process similar to cold-welding. Unlike external connections, in which the occlusal force is concentrated mainly on the abutment screw, the occlusal force is transmitted to the implant inner wall through the abutment–implant connection in internal connection-type implants. Therefore, less screw loosening occurs in this type of implant. In addition, the abutment–implant contact area is wider internal connection-type implants, and this prevents stress from concentrating at specific sites such as the abutment screw, and contributes to the stability of the soft tissue seal.

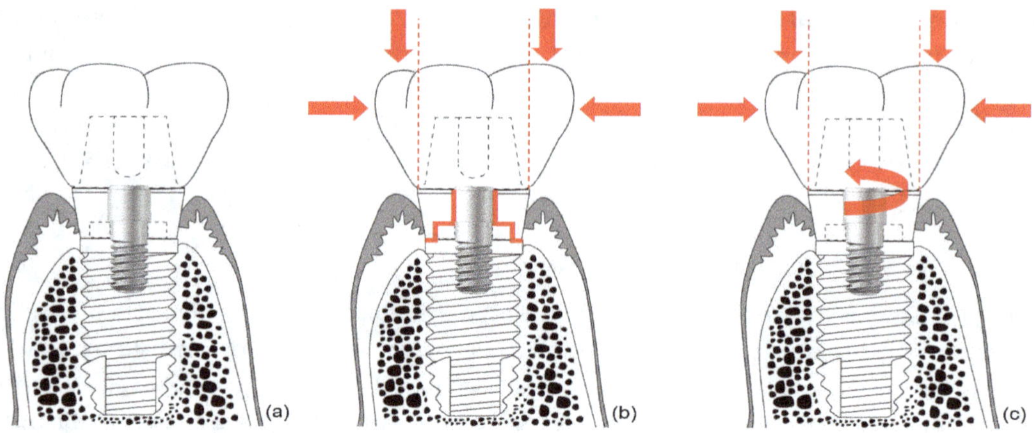

Figure 4. Schematic illustration of the 'soft tissue seal' theory. Micromobility of the abutment in external connection-type implants disrupts the surrounding soft tissue seal, which plays an important role in preventing external irritants from penetrating into the body. (**a**) External connection-type implant. (**b**) Parts experiencing the greatest stress (red lines) from eccentric forces (red arrows). (**c**) Abutment screw-loosening (red rotated arrow) by eccentric forces (red arrows).

3.4. Submerged and Nonsubmerged Implants

Depending on whether the top of the implant is at the alveolar bone or gingival level, implants can be divided into submerged-type and nonsubmerged-type. For submerged implants, the soft tissue seal is formed at the abutment area, rather than at the neck part for the nonsubmerged type. Histologically, there are no significant differences in the degree and pattern of soft tissue attachment to implants between submerged and nonsubmerged types [38]. When nonsubmerged implants are placed at the proper vertical position of the alveolar bone, the mobility of the abutment does not interfere with the soft tissue seal, or cause marginal bone resorption, because the interface between the abutment and the implant is positioned outside the soft tissue [34,35].

When this design was first developed, microgap bacteria residing between the abutment and implant were considered to be the cause of marginal bone resorption [39–41]. Therefore, a design was developed to export the position of this microgap outside the body [42]. However, such a design limits the customization of the patient's emergence profile, resulting in difficulties in terms of long-term clinical results for aesthetically acceptable implant prostheses.

To maintain an adequate soft tissue seal, there must be a proper foundation of underlying bone. However, nonsubmerged-type implants can be susceptible to marginal bone resorption due to the concentration of stress at the top of the implant [43].

3.5. Materials for Abutment

Achieving soft tissue seals may also depend on the type of material used for the abutment. Abrahamsson et al. (1998) investigated the stability of soft tissue seals attached via gold alloy, dental porcelain, titanium, and aluminum oxide. In this study, marginal bone resorption occurred when seals were attached to surfaces composed of gold alloy and dental porcelain, because no soft tissue seal formed. However, when titanium and aluminum oxide were used, a soft tissue seal was achieved, and marginal bone was not absorbed [44]. Welander et al. (2008) also reported that epithelial adhesions receded around abutments attached via gold alloy [45]. Therefore, when using a UCLA abutment, the transmucosal area of the abutment is made of gold or dental porcelain, and a soft tissue seal may not be properly achieved, resulting in marginal bone resorption.

More recently, titanium and zirconia have been used as materials for abutments. One advantage of zirconia is that it is more aesthetic than titanium. While several studies show that there are no significant differences in the soft tissue seal between these two materials, zirconia has a lower fracture strength than titanium, and is thus more likely to be associated with mechanical complications [45–47]. In addition, adhesion of bacteria to titanium occurs less readily than to zirconia [48].

Recent advances in digital dentistry have made it possible to fabricate and restore implant-supported restorations in just a single visit. To this end, lithium disilicate and polymer-infiltrated ceramic network (PICN), which are easy to process on the day, are used as abutment material. These materials are used as implant abutments after cementing to the prefabricated titanium base with adhesive resin cement. Although little research has been conducted on the soft tissue seal of these new materials, Smallidge et al. have reported favorable epithelial cell growth on the PICN surface when PICN has a relatively low surface roughness (Ra < 0.254 μm) [49]. Another recent study reported that the surface roughness of lithium disilicate was smoother than that of PICN after the same polishing process with 6 μm diamond slurry, and the surface roughness of both of materials was unaffected by the ultrasonic scaling procedure [50]. Mehl et al. found that the adhesive resin joint connecting the titanium base and the abutment materials had neither influence on soft tissue anatomy nor on bone loss in the animal study [51]. In zirconia abutments, however, junctional epithelium was significantly shorter than titanium one-piece abutments [51]. Ongun et al. measured the mechanical properties of these hybrid-type abutments including titanium bases, showing that PICN had lower fracture resistance and weaker adhesion to resin cements compared with lithium disilicate ceramic [52]. Such mechanical failure of PICN hybrid-type abutments could also cause the soft tissue seal to break.

3.6. *Detachment of Abutments*

When the abutment becomes disconnected from a submerged-type implant, the soft tissue seal is broken, and microorganisms in the oral cavity can then penetrate into the tissues surrounding the implant [53]. This may result in the loss of marginal bone. Abrahamsson et al. reported that the absorption of marginal bone is doubled when the abutment is detached five times [54]. For these reasons, some clinicians have proposed the 'one abutment-one time (OAOT)' concept to prevent marginal bone loss [55,56]. Clinicians should be aware that during a prosthetic restoration procedure, or during the postrestoration maintenance period, it may be advantageous to minimize the process of removing the abutment.

A systematic review suggested that the OAOT protocol might preserve peri-implant bone loss and soft tissue changes for two reasons [57]. First of all, the micro-gap between abutment and implant could cause to bacterial leakage and micromotion, and this might lead to the inflammation of peri-implant soft tissue and bone resorption. The OAOT protocol could provide less micro-gap because healing or temporary abutments were installed by less preloading force (<10 Ncm) than final abutments (about 30 Ncm) [57]. Second, the OAOT protocol could reduce the disruption of the soft tissue seal around the implant abutment complex to avoid repeated the dis/reconnection of abutments [57].

3.7. *Surface Modification of Abutments*

Various technologies have been explored for improving the soft tissue seal at the transmucosal part of the abutment, including surface treatments, such as coating, machining, blasting, plasma spraying, etching, and laser processing [58].

Yang et al. reported that, when ultraviolet light is applied to surfaces, gingival fibroblasts proliferate more readily on surfaces made of zirconia [59]. Several studies showed that, when an abutment is laser-treated, the connective tissue is directly attached to the surface of the abutment by perpendicular fibers [60–62]. In addition, as the surface roughness of the transmucosal part of the abutment increases, the soft tissue seal improves. This may be because a rougher surface has a larger surface area to which the soft tissue can attach [63]. A previous study also suggested that hydrothermal treatment on titanium alloy could change minimally surface topography to enhance hydrophilicity [64].

Subsequently, the treatment contributed to the integration of epithelial cells to the surface and might facilitate the healthy epithelial tissue sealing around the transmucosal part of the implant [64].

The surface of the abutment can be modified to change the surface roughness or the free energy. While this may enhance the soft tissue seal, it can also increase plaque accumulation and the tendency for bacterial colonization to occur [65,66]. Thus, surface treatments applied to abutments should be carefully selected.

4. Hard Tissue Responses to Implant System Materials and Structures

4.1. The Bone Stimulation Theory

The soft and hard tissues surrounding the implant play complementary roles. Alveolar bone is a hard tissue that withstands the masticatory force applied to the implant, and serves to transmit it to the jawbone. The soft tissue, gingiva, and mucosa protect the alveolar bone from external irritants such as bacteria. The condition of the soft tissue is maintained by the underlying alveolar bone, and the alveolar bone is protected by the overlying soft tissue.

In general, after the restoration of an implant, between 1 and 1.5 mm of the marginal bone around the implant is absorbed during the first year owing to the application of occlusal force, and 0.2 mm is absorbed per year thereafter [67]. On the basis of the results of studies showing that marginal bone is steadily absorbed every year, it was thought that long-length implants should be beneficial for long-term predictability [67]. This was observed in long-term studies of the Brånemark system using an external connection-type implant, which is limited and inapplicable to some internal friction connections [14,68,69]. By contrast, several studies on a certain implant connection system reported that peri-implant marginal bone is increased by occlusal loading [68,69]. Because the use of long implants is likely to cause damage to important anatomical structures such as nerves, it may be more advantageous to insert short implants if warranted for long-term prognosis without marginal bone resorption.

In natural dentition, when periodontal disease occurs or a natural tooth is lost, the alveolar bone of the corresponding region is resorbed. However, when the natural tooth and the periodontal tissue are healthy, the alveolar bone is well-maintained. Except for a small amount of loss due to mechanical degeneration or aging, the alveolar bone should be well-maintained throughout life, as periodontal ligaments have been shown to transfer adequate stimulation to alveolar bone. Otherwise, disuse atrophy of the bone can occur. From this point of view, if the peri-implant bone is appropriately stimulated by the implant, the peri-implant marginal bone will not be resorbed, and the quantity and quality of the bone are likely to be preserved.

The Astra implant system (Dentsply Sirona, Charlotte, NC, United States) involves an internal friction connection type, and was the first connection system to embody this concept. The implant–abutment connection of this system improves the amount and quality of peri-implant bone by properly transmitting the masticatory force to the surrounding alveolar bone. This hypothesis was reported by Frost [70] and can be applied to alveolar bone as well as to other bones in the human body [70]. Hence, under conditions involving the application of appropriate strain to human bone, osteoblasts are activated, which increases the amount and quality of the bone.

Before existing implant systems were widely used in clinical practice, various types and shapes of implants were developed, and most disappeared without displaying any ability to withstand mechanical or biological complications [71,72]. The Brånemark system was the first to achieve successful long-term predictable prognosis, and the consequential popularization of implants. Unlike previous plain-shaped systems, this system can deliver occlusal force to the alveolar bone because it has a thread on the implant surface [71,72]. The thread of the implant transforms the shear stress generated at the interface between the implant and the bone into compressive stress so that the appropriate stimulus can be transmitted to the bone (Figure 5). This stimulation is one of the factors that allows the bone to remain stable over the long term.

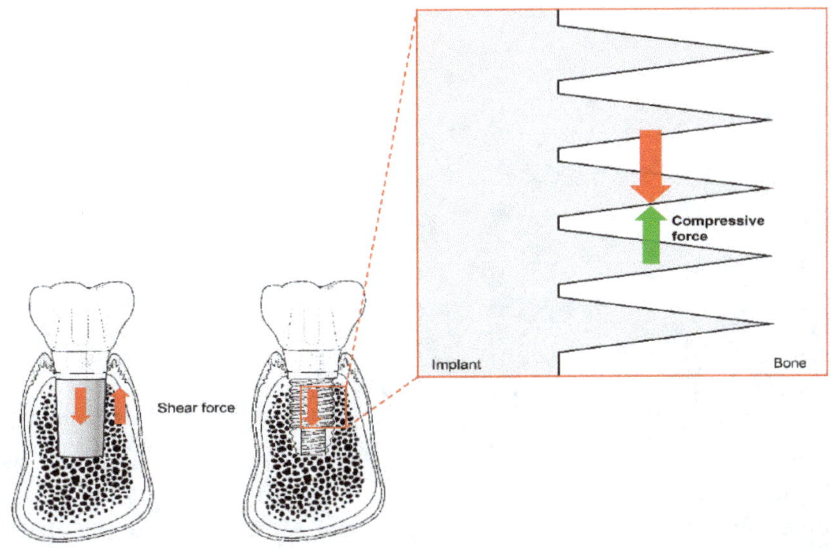

Figure 5. The thread function of non-threaded (**left**) and threaded (**right**) dental implants. Shear force (red arrows) is transformed into compressive force (green arrow) by the threads. Note the reduction of shear force due to the partial switch to compressive force in the magnified diagram (vertically and horizontally; not marked).

A disadvantage of these external connection-type implants is that the soft tissue seal formed around the abutment is destroyed by micromobility at the connection. The Brånemark implant represents the beginning of modern implants, and was the first system to perform well in clinical practice. However, marginal bone resorption was found to be caused by the destruction of the soft-tissue seal. To prevent such marginal bone loss, an Astra internal connection implant system was developed. This internal friction system maintains bone by applying appropriate stimulation to the bone around the implant without loss of the soft tissue seal around the implant.

4.2. *Mechanism of Bone Stimulation*

The connection of the Astra implant system has an internal conical shape with a slope of 11 degrees. The occlusal force applied to the abutment is transmitted to the implant through this conical connection. The masticatory force delivered to the implant thus becomes the source of the stain to stimulate the alveolar bone [73]. Thus, when the abutment receives occlusal force and sinks downward, the conical opening of the implant is opened wider, and the bone around the implant is consequentially stimulated (Figure 6). This stimulation activates osteoblasts in the alveolar bone, thereby increasing the amount and quality of alveolar bone. This increase in alveolar bone can lead to a positive change in the results of clinical procedures. This reduces the need for invasive bone grafting or the placement of excessively long implants during implant surgery. This represents a positive result for both the patient and the surgeon.

4.3. *Prevention of Hard Tissue Loss*

The marginal bone loss that occurs in the mobile connection of external connection-type implants does not lead directly to the failure of the implant. However, it can cause considerable complications in the tissue surrounding the implant. In general, these external connection implants are known to lose marginal bone up to the second or third thread level of the implant [74]. This bone loss can alter the properties of the overlying soft tissue, resulting in a reduction in the attached gingiva. This weakens the soft tissue seal and increases the likelihood of bacterial invasion and peri-implantitis. A detailed periodical examination of the condition of tissues around the implant is thus essential for long-term success when external connection-type implants are used.

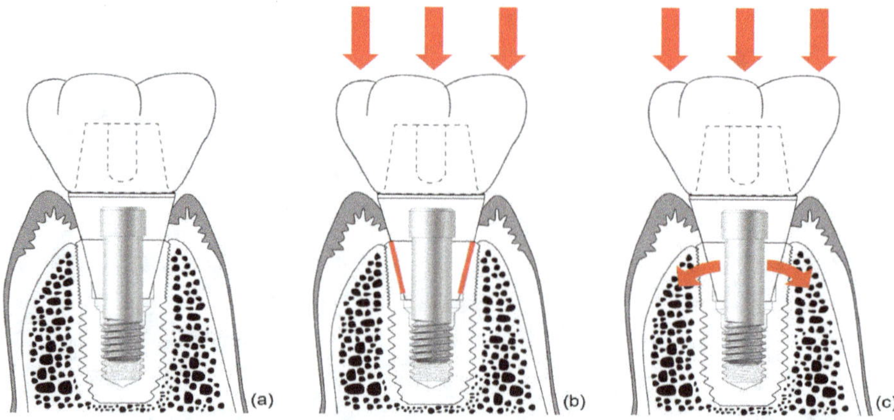

Figure 6. Schematic drawing of bone stimulation. When occlusal force is applied to an internal connection-type implant, the implant around the connection expands and stimulates the surrounding bone to induce bone proliferation. (**a**) Internal friction connection-type implant. (**b**) The occlusal force is transmitted to the implant through the conical connection parts (red lines). (**c**) The coronal expansion of the implant (curved red arrows) becomes the source of the strain that stimulates the alveolar bone.

The issue of whether gingiva must be present for the health of natural teeth has been investigated. Clinically, even if the gingiva cannot completely wrap the tooth, it should be able to prevent the movement of the surrounding soft tissue from being transmitted to the free gingiva [75]. In other words, cheek, lip, and mandibular movements should not be transferred to the marginal gingiva. To achieve this, a certain amount of attached gingiva must be present to prevent the penetration of bacteria into the periodontal tissue [76].

This principle of natural dentition should also be borne in mind when considering implant restorations [77]. An appropriate amount of attached gingiva should be present, rather than free gingiva alone, to prevent microbial invasion into tissue surrounding the implant. According to the systematic review in 2018, if there is the insufficient attached gingiva around implant, the apically positioned flap with autogenous graft is suggested to increase the width of the gingiva [78]. However, it is not enough simply to increase the width of attached gingiva, because this surgical procedure is unable to alter the level of mucogingival junction [79]. Additional vestibuloplasty is, therefore, recommended to create "new" mucogingival junction by preventing the movement of the lips and cheeks from affecting the free gingiva.

In addition, abutment and restoration contour have been recently reported to have effects on marginal bone loss. An emergence angle of more than 30 degrees and a convex emergence profile may increase the risk of peri-implantitis [80]. The association between the restoration contour and the soft tissue seal remains uncertain. However, in order to prevent the bone loss, it is important to maintain the favorable soft tissue environment by adjusting the emergence angle, the emergence profile, the position of a restoration margin, and the removal of excess cement [80–82].

5. Summary

Dental implants should be capable of performing dental functions for a prolonged period of time. For this to be possible, the health of the surrounding soft and hard tissues is essential. Alveolar bone must be able to withstand masticatory force, and the overlying soft tissue should be able to protect the alveolar bone from external irritants.

The soft tissue seal is weaker around implants than around natural teeth. Thus, to avoid damage, the peri-implant soft tissue seal should not be mobile. Free and abutment-attached gingiva cannot prevent the destruction of the soft tissue seal that results from the movements of the lips and cheeks. Additionally, it is impossible to prevent all micromobility of the abutment in external connection-type implants. Hence, it is necessary to secure sufficient bone-attached gingiva, or use an implant system with extensive and deep connections, such as internal connection-type implants. The resulting immobility contributes to the maintenance of a healthy soft tissue seal, and prevents bacterial invasion into the peri-implant tissue. In addition, internal connection-type implants can transform occlusal load into strain that stimulates the surrounding bone through the abutment–implant connection. This strain enhances the amount and quality of peri-implant bone.

Taking these findings into account, clinicians may find it advantageous to select internal conical connection-type implants rather than external connection-type implants, to allow dental implants to function properly as artificial organs with long-term predictability.

Author Contributions: All authors have read and agree to the published version of the manuscript. Conceptualization, J.-J.K., J.-H.L., and I.-S.L.Y.; data curation, J.-J.K. and J.-H.L.; formal analysis, J.-J.K. and J.-H.L.; funding acquisition, I.-S.L.Y.; investigation, J.-J.K., J.-H.L., and J.-B.L.; methodology, J.-J.K., J.-H.L., J.C.K., J.-B.L., and I.-S.L.Y.; project administration, I.-S.L.Y.; resources, J.C.K. and I.-S.L.Y.; software, J.-H.L.; supervision, I.-S.L.Y.; validation, J.-J.K. and J.C.K.; visualization, J.-H.L. and J.C.K.; writing—original draft, J.-H.L., J.-J.K., and I.-S.L.Y.; writing—review and editing, J.-H.L., J.-J.K., J.C.K., J.-B.L., and I.-S.L.Y. All authors have read and agreed to the published version of the manuscript.

References

1. Pjetursson, B.E.; Heimisdottir, K. Dental implants—Are they better than natural teeth? *Eur. J. Oral Sci.* **2018**, *126*, 81–87. [CrossRef] [PubMed]
2. Albrektsson, T.; Chrcanovic, B.; Ostman, P.O.; Sennerby, L. Initial and long-term crestal bone responses to modern dental implants. *Periodontology 2000* **2017**, *73*, 41–50. [CrossRef] [PubMed]
3. De Bruyn, H.; Christiaens, V.; Doornewaard, R.; Jacobsson, M.; Cosyn, J.; Jacquet, W.; Vervaeke, S. Implant surface roughness and patient factors on long-term peri-implant bone loss. *Periodontology 2000* **2017**, *73*, 218–227. [CrossRef] [PubMed]
4. Howe, M.S.; Keys, W.; Richards, D. Long-term (10-year) dental implant survival: A systematic review and sensitivity meta-analysis. *J. Dent.* **2019**, *84*, 9–21. [CrossRef] [PubMed]
5. Srinivasan, M.; Meyer, S.; Mombelli, A.; Muller, F. Dental implants in the elderly population: A systematic review and meta-analysis. *Clin. Oral Implant. Res.* **2017**, *28*, 920–930. [CrossRef] [PubMed]
6. Starch-Jensen, T.; Aludden, H.; Hallman, M.; Dahlin, C.; Christensen, A.E.; Mordenfeld, A. A systematic review and meta-analysis of long-term studies (five or more years) assessing maxillary sinus floor augmentation. *Int. J. Oral Maxillofac. Surg.* **2018**, *47*, 103–116. [CrossRef] [PubMed]
7. De Kok, I.J.; Duqum, I.S.; Katz, L.H.; Cooper, L.F. Management of Implant/Prosthodontic Complications. *Dent. Clin. North Am.* **2019**, *63*, 217–231. [CrossRef]
8. Esposito, M.; Hirsch, J.; Lekholm, U.; Thomsen, P. Differential diagnosis and treatment strategies for biologic complications and failing oral implants: A review of the literature. *Int. J. Oral Maxillofac. Implant.* **1999**, *14*, 473–490.
9. Hsu, Y.T.; Mason, S.A.; Wang, H.L. Biological implant complications and their management. *J. Int. Acad. Periodontol.* **2014**, *16*, 9–18.
10. Lang, N.P.; Wilson, T.G.; Corbet, E.F. Biological complications with dental implants: Their prevention, diagnosis and treatment. *Clin. Oral Implant. Res.* **2000**, *11*, 146–155. [CrossRef]
11. Sadid-Zadeh, R.; Kutkut, A.; Kim, H. Prosthetic failure in implant dentistry. *Dent. Clin. North Am.* **2015**, *59*, 195–214. [CrossRef] [PubMed]
12. Vetromilla, B.M.; Brondani, L.P.; Pereira-Cenci, T.; Bergoli, C.D. Influence of different implant-abutment connection designs on the mechanical and biological behavior of single-tooth implants in the maxillary esthetic zone: A systematic review. *J. Prosthet. Dent.* **2019**, *121*, 398–403.e3. [CrossRef] [PubMed]
13. Lemos, C.A.A.; Verri, F.R.; Bonfante, E.A.; Santiago Junior, J.F.; Pellizzer, E.P. Comparison of external and internal implant-abutment connections for implant supported prostheses. A systematic review and meta-analysis. *J. Dent.* **2018**, *70*, 14–22. [CrossRef] [PubMed]
14. de Medeiros, R.A.; Pellizzer, E.P.; Vechiato Filho, A.J.; Dos Santos, D.M.; da Silva, E.V.; Goiato, M.C. Evaluation of marginal bone loss of dental implants with internal or external connections and its association with other variables: A systematic review. *J. Prosthet. Dent.* **2016**, *116*, 501–506. [CrossRef]
15. Gracis, S.; Michalakis, K.; Vigolo, P.; Vult von Steyern, P.; Zwahlen, M.; Sailer, I. Internal vs. external connections for abutments/reconstructions: A systematic review. *Clin. Oral Implant. Res.* **2012**, *23*, 202–216. [CrossRef]

16. Bozkaya, D.; Muftu, S. Mechanics of the tapered interference fit in dental implants. *J. Biomech.* **2003**, *36*, 1649–1658. [CrossRef]
17. Jeong, C.G.; Kim, S.K.; Lee, J.H.; Kim, J.W.; Yeo, I.S.L. Clinically available preload prediction based on a mechanical analysis. *Arch. Appl. Mech.* **2017**, *87*, 2003–2009. [CrossRef]
18. Michalakis, K.X.; Calvani, P.L.; Muftu, S.; Pissiotis, A.; Hirayama, H. The effect of different implant-abutment connections on screw joint stability. *J. Oral Implantol.* **2014**, *40*, 146–152. [CrossRef]
19. Lee, J.H.; Huh, Y.H.; Park, C.J.; Cho, L.R. Effect of the Coronal Wall Thickness of Dental Implants on the Screw Joint Stability in the Internal Implant-Abutment Connection. *Int. J. Oral Maxillofac. Implant.* **2016**, *31*, 1058–1065. [CrossRef]
20. Mishra, S.K.; Chowdhary, R.; Kumari, S. Microleakage at the Different Implant Abutment Interface: A Systematic Review. *J. Clin. Diagn. Res.* **2017**, *11*, ZE10–ZE15. [CrossRef]
21. Yilmaz, B.; Gilbert, A.B.; Seidt, J.D.; McGlumphy, E.A.; Clelland, N.L. Displacement of Implant Abutments Following Initial and Repeated Torqueing. *Int. J. Oral Maxillofac. Implant.* **2015**, *30*, 1011–1018. [CrossRef] [PubMed]
22. Saleh Saber, F.; Abolfazli, N.; Jannatii Ataei, S.; Taghizade Motlagh, M.; Gharekhani, V. The effect of repeated torque tightening on total lengths of implant abutments in different internal implantabutment connections. *J. Dent. Res. Dent. Clin. Dent. Prospect.* **2017**, *11*, 110–116. [CrossRef] [PubMed]
23. Bartold, P.M.; Walsh, L.J.; Narayanan, A.S. Molecular and cell biology of the gingiva. *Periodontology 2000* **2000**, *24*, 28–55. [CrossRef] [PubMed]
24. Berglundh, T.; Lindhe, J.; Ericsson, I.; Marinello, C.P.; Liljenberg, B.; Thomsen, P. The soft tissue barrier at implants and teeth. *Clin. Oral Implant. Res.* **1991**, *2*, 81–90. [CrossRef] [PubMed]
25. Moon, I.S.; Berglundh, T.; Abrahamsson, I.; Linder, E.; Lindhe, J. The barrier between the keratinized mucosa and the dental implant. An experimental study in the dog. *J. Clin. Periodontol.* **1999**, *26*, 658–663. [CrossRef] [PubMed]
26. Atsuta, I.; Ayukawa, Y.; Furuhashi, A.; Yamaza, T.; Tsukiyama, Y.; Koyano, K. Promotive effect of insulin-like growth factor-1 for epithelial sealing to titanium implants. *J. Biomed. Mater. Res. A* **2013**, *101*, 2896–2904. [CrossRef] [PubMed]
27. Donley, T.G.; Gillette, W.B. Titanium endosseous implant-soft tissue interface: A literature review. *J. Periodontol.* **1991**, *62*, 153–160. [CrossRef]
28. Gould, T.R.; Westbury, L.; Brunette, D.M. Ultrastructural study of the attachment of human gingiva to titanium in vivo. *J. Prosthet. Dent.* **1984**, *52*, 418–420. [CrossRef]
29. Ikeda, H.; Shiraiwa, M.; Yamaza, T.; Yoshinari, M.; Kido, M.A.; Ayukawa, Y.; Inoue, T.; Koyano, K.; Tanaka, T. Difference in penetration of horseradish peroxidase tracer as a foreign substance into the peri-implant or junctional epithelium of rat gingivae. *Clin. Oral Implant. Res.* **2002**, *13*, 243–251. [CrossRef]
30. Atsuta, I.; Ayukawa, Y.; Kondo, R.; Oshiro, W.; Matsuura, Y.; Furuhashi, A.; Tsukiyama, Y.; Koyano, K. Soft tissue sealing around dental implants based on histological interpretation. *J. Prosthodont. Res.* **2016**, *60*, 3–11. [CrossRef]
31. Atsuta, I.; Yamaza, T.; Yoshinari, M.; Goto, T.; Kido, M.A.; Kagiya, T.; Mino, S.; Shimono, M.; Tanaka, T. Ultrastructural localization of laminin-5 (gamma2 chain) in the rat peri-implant oral mucosa around a titanium-dental implant by immuno-electron microscopy. *Biomaterials* **2005**, *26*, 6280–6287. [CrossRef]
32. Ikeda, H.; Yamaza, T.; Yoshinari, M.; Ohsaki, Y.; Ayukawa, Y.; Kido, M.A.; Inoue, T.; Shimono, M.; Koyano, K.; Tanaka, T. Ultrastructural and immunoelectron microscopic studies of the peri-implant epithelium-implant (Ti-6Al-4V) interface of rat maxilla. *J. Periodontol.* **2000**, *71*, 961–973. [CrossRef] [PubMed]
33. Abdallah, M.N.; Badran, Z.; Ciobanu, O.; Hamdan, N.; Tamimi, F. Strategies for Optimizing the Soft Tissue Seal around Osseointegrated Implants. *Adv. Healthc. Mater.* **2017**, *6*, 1700549. [CrossRef] [PubMed]
34. Hermann, J.S.; Buser, D.; Schenk, R.K.; Cochran, D.L. Crestal bone changes around titanium implants. A histometric evaluation of unloaded non-submerged and submerged implants in the canine mandible. *J. Periodontol.* **2000**, *71*, 1412–1424. [CrossRef] [PubMed]
35. Hermann, J.S.; Schoolfield, J.D.; Schenk, R.K.; Buser, D.; Cochran, D.L. Influence of the size of the microgap on crestal bone changes around titanium implants. A histometric evaluation of unloaded non-submerged implants in the canine mandible. *J. Periodontol.* **2001**, *72*, 1372–1383. [CrossRef] [PubMed]

36. Monje, A.; Insua, A.; Wang, H.L. Understanding Peri-Implantitis as a Plaque-Associated and Site-Specific Entity: On the Local Predisposing Factors. *J. Clin. Med.* **2019**, *8*, 279. [CrossRef]
37. Liu, Y.; Wang, J. Influences of microgap and micromotion of implant-abutment interface on marginal bone loss around implant neck. *Arch. Oral Biol.* **2017**, *83*, 153–160. [CrossRef]
38. Abrahamsson, I.; Berglundh, T.; Wennstrom, J.; Lindhe, J. The peri-implant hard and soft tissues at different implant systems. A comparative study in the dog. *Clin. Oral Implant. Res.* **1996**, *7*, 212–219. [CrossRef]
39. D'Ercole, S.; Scarano, A.; Perrotti, V.; Mulatinho, J.; Piattelli, A.; Iezzi, G.; Tripodi, D. Implants with internal hexagon and conical implant-abutment connections: An in vitro study of the bacterial contamination. *J. Oral Implantol.* **2014**, *40*, 30–36. [CrossRef]
40. Koutouzis, T.; Mesia, R.; Calderon, N.; Wong, F.; Wallet, S. The effect of dynamic loading on bacterial colonization of the dental implant fixture-abutment interface: An in vitro study. *J. Oral Implantol.* **2014**, *40*, 432–437. [CrossRef]
41. Piattelli, A.; Vrespa, G.; Petrone, G.; Iezzi, G.; Annibali, S.; Scarano, A. Role of the microgap between implant and abutment: A retrospective histologic evaluation in monkeys. *J. Periodontol.* **2003**, *74*, 346–352. [CrossRef] [PubMed]
42. Buser, D.; Mericske-Stern, R.; Dula, K.; Lang, N.P. Clinical experience with one-stage, non-submerged dental implants. *Adv. Dent. Res.* **1999**, *13*, 153–161. [CrossRef] [PubMed]
43. Hansson, S. A conical implant-abutment interface at the level of the marginal bone improves the distribution of stresses in the supporting bone. An axisymmetric finite element analysis. *Clin. Oral Implant. Res.* **2003**, *14*, 286–293. [CrossRef] [PubMed]
44. Abrahamsson, I.; Berglundh, T.; Lindhe, J. Soft tissue response to plaque formation at different implant systems. A comparative study in the dog. *Clin. Oral Implant. Res.* **1998**, *9*, 73–79. [CrossRef] [PubMed]
45. Welander, M.; Abrahamsson, I.; Berglundh, T. The mucosal barrier at implant abutments of different materials. *Clin. Oral Implant. Res.* **2008**, *19*, 635–641.
46. Kohal, R.J.; Weng, D.; Bachle, M.; Strub, J.R. Loaded custom-made zirconia and titanium implants show similar osseointegration: An animal experiment. *J. Periodontol.* **2004**, *75*, 1262–1268. [CrossRef] [PubMed]
47. Soo, S.Y.; Silikas, N.; Satterthwaite, J. Measurement of Fracture Strength of Zirconia Dental Implant Abutments with Internal and External Connections Using Acoustic Emission. *Materials* **2019**, *12*, 2009. [CrossRef]
48. de Avila, E.D.; de Molon, R.S.; Lima, B.P.; Lux, R.; Shi, W.; Junior, M.J.; Spolidorio, D.M.; Vergani, C.E.; de Assis Mollo Junior, F. Impact of Physical Chemical Characteristics of Abutment Implant Surfaces on Bacteria Adhesion. *J. Oral Implantol.* **2016**, *42*, 153–158. [CrossRef]
49. Smallidge, M.J.; Sabol, J.V.; Aita-Holmes, C.; Chuang, H.; Dickinson, D.P. Human Gingival Epithelial Growth In Vitro on a Polymer-Infiltrated Ceramic Network Restorative Material. *J. Prosthodont.* **2019**, *28*, 541–546. [CrossRef]
50. Lee, J.H.; Kim, S.H.; Han, J.S.; Yeo, I.S.L.; Yoon, H.I.; Lee, J. Effects of ultrasonic scaling on the optical properties and surface characteristics of highly translucent CAD/CAM ceramic restorative materials: An in vitro study. *Ceram. Int.* **2019**, *45*, 14594–14601. [CrossRef]
51. Mehl, C.; Gassling, V.; Schultz-Langerhans, S.; Acil, Y.; Bahr, T.; Wiltfang, J.; Kern, M. Influence of Four Different Abutment Materials and the Adhesive Joint of Two-Piece Abutments on Cervical Implant Bone and Soft Tissue. *Int. J. Oral Maxillofac. Implant.* **2016**, *31*, 1264–1272. [CrossRef] [PubMed]
52. Ongun, S.; Kurtulmus-Yilmaz, S.; Meric, G.; Ulusoy, M. A Comparative Study on the Mechanical Properties of a Polymer-Infiltrated Ceramic-Network Material Used for the Fabrication of Hybrid Abutment. *Materials* **2018**, *11*, 1681. [CrossRef] [PubMed]
53. Rodriguez, X.; Vela, X.; Mendez, V.; Segala, M.; Calvo-Guirado, J.L.; Tarnow, D.P. The effect of abutment dis/reconnections on peri-implant bone resorption: A radiologic study of platform-switched and non-platform-switched implants placed in animals. *Clin. Oral Implant. Res.* **2013**, *24*, 305–311. [CrossRef] [PubMed]
54. Abrahamsson, I.; Berglundh, T.; Lindhe, J. The mucosal barrier following abutment dis/reconnection. An experimental study in dogs. *J. Clin. Periodontol.* **1997**, *24*, 568–572. [CrossRef] [PubMed]
55. Canullo, L.; Bignozzi, I.; Cocchetto, R.; Cristalli, M.P.; Iannello, G. Immediate positioning of a definitive abutment versus repeated abutment replacements in post-extractive implants: 3-year follow-up of a randomised multicentre clinical trial. *Eur. J. Oral Implantol.* **2010**, *3*, 285–296.

56. Degidi, M.; Nardi, D.; Piattelli, A. One abutment at one time: Non-removal of an immediate abutment and its effect on bone healing around subcrestal tapered implants. *Clin. Oral Implant. Res.* **2011**, *22*, 1303–1307. [CrossRef]
57. Wang, Q.Q.; Dai, R.; Cao, C.Y.; Fang, H.; Han, M.; Li, Q.L. One-time versus repeated abutment connection for platform-switched implant: A systematic review and meta-analysis. *PLoS ONE* **2017**, *12*, e0186385. [CrossRef]
58. Ghensi, P.; Bettio, E.; Maniglio, D.; Bonomi, E.; Piccoli, F.; Gross, S.; Caciagli, P.; Segata, N.; Nollo, G.; Tessarolo, F. Dental Implants with Anti-Biofilm Properties: A Pilot Study for Developing a New Sericin-Based Coating. *Materials* **2019**, *12*, 2429. [CrossRef]
59. Yang, Y.; Zhou, J.; Liu, X.; Zheng, M.; Yang, J.; Tan, J. Ultraviolet light-treated zirconia with different roughness affects function of human gingival fibroblasts in vitro: The potential surface modification developed from implant to abutment. *J. Biomed. Mater. Res. B Appl. Biomater.* **2015**, *103*, 116–124. [CrossRef]
60. Iglhaut, G.; Becker, K.; Golubovic, V.; Schliephake, H.; Mihatovic, I. The impact of dis-/reconnection of laser microgrooved and machined implant abutments on soft- and hard-tissue healing. *Clin. Oral Implant. Res.* **2013**, *24*, 391–397. [CrossRef]
61. Nevins, M.; Camelo, M.; Nevins, M.L.; Schupbach, P.; Kim, D.M. Connective tissue attachment to laser-microgrooved abutments: A human histologic case report. *Int. J. Periodontics Restor. Dent.* **2012**, *32*, 385–392.
62. Nevins, M.; Kim, D.M.; Jun, S.H.; Guze, K.; Schupbach, P.; Nevins, M.L. Histologic evidence of a connective tissue attachment to laser microgrooved abutments: A canine study. *Int. J. Periodontics Restor. Dent.* **2010**, *30*, 245–255.
63. Guida, L.; Oliva, A.; Basile, M.A.; Giordano, M.; Nastri, L.; Annunziata, M. Human gingival fibroblast functions are stimulated by oxidized nano-structured titanium surfaces. *J. Dent.* **2013**, *41*, 900–907. [CrossRef] [PubMed]
64. Sakamoto, Y.; Ayukawa, Y.; Furuhashi, A.; Kamo, M.; Ikeda, J.; Atsuta, I.; Haraguchi, T.; Koyano, K. Effect of Hydrothermal Treatment with Distilled Water on Titanium Alloy for Epithelial Cellular Attachment. *Materials* **2019**, *12*, 2748. [CrossRef]
65. Albouy, J.P.; Abrahamsson, I.; Berglundh, T. Spontaneous progression of experimental peri-implantitis at implants with different surface characteristics: An experimental study in dogs. *J. Clin. Periodontol.* **2012**, *39*, 182–187. [CrossRef]
66. Yeo, I.S.; Kim, H.Y.; Lim, K.S.; Han, J.S. Implant surface factors and bacterial adhesion: A review of the literature. *Int. J. Artif. Organs* **2012**, *35*, 762–772. [CrossRef]
67. Albrektsson, T.; Zarb, G.; Worthington, P.; Eriksson, A.R. The long-term efficacy of currently used dental implants: A review and proposed criteria of success. *Int. J. Oral Maxillofac. Implant.* **1986**, *1*, 11–25.
68. Palmer, R.M.; Palmer, P.J.; Smith, B.J. A 5-year prospective study of Astra single tooth implants. *Clin. Oral Implant. Res.* **2000**, *11*, 179–182. [CrossRef]
69. Puchades-Roman, L.; Palmer, R.M.; Palmer, P.J.; Howe, L.C.; Ide, M.; Wilson, R.F. A clinical, radiographic, and microbiologic comparison of Astra Tech and Branemark single tooth implants. *Clin. Implant. Dent. Relat. Res.* **2000**, *2*, 78–84. [CrossRef]
70. Frost, H.M. Perspectives: bone's mechanical usage windows. *Bone Miner.* **1992**, *19*, 257–271. [CrossRef]
71. Buser, D.; Sennerby, L.; De Bruyn, H. Modern implant dentistry based on osseointegration: 50 years of progress, current trends and open questions. *Periodontology 2000* **2017**, *73*, 7–21. [CrossRef] [PubMed]
72. Taylor, T.D.; Agar, J.R. Twenty years of progress in implant prosthodontics. *J. Prosthet. Dent.* **2002**, *88*, 89–95. [CrossRef] [PubMed]
73. de Vasconcellos, L.G.; Kojima, A.N.; Nishioka, R.S.; de Vasconcellos, L.M.; Balducci, I. Axial loads on implant-supported partial fixed prostheses for external and internal hex connections and machined and plastic copings: Strain gauge analysis. *J. Oral Implantol.* **2015**, *41*, 149–154. [CrossRef] [PubMed]
74. Tarnow, D.P.; Cho, S.C.; Wallace, S.S. The effect of inter-implant distance on the height of inter-implant bone crest. *J. Periodontol.* **2000**, *71*, 546–549. [CrossRef]
75. Friedman, M.T.; Barber, P.M.; Mordan, N.J.; Newman, H.N. The "plaque-free zone" in health and disease: A scanning electron microscope study. *J. Periodontol.* **1992**, *63*, 890–896. [CrossRef]
76. Lang, N.P.; Loe, H. The relationship between the width of keratinized gingiva and gingival health. *J. Periodontol.* **1972**, *43*, 623–627. [CrossRef]

77. Thoma, D.S.; Muhlemann, S.; Jung, R.E. Critical soft-tissue dimensions with dental implants and treatment concepts. *Periodontology 2000* **2014**, *66*, 106–118. [CrossRef]
78. Giannobile, W.V.; Jung, R.E.; Schwarz, F.; Groups of the 2nd Osteology Foundation Consensus, M. Evidence-based knowledge on the aesthetics and maintenance of peri-implant soft tissues: Osteology Foundation Consensus Report Part 1-Effects of soft tissue augmentation procedures on the maintenance of peri-implant soft tissue health. *Clin. Oral Implant. Res.* **2018**, *29*, 7–10. [CrossRef]
79. Ainamo, A.; Bergenholtz, A.; Hugoson, A.; Ainamo, J. Location of the mucogingival junction 18 years after apically repositioned flap surgery. *J. Clin Periodontol.* **1992**, *19*, 49–52.
80. Katafuchi, M.; Weinstein, B.F.; Leroux, B.G.; Chen, Y.W.; Daubert, D.M. Restoration contour is a risk indicator for peri-implantitis: A cross-sectional radiographic analysis. *J. Clin Periodontol.* **2018**, *45*, 225–232. [CrossRef]
81. Canullo, L.; Schlee, M.; Wagner, W.; Covani, U.; Montegrotto Group for the Study of Peri-implant, D. International Brainstorming Meeting on Etiologic and Risk Factors of Peri-implantitis, Montegrotto (Padua, Italy), August 2014. *Int. J. Oral Maxillofac. Implant.* **2015**, *30*, 1093–1104. [CrossRef] [PubMed]
82. Derks, J.; Schaller, D.; Hakansson, J.; Wennstrom, J.L.; Tomasi, C.; Berglundh, T. Effectiveness of Implant Therapy Analyzed in a Swedish Population: Prevalence of Peri-implantitis. *J. Dent. Res.* **2016**, *95*, 43–49. [CrossRef] [PubMed]

8

A Vitronectin-Derived Bioactive Peptide Improves Bone Healing Capacity of SLA Titanium Surfaces

Chang-Bin Cho [1,†], Sung Youn Jung [2,†], Cho Yeon Park [2], Hyun Ki Kang [2], In-Sung Luke Yeo [1,*] and Byung-Moo Min [2,*]

1 Department of Prosthodontics, Seoul National University School of Dentistry, and Dental Research Institute, 101 Daehak-Ro, Jongno-Gu, Seoul 03080, Korea; istardental@naver.com

2 Department of Oral Biochemistry and Program in Cancer and Developmental Biology, Seoul National University School of Dentistry, and Dental Research Institute, 101 Daehak-Ro, Jongno-Gu, Seoul 03080, Korea; jsy1618@snu.ac.kr (S.Y.J.); choyeon94@snu.ac.kr (C.Y.P.); kang1978@snu.ac.kr (H.K.K.)

* Correspondence: pros53@snu.ac.kr (I.-S.L.Y.); bmmin@snu.ac.kr (B.-M.M.)

† These authors contributed equally to this work.

Abstract: In this study, we evaluated early bone responses to a vitronectin-derived, minimal core bioactive peptide, RVYFFKGKQYWE motif (VnP-16), both in vitro and in vivo, when the peptide was treated on sandblasted, large-grit, acid-etched (SLA) titanium surfaces. Four surface types of titanium discs and of titanium screw-shaped implants were prepared: control, SLA, scrambled peptide-treated, and VnP-16-treated surfaces. Cellular responses, such as attachment, spreading, migration, and viability of human osteoblast-like HOS and MG63 cells were evaluated in vitro on the titanium discs. Using the rabbit tibia model with the split plot design, the implants were inserted into the tibiae of four New Zealand white rabbits. After two weeks of implant insertion, the rabbits were sacrificed, the undecalcified specimens were prepared for light microscopy, and the histomorphometric data were measured. Analysis of variance tests were used for the quantitative evaluations in this study. VnP-16 was non-cytotoxic and promoted attachment and spreading of the human osteoblast-like cells. The VnP-16-treated SLA implants showed no antigenic activities at the interfaces between the bones and the implants and indicated excellent bone-to-implant contact ratios, the means of which were significantly higher than those in the SP-treated implants. VnP-16 reinforces the osteogenic potential of the SLA titanium dental implant.

Keywords: vitronectin; RVYFFKGKQYWE motif; cellular responses; dental implants; osseointegration

1. Introduction

Attachment of cells is the first step in cell–biomaterial interactions [1]. The transmembrane proteins on the cell membrane recognize and bind biomacromolecules adsorbed on the surface of the biomaterial [1]. These biomacromolecules are from the extracellular matrix (ECM), controlling cellular behaviors such as attachment, spreading, proliferation, and differentiation depending on the interacting transmembrane receptors [2]. Therefore, these ECM biomolecules, if applied to the titanium dental implant surface, are anticipated to have potential in reinforcing osseointegration [3–5]. One candidate molecule is vitronectin.

Vitronectin, one of the ECM proteins, is an abundant multifunctional glycoprotein found in serum, the extracellular matrix, and bone, and is involved in various physiological processes such as cell attachment, spreading, and migration [6–8]. Vitronectin contributes to healing of the bone surrounding a dental implant by promoting the attachment and spreading of the osteogenic cells [9,10]. This ECM protein appears to play a major role in initial bone healing by reorganizing the intracellular microfilaments and microtubules, which facilitates cell attachment and spreading [11–13]. However, the use of such an original protein has several critical limitations: a high cost for synthesis, antigenicity and instability of the molecule, and steric hindrance of this macromolecule in focal adhesion [5,14,15]. A functional peptide derived from the parent protein is a notable alternative, overcoming these limitations and maintaining the original biological activity [3,5,9,14,16,17]. In addition, bioactive peptides have advantages over larger protein molecules due to their robustness and sterilizability [18]. Recently, a vitronectin-derived functional peptide sequence, RVYFFKGKQYWE (VnP-16), has shown a Janus regulation for bone formation: promotion of osteoblast activity and inhibition of osteoclast activity, which is a desirable effect for osteogenesis that vitronectin does not have [9]. The VnP-16 peptide promoted bone formation by accelerating osteoblast differentiation and activity through direct interaction with β1 integrin followed by focal adhesion kinase (FAK) activation. Concomitantly, the peptide inhibited bone resorption by restraining Janus N-terminal Kinase (JNK)-c-Fos-nuclear factor of activated T cells, cytoplasmic 1 (NFATc1)-induced osteoclast differentiation and αvβ3 integrin-c-Src-proline-rich tyrosine kinase 2 (PYK2)-mediated resorptive function. Moreover, VnP-16 peptide decreased the bone resorbing activity of pre-existing mature osteoclasts without changing their survival rate [9].

The functionalization of a titanium implant via the immobilization of desirable proteins or their bioactive peptides in their native conformations is a promising approach to overcome the bioinertness of the surface, leading to improved osseointegration [18,19]. Several methodologies, including physical adsorption, covalent immobilization via chemical methods, and covalent immobilization via physical methods, have been investigated since the inception of protein functionalization on titanium substrates [19]. Physical adsorption is the simplest method to immobilize proteins on titanium substrates. Chemical immobilization, the most established of the protein functionalization approaches, proved that it was possible to covalently immobilize proteins to titanium substrates, overcoming the unintentional protein release observed in adsorption approaches. Physical covalent immobilization of biomolecules is the most recent approach to dental and orthopedic biomimetic functionalization, and possesses advantages over adsorption and chemical covalent immobilization [19]. Other methods on peptide-functionalization of titanium surfaces are also reported. Control of both peptide orientation and surface concentration is achieved by varying the solution pH or by applying an electric field [18]. In addition, multifunctional coating improves cell adhesion on titanium surfaces by using cooperatively acting peptides [20].

A micro-roughened surface of commercially pure titanium has been clinically used in the field of implant dentistry [10]. A sandblasted large-grit acid-etched (SLA) surface with approximately 1.5 μm of arithmetic mean deviation is known to accelerate osseointegration at the bone-implant interface, compared to the turned surface with no modification at the micro-level [10,21,22]. The application of VnP-16 to the SLA surface increases clinical relevance in the further enhancement of bone formation and makes use of dental implants extended to patients suffering from bone metabolic weaknesses, like osteoporosis. The VnP-16-treated SLA titanium surface has not been investigated yet.

This study aimed to evaluate the early bone response to the VnP-16-treated SLA titanium surface in vivo. In vitro tests were also performed using osteoblast-like cells. The hypothesis underlying this study was that the application of VnP-16 would further reinforce the osteogenic potential of the SLA surface.

2. Materials and Methods

2.1. Cells, Peptides, and Reagents

HOS and MG-63 cells, lines derived from human osteosarcomas, were purchased from the American Type Culture Collection (Rockville, MD, USA) and cultured in Dulbecco's modified Eagle's medium (Gibco BRL, Carlsbad, CA, USA) supplemented with 10% fetal bovine serum. Each peptide was synthesized using the 9-fluorenylmethoxycarbonyl-based solid-phase method with a C-terminal amide using a Pioneer Peptide Synthesizer (Applied Biosystems, Foster City, CA, USA) in the Peptron (Daejeon, Korea). The synthetic peptides used in the study had a purity greater than 95%, as determined using high-performance liquid chromatography. Human plasma vitronectin was obtained from Millipore (Bedford, MA, USA).

2.2. Disc Preparation and Surface Characterization

Titanium disc specimens, which were 0.5 mm thick and 10 mm in radius, were made of commercially pure grade 4 titanium. The discs, serving as control, were prepared by polishing with #600 and #1200 sandpaper. The other discs were subjected to sandblasting with large alumina particles and etched with a hydrochloric acid solution to generate the SLA surface (Deep Implant System, Seongnam, Korea). The SLA titanium discs were rinsed, ultrasonically washed, and dried. One group of the SLA discs was left untreated, another was treated with a scrambled peptide (SP; 10.5 $\mu g/cm^2$), and the other was treated with VnP-16 (10.5 $\mu g/cm^2$).

The surfaces of the four types of disc were imaged using field emission-scanning electron microscopy (FE-SEM; S-4700, Hitachi, Tokyo, Japan). The element composition of each group was analyzed by electron spectroscopy for the chemical analysis (ESCA; Sigma Probe, Thermo Scientific, Waltham, MA, USA). Confocal laser scanning microscopy (CLSM; LSM 800, Carl Zeiss AG, Oberkochen, Germany) calculated two surface parameters for surface topography of the investigated discs; arithmetic mean deviation (Ra) and the developed surface area ratio (Sdr) [23].

2.3. Cell Attachment and Spreading Assays

The cell attachment assay was performed as described previously [9]. The physical adsorption method was used for the application of peptides. Twenty-four-well culture plates were coated with 0.26 $\mu g/cm^2$ human plasma vitronectin for 24 h at 4 °C or 10.5 $\mu g/cm^2$ synthetic peptides for 24 h at room temperature, blocked with 1% heat-inactivated bovine serum albumin (BSA) in phosphate-buffered saline (PBS) for 1 h at 37 °C, and then washed with PBS. Cells (1×10^5 cells/500 µL) were added to each plate and incubated in serum-free culture medium for 1 h at 37 °C. After incubation period, unattached cells were removed by rinsing twice with PBS. Attached cells were fixed with 10% formalin for 15 min, stained with 0.5% crystal violet for 1 h, gently washed with distilled water three times, and dissolved with 2% sodium dodecyl sulfate for 5 min. Absorbance was measured at 570 nm using a microplate reader. For cell-spreading assay, cells (7×10^4 cells/500 µL) were added to each substrate-coated plate and incubated for 3 h at 37 °C. To determine cell spreading, formalin-fixed and crystal violet-stained cell surface area was measured with Image-Pro plus software (Version 4.5; Media Cybernetics, Silver Spring, MD, USA).

2.4. Migration Assay

Migration assays were performed using a transwell migration chamber (Corning, Pittston, PA, USA) possessing 8 µm pores as described previously [24]. The lower side of each transwell filter was coated with vitronectin (0.26 $\mu g/cm^2$), or synthetic peptides (10.5 $\mu g/cm^2$) by drying for 24 h at 4 °C (vitronectin) or for 24 h at room temperature (peptides). Cells (2×10^4 cells/24-well) were seeded in the upper chamber of a transwell filter and allowed to migrate for 24 h at 37 °C. Cells were then fixed with 10% formalin for 15 min and stained with 0.5% crystal violet. Unmigrated cells in the upper side of the transwell filter were removed with a cotton swab, and cell migration was quantified by counting the number of cells that had migrated through the filter. Human placental laminin was used as the positive controls and SP was used as the negative control.

2.5. Cell Viability Assay

The viabilities of cells were investigated using the EZ-Cytox Cell Viability Assay kit (water-soluble tetrazolium salt method; Daeil Lab Service, Seoul, Korea). A 96-well microplate was coated with VnP-16 peptide (0, 10.6, 21.2, or 42.4 $\mu g/cm^2$) by drying for 24 h at room temperature. Cells (1.5 ×

10^4 cells/100 μL) were seeded onto a 96-well microplate and then cultured for 24 h or 48 h at 37 °C. The water-soluble tetrazolium salt reagent solution (10 μL) was added to each well, and the plate was incubated for 2 h at 37 °C. The absorbance at 450 nm was then measured using a microplate reader.

2.6. *In Vivo Experiment*

Sixteen screw-shaped grade 4 titanium implants were made, which were 3.5 mm in major diameter and 11 mm in length (Warantec, Seongnam, Korea). Four implants were used as they were without any surface modification and designated as turned surface (control). The surface of another four implants was SLA (Deep Implant System, Seongnam, Korea). Half of the rest of the eight implants were treated with SP while the other half were treated with VnP-16 (1.0 mg/cm^2). Using the physical adsorption method, the Ti implants were placed on 0.2 ml PCR tubes and coated with the synthetic peptides by drying for 7 d in a vacuum at room temperature.

All the animal experiments performed in this study were approved by the Ethics Committee of Animal Experimentation of the Institutional Animal Care and Use Committee (CRONEX-IACUC 201705001; Cronex, Hwasung, Korea). These experiments were conducted following the Animal Research: Reporting In Vivo Experiments (ARRIVE) guidelines for the care and use of laboratory animals [25]. Four New Zealand white rabbits were used in this study, which were male, approximately five to six months in age and 2.5 to 3.0 kg in weight. The experimental animals were intramuscularly anesthetized with a dose of 15 mg/kg tiletamine hydrochloride and zolazepam hydrochloride (Zoletil, Virbac, Carros, France) and 5 mg/kg xylazine (Rompun, Bayer AG, Leverkusen, Germany). The skin hair was shaved at the tibial area of the rabbits, which was disinfected with aqueous iodine. A full-thickness incision from the skin to the periosteum of the tibiae was made, and the flaps were elevated to expose the medial surfaces of the tibiae. Drilling was conducted for to make the holes on the medial surfaces for implant insertion. The final diameter of the holes was 3.2 mm. Two implants were inserted into each tibia and arranged according to the split plot design. The periosteum and fascia were sutured with 4-0 polyglactin 910 (Vicryl, Ethicon, Somerville, NJ, USA) while the skin was sutured with 4-0 Nylon (Ethilon, Ethicon, Somerville, NJ, USA). Each experimental animal was housed in a separate cage and an antibiotic, enrofloxacin, (Biotril, Komipharm International, Siheung, Korea) was administered to prevent infection.

2.7. *Light Microscopic Evaluation*

The rabbits were sacrificed under general anesthesia with the intravenous administration of potassium chloride at 14 days after implant insertion. The implants were removed en bloc with the surrounding bones and fixed in 10% neutral buffered formalin for 2 weeks. After formalin fixation, each implant-bone block was dehydrated with ethanol. Then, the blocks were resin-embedded (Technovit 7200, Heraeus Kulzer, Hanau, Germany) and ground for light microscopy using an EXAKT system (EXAKT Apparatebau, Norderstedt, Germany), according to the methods described in the previous studies [23,26]. Sections of the implant-bone blocks were prepared with a final thickness of approximately 50 μm and modified Goldner's Masson trichrome staining [27]. The interfacial areas between the bones and implants were observed and evaluated from the bone crests to 2 mm in depth for histomorphometry, where bone-to-implant contact (BIC) and bone area (BA) ratios were calculated. The image analyses and the histomorphometric calculations were performed on ×100 magnified images using a light microscope (BX51, Olympus, Tokyo, Japan), SPOT version 4.0 software (Diagnostic Instruments, Sterling Heights, MI, USA) and Image-Pro Plus (Media Cybernetics, Rockville, MD, USA).

2.8. *Statistics*

Descriptive statistics for the data were presented as the mean ± standard deviation (SD). The statistical analyses were performed with R software (version 3.6.1, R Foundation for Statistical Computing, Vienna, Austria). All the data obtained in this study were confirmed to be normally distributed by the Shapiro–Wilk test. Analysis of variance tests were used for comparisons among the groups. When a significant difference was found, Tukey's honestly significant difference test was further applied for pairwise comparison. The level of significance was 0.05 in this study.

3. Results

3.1. Surface Characteristics

The FE-SEM images of the specimens showed very different topographical features between the polished and SLA surfaces (Figure 1A). Some grooves on the overall flat surfaces were found for the polished specimens, while a honeycomb-like irregular topography was observed for the SLA specimens. The treatments of SP and VnP-16 had little effect on the surface physical features of the specimens (Figure 1A). There was no significant difference in either the Ra or Sdr among the SLA titanium discs, regardless of the peptide treatment ($p > 0.05$) (Figure 1B). However, in surface chemistry, the treatments of the functional peptides were confirmed from the results of higher nitrogen contents for the SP- and VnP-16-treated surfaces, compared to those for the other groups (polished and SLA titanium surfaces) ($p < 0.05$) (Figure 1C). The highest content element was carbon for every group.

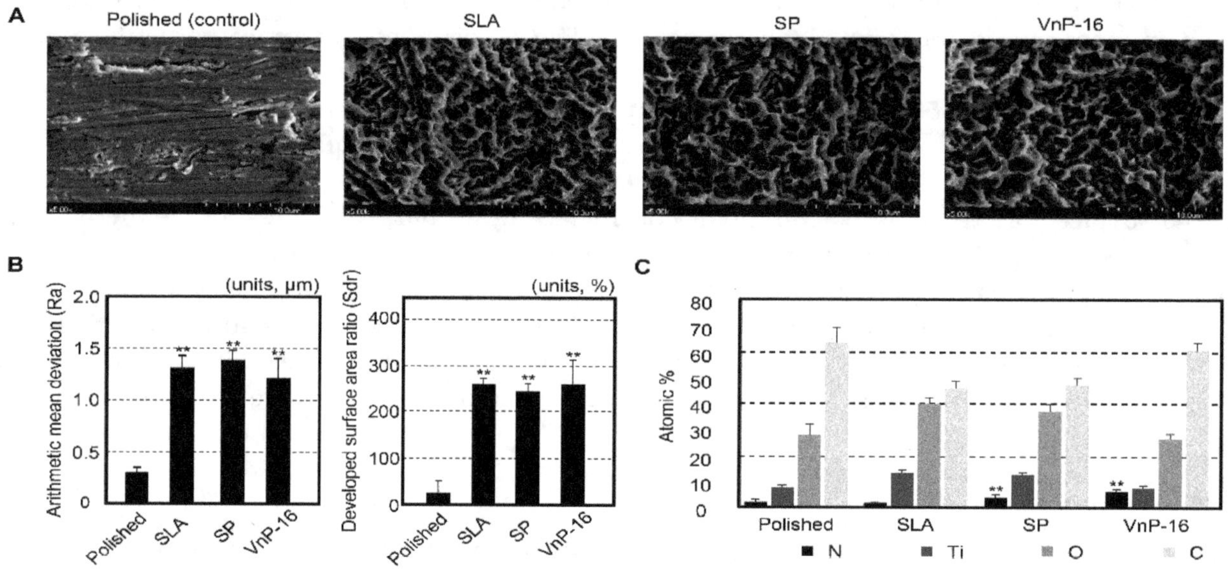

Figure 1. Surface characteristics of the titanium specimens investigated in this study. (**A**) Field emission scanning electron microscopy definitely shows different topographical features between the polished and sandblasted, large-grit, acid-etched (SLA) surfaces. (**B**) The mean values of the measured surface parameters indicated that the peptide treatment did not change the surfaces physically at the micro level. Note the significant differences in the surface parameters between the polished and the other SLA surfaces. ** $p < 0.01$ vs. the polished surface. (**C**) Electron spectroscopy for chemical analysis detected high nitrogen content on the peptide-treated surfaces. Almost no nitrogen was found in the other groups. ** $p < 0.01$ vs. the polished and SLA surfaces (significant differences are marked only for the nitrogen content).

3.2. Effects of VnP-16 Peptide on Cellular Responses of Human Osteoblast-Like Cells

To investigate whether a human vitronectin-derived peptide, VnP-16, could mediate cell behavior of osteoblasts, cell attachment, spreading, and migration of human osteoblast-like cells, including HOS and MG-63, were assayed. The attachment of osteoblast-like cells was evaluated using a cell adhesion assay in a serum-free medium. Human plasma vitronectin strongly promoted cell attachment (Figure 2A upper, B) and spreading (Figure 2A lower, C) in osteoblast-like HOS cells. The VnP-16 peptide also promoted greater cell attachment (Figure 2A upper, B) and spreading (Figure 2A lower, C) than the BSA or SP control, and its attachment and spreading activities were comparable to those of vitronectin (Figure 2A–C). In addition, vehicle and SP did not participate in cell migration in HOS cells. On the other hand, vitronectin and the VnP-16 peptide promoted cell migration in HOS cells, while the VnP-16 peptide was significantly less effective than vitronectin (Figure 2D). The VnP-16 peptide did not affect the proliferation or viability of HOS cells (Figure 2E), indicating that its stimulatory effect on the cell behavior of HOS cells was not due to cytotoxicity or enhanced cell proliferation. These results support that VnP-16 is functionally active in promoting osteoblastic responses.

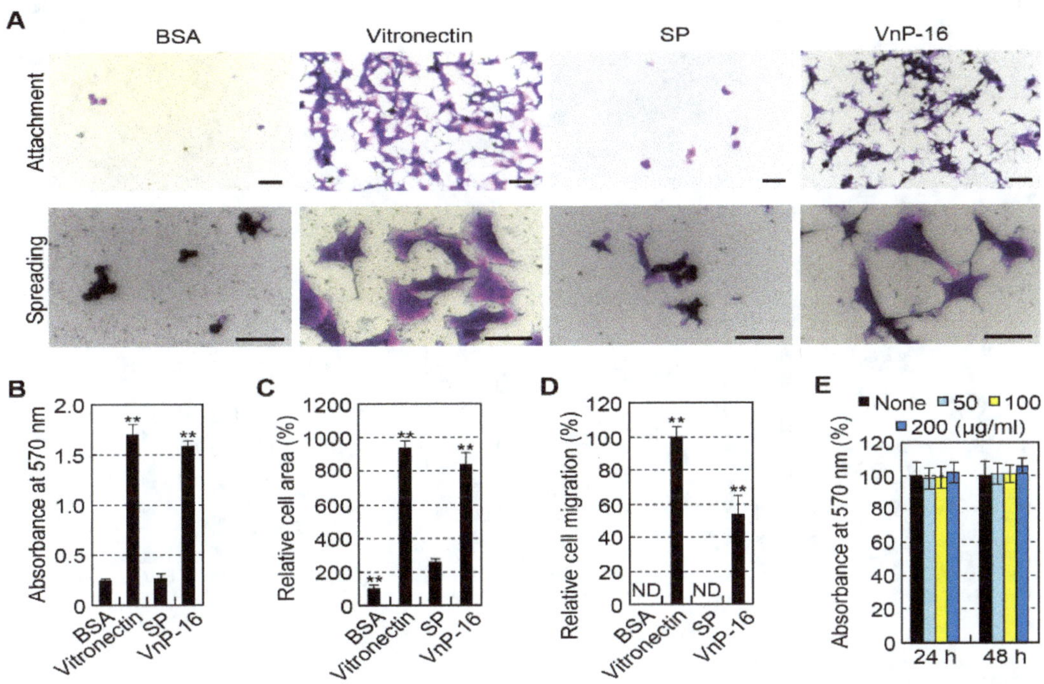

Figure 2. Cell attachment, spreading, and migration of osteoblast like HOS cells seeded on culture plates treated with vitronectin and synthetic peptides. (**A**) Photographs of osteoblast-like HOS cells adhering (upper panel) and spreading (lower panel) to culture plates treated with 1% bovine serum albumin (BSA), vitronectin (0.26 µg/cm^2), scrambled peptide (SP), and VnP-16 peptide (10.5 µg/cm^2). Bar = 100 µm. (**B**,**C**) Cell attachment (**B**) and spreading (**C**) to immobilized synthetic peptides. HOS cells were allowed to adhere to peptide-treated plates for 1 h (**B**) or 3 h (**C**) in serum-free medium. (**D**) Migration of osteoblast-like HOS cells induced by vitronectin and synthetic peptides. HOS cells were seeded into the upper chambers of transwell filters coated with vitronectin (0.26 µg/cm^2), SP, or VnP-16 (10.5 µg/cm^2) and were incubated for 24 h. ND, not detected. (**E**) The viabilities of osteoblast-like HOS cells treated with VnP-16 for 24 or 48 h. ** $p < 0.01$ vs. the SP-treated control group. Data in (**B**–**E**) (n = 4) represent the mean ± SD.

Next, to determine whether the effects of the VnP-16 peptide on the cell behavior of HOS cells were similar to those of other human osteoblast-like cells, we used human osteoblast-like MG-63 cells. Similar, but not identical, results were obtained for cell behavior in MG-63 cells. Human plasma vitronectin and VnP-16 peptide strongly promoted cell attachment (Figure 3A upper, B) and spreading (Figure 3A lower, C) in MG-63 cells compared to the BSA or SP control. In addition, the cell attachment and spreading activities of VnP-16 peptide were comparable to those of vitronectin (Figure 3A–C). Similarly, VnP-16 peptide did not affect the proliferation or viability of MG-63 cells (Figure 3D). However, the cell migration activities of vitronectin and the VnP-16 peptide were different between HOS and MG-63 cells. In other words, vitronectin and the VnP-16 peptide had no effect on cell migration in MG-63 cells (data not shown). Therefore, the cellular responses of the VnP-16 peptide to the human osteoblast-like cells HOS and MG-63 had different effects on cell migration but had similar effects on cell attachment, spreading, and viability.

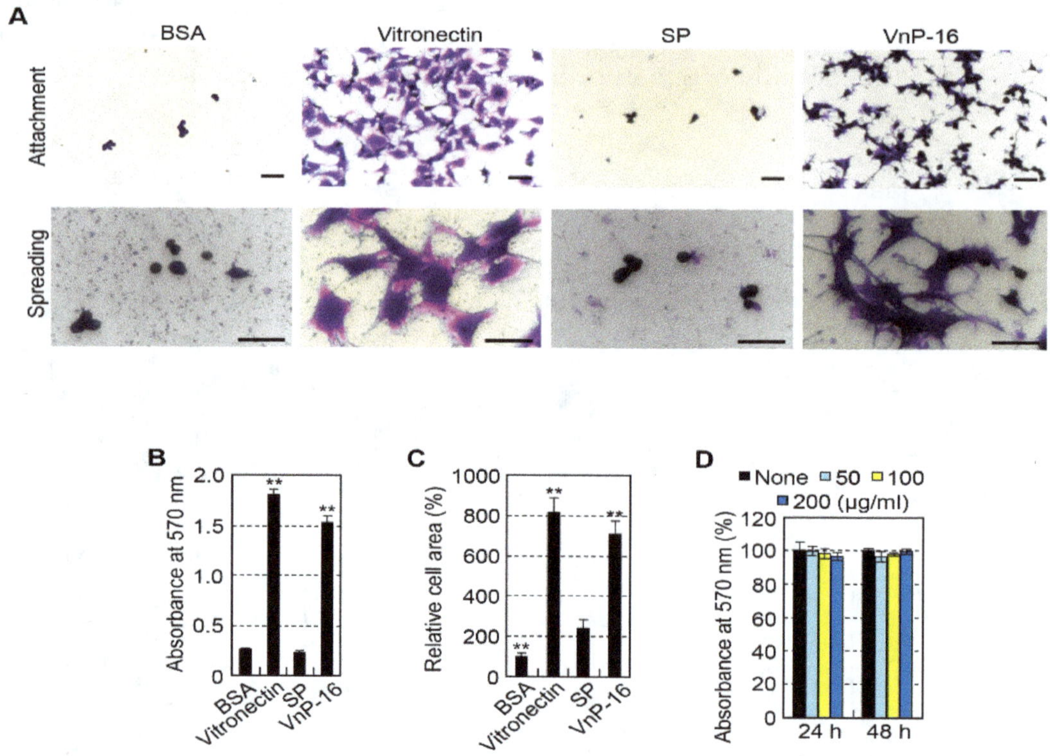

Figure 3. Cell attachment and spreading of osteoblast-like MG-63 cells seeded on culture plates treated with vitronectin and synthetic peptides. (**A**) Photographs of osteoblast-like MG-63 cells adhering (upper panel) and spreading (lower panel) to culture plates treated with 1% bovine serum albumin (BSA), vitronectin (0.26 μg/cm^2), scrambled peptide (SP), and VnP-16 peptide (10.5 μg/cm^2). Bar = 100 μm. (**B–C**) Cell attachment (**B**) and spreading (**C**) to immobilized synthetic peptides. MG-63 cells were allowed to adhere to peptide-treated plates for 1 h (**B**) or 3 h (**C**) in serum-free medium. (**D**) The viabilities of osteoblast-like MG-63 cells treated with VnP-16 for 24 or 48 h. ** $p < 0.01$ vs. the SP-treated control group. Data in (**B–D**) ($n = 4$) represent the mean ± SD.

3.3. Histomorphometry

Every experimental animal was healthy, and no signs of diseases or pathologic states were found until the sacrifice. There were no special inflammatory or immune cells found in the light microscopic view of the specimens. After 14 days of implant insertion, sufficient mineralization was observed in each section (Figure 4A). The mean value and standard deviation of each group were 47.0% ± 7.5% for the turned surface, 64.4% ± 8.6% for SLA, 42.1% ± 18.1% for SP-treated and 65.0% ± 7.2% for the VnP-16-treated surface. The histomorphometric data showed significant differences in BIC ($p = 0.027$). However, the pairwise comparisons between the groups found no significant differences in BIC (Figure 4B). The mean values and standard deviation in the BA were 58.8% ± 6.0% for the turned group, 56.8% ± 6.4% for SLA, 56.6% ± 8.4% for the SP-treated group, and 61.5% ± 10.6% for the VnP-16-treated group (Figure 4C). There were no significant differences in BA among the groups.

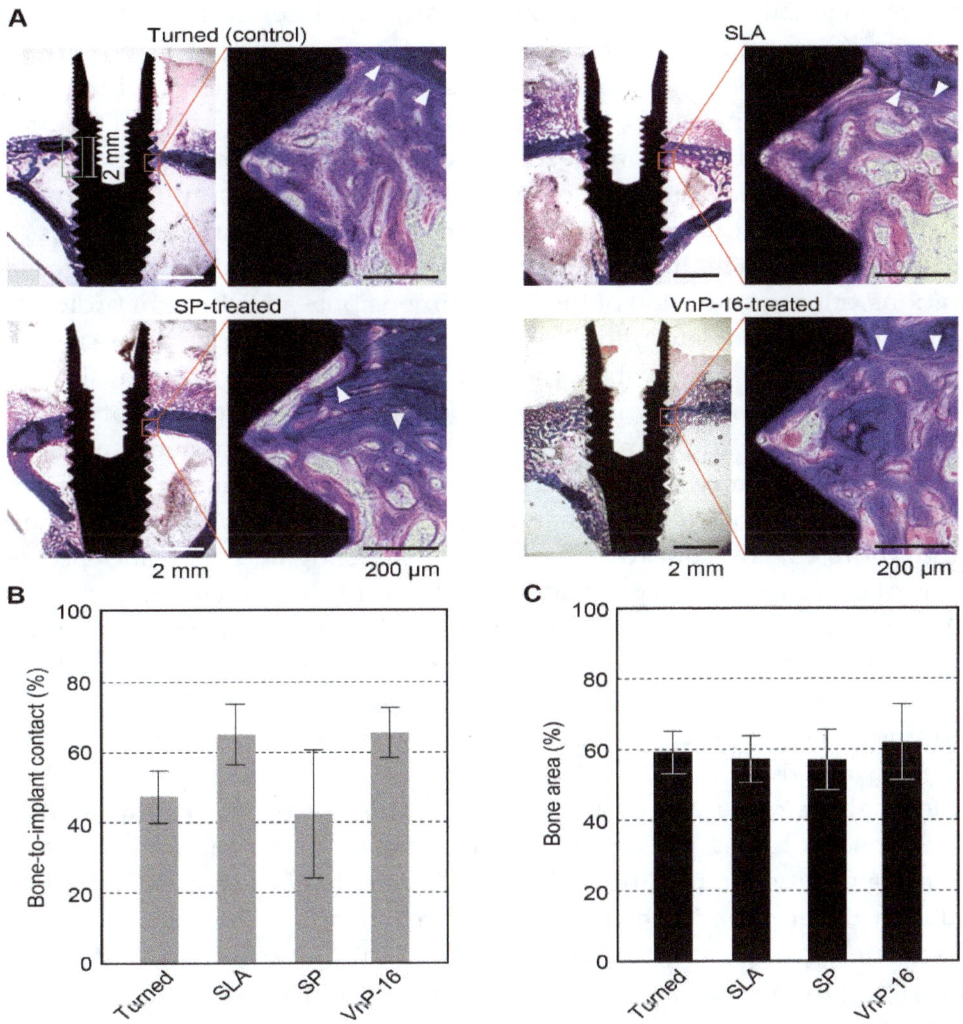

Figure 4. The histologic views and histomorphometric data for bone responses to the turned, SLA, SP-treated SLA, and VnP-16-treated SLA titanium implant surfaces. (**A**) The demarcation lines (white arrowheads), difference in stained colors and maturity of the bone (cancellous or cortical) differentiate the new bone from the existing old bone. Here, the new bone is stained more reddish while the old bone is stained more blueish. (**B**) Bone-to-implant contact ratios were measured, which are defined as the percentage of the implant surface in contact with bone to the total implant surface at the region of interest, which was the area ranging from the bone crest to 2 mm in depth in this study (green edged rectangle in (**A**)). (**C**) The ratio of the area filled with bone to the total area of the region of interest (bone area, or BA ratio) was also measured for each implant.

4. Discussion

The results of these in vitro and in vivo studies indicated that the VnP-16-treated SLA titanium surface augments the initial bone response to a dental implant. The VnP-16 bioactive peptide is expected to accelerate early bone healing further when this peptide is applied to the SLA titanium dental implant. VnP-16 is another candidate biomolecule for stronger osseointegration into a dental implant that is clinically applicable, together with some laminin-derived peptides [3,5,23]. Because VnP-16 has both the upregulation of osteoblast activity and the downregulation of osteoclast activity, different from other peptides, the clinical applicability of this material is considered to be higher [9].

Since VnP-16 downregulates osteoclast activity, this vitronectin-derived peptide is applicable to osteoporotic patients as well as to normal patients. A previous study has already shown the improved bone healing capacity of VnP-16 in an in vivo experiment using ovariectomized rats [9]. The SLA titanium implant is well-known to have long-term clinical performance with high survival rates (higher than 95%) [28,29]. However, this micro-roughened titanium surface has some limitations in the use for patients with a problem in bone metabolism, including osteoporosis [30]. The cell adhesion molecules can potentiate the bone healing capacities of the modified titanium surfaces used in dental clinics without immune responses, which is shown in this study. The effect of VnP-16 on osseointegration of the SLA dental implant needs to be evaluated for normal and osteoporotic patients.

This study used the physical adsorption method for the VnP-16 application to titanium surface. One of the main advantages of this method is the simplicity, that is, an easy process to functionalize the titanium implant surface while this method has several important disadvantages like low effective peptide concentrations, and denaturation of the three dimensional structures of proteins or peptides [19]. The concentration of VnP-16 was determined from a dose-response curve through the cell attachment assay, as in a previous study (data not shown) [9]. The lowest concentration, showing the maximal effect in cell attachment, was used in this study, which solved the problem of low effective peptide concentration. VnP-16 is a peptide composed of 12 amino acids, which are considered to have no specific three dimensional structure [5]. Furthermore, the other approaches to peptide immobilization require additional reactions and costs [19]. Therefore, physical adsorption was the method of choice in this study although more effective approach needs to be investigated continuously.

In the analysis of surface chemistry of this study, higher nitrogen contents on the peptide-treated surfaces imply the applications of the peptides to the titanium implant surfaces. However, the results of the amounts of carbon detected on the surfaces were hard to interpret, despite that carbon was the most abundant on all the surfaces investigated in this study. These unclear results are considered to be from the phenomenon of hydrocarbon contamination on titanium surface, which is usual when titanium is exposed to air [31,32].

Although the analysis of variance test for BIC in this study showed a p-value less than 0.05, the pairwise comparisons found no significant differences between the groups. Perhaps, large standard deviation, especially obtained from the measurements of the turned and SP-treated implants, caused no significant differences in the pairwise comparisons. The high mean BIC ratios in the SLA and VnP-16-treated groups and the low mean BIC in the turned and SP-treated groups were considered to contribute to the significant difference in the analysis of variance test for all the groups. The large standard deviation of the data occurred because of the small sample size in this study. Another reason for the large deviation might be the difficulty in displaying the entire three-dimensional bone-implant interface in light microscopic histology. The selection of one cross-sectional plane for light microscopy is arbitrary, and the data from the cross-section are poorly correlated with the data measured on the whole three dimensional image [33]. In order to obtain the similar data between two- and three-dimensional images, three to four histologic sections for each specimen are needed, which are extremely difficult to prepare from a undecalcified specimen, including a titanium implant [34]. Methodological advancements, like three dimensional imaging analysis by micro-computed tomography, and a technique to make more histologic sections from a hard specimen are needed for more obvious in vivo results.

5. Conclusions

A human vitronectin-derived peptide, VnP-16 (RVYFFKGKQYWE motif), showed excellent histomorphometric osseointegration data without any special antigen–antibody reaction when this peptide was treated on an SLA titanium dental implant, which has been successfully used in clinics. From the in vitro results of this study, VnP-16 promotes the attachment of osteogenic cells and differentiation into osteoblasts, which may increase the bone healing capacity of the SLA's titanium surface. Considering both the in vitro and in vivo results of this study, VnP-16 reinforces the osteogenic potential of the SLA titanium dental implant when this peptide is applied to the SLA surface. In the future, VnP-16 may expand the clinical indications of SLA titanium dental implants.

Author Contributions: Conceptualization, I.-S.L.Y. and B.-M.M.; methodology, I.-S.L.Y. and B.-M.M.; software, C.-B.C., S.Y.J., C.Y.P., and H.K.K.; validation, I.-S.L.Y. and B.-M.M.; formal analysis, C.-B.C. and S.Y.J.; Investigation,

C.-B.C., S.Y.J., C.Y.P., and H.K.K.; resources, I.-S.L.Y. and B.-M.M.; data curation, C.-B.C. and S.Y.J.; writing—original draft preparation, C.-B.C. and S.Y.J.; writing—review and editing, C.Y.P., H.K.K., I.-S.L.Y., and B.-M.M.; visualization, C.-B.C. and S.Y.J.; supervision, I.-S.L.Y. and B.-M.M.; project administration, I.-S.L.Y. and B.-M.M.; funding acquisition, I.-S.L.Y. and B.-M.M.

References

1. Anderson, J.M.; Rodriguez, A.; Chang, D.T. Foreign body reaction to biomaterials. *Semin. Immunol.* **2008**, *20*, 86–100. [CrossRef]
2. Ravanetti, F.; Gazza, F.; D'Arrigo, D.; Graiani, G.; Zamuner, A.; Zedda, M.; Manfredi, E.; Dettin, M.; Cacchioli, A. Enhancement of peri-implant bone osteogenic activity induced by a peptidomimetic functionalization of titanium. *Ann. Anat.* **2018**, *218*, 165–174. [CrossRef]
3. Kang, H.K.; Kim, O.B.; Min, S.K.; Jung, S.Y.; Jang, D.H.; Kwon, T.K.; Min, B.M.; Yeo, I.S. The effect of the DLTIDDSYWYRI motif of the human laminin alpha2 chain on implant osseointegration. *Biomaterials* **2013**, *34*, 4027–4037. [CrossRef]
4. Shekaran, A.; Garcia, A.J. Extracellular matrix-mimetic adhesive biomaterials for bone repair. *J. Biomed. Mater. Res. A* **2011**, *96*, 261–272. [CrossRef]
5. Yeo, I.S.; Min, S.K.; Kang, H.K.; Kwon, T.K.; Jung, S.Y.; Min, B.M. Identification of a bioactive core sequence from human laminin and its applicability to tissue engineering. *Biomaterials* **2015**, *73*, 96–109. [CrossRef]
6. Boron, W.F.; Boulpaep, E.L. *Medical Physiology E-Book*; Elsevier Health Sciences: Kidlington, Oxford, UK, 2016.
7. Cherny, R.C.; Honan, M.A.; Thiagarajan, P. Site-directed mutagenesis of the arginine-glycine-aspartic acid in vitronectin abolishes cell adhesion. *J. Biol. Chem.* **1993**, *268*, 9725–9729.
8. Shin, T.M.; Isas, J.M.; Hsieh, C.L.; Kayed, R.; Glabe, C.G.; Langen, R.; Chen, J. Formation of soluble amyloid oligomers and amyloid fibrils by the multifunctional protein vitronectin. *Mol. Neurodegener.* **2008**, *3*, 16. [CrossRef]
9. Min, S.K.; Kang, H.K.; Jung, S.Y.; Jang, D.H.; Min, B.M. A vitronectin-derived peptide reverses ovariectomy-induced bone loss via regulation of osteoblast and osteoclast differentiation. *Cell Death Differ.* **2018**, *25*, 268–281. [CrossRef]
10. Yeo, I.S. Surface modification of dental biomaterials for controlling bone response. In *Bone Response to Dental Implant Materials*; Elsevier: Kidlington, Oxford, UK, 2017; pp. 43–46.
11. Howlett, C.R.; Evans, M.D.; Walsh, W.R.; Johnson, G.; Steele, J.G. Mechanism of initial attachment of cells derived from human bone to commonly used prosthetic materials during cell culture. *Biomaterials* **1994**, *15*, 213–222. [CrossRef]
12. Rivera-Chacon, D.M.; Alvarado-Velez, M.; Acevedo-Morantes, C.Y.; Singh, S.P.; Gultepe, E.; Nagesha, D.; Sridhar, S.; Ramirez-Vick, J.E. Fibronectin and vitronectin promote human fetal osteoblast cell attachment and proliferation on nanoporous titanium surfaces. *J. Biomed. Nanotechnol.* **2013**, *9*, 1092–1097. [CrossRef]
13. Scotchford, C.A.; Ball, M.; Winkelmann, M.; Voros, J.; Csucs, C.; Brunette, D.M.; Danuser, G.; Textor, M. Chemically patterned, metal-oxide-based surfaces produced by photolithographic techniques for studying protein- and cell-interactions. II: Protein adsorption and early cell interactions. *Biomaterials* **2003**, *24*, 1147–1158. [CrossRef]
14. Cacchioli, A.; Ravanetti, F.; Bagno, A.; Dettin, M.; Gabbi, C. Human Vitronectin-Derived Peptide Covalently Grafted onto Titanium Surface Improves Osteogenic Activity: A Pilot In Vivo Study on Rabbits. *Tissue Eng. Part. A* **2009**, *15*, 2917–2926. [CrossRef]
15. Petrie, T.A.; Raynor, J.E.; Dumbauld, D.W.; Lee, T.T.; Jagtap, S.; Templeman, K.L.; Collard, D.M.; Garcia, A.J. Multivalent integrin-specific ligands enhance tissue healing and biomaterial integration. *Sci. Transl. Med.* **2010**, *2*, 45ra60. [CrossRef]
16. Rezania, A.; Healy, K.E. Biomimetic peptide surfaces that regulate adhesion, spreading, cytoskeletal organization, and mineralization of the matrix deposited by osteoblast-like cells. *Biotechnol. Prog.* **1999**, *15*, 19–32. [CrossRef]
17. Vukicevic, S.; Luyten, F.P.; Kleinman, H.K.; Reddi, A.H. Differentiation of canalicular cell processes in bone cells by basement membrane matrix components: Regulation by discrete domains of laminin. *Cell* **1990**, *63*, 437–445. [CrossRef]
18. Martin, L.J.; Akhavan, B.; Bilek, M.M.M. Electric fields control the orientation of peptides irreversibly immobilized on radical-functionalized surfaces. *Nat. Commun.* **2018**, *9*, 357. [CrossRef]

19. Stewart, C.; Akhavan, B.; Wise, S.G.; Bilek, M.M. A review of biomimetic surface functionalization for bone-integrating orthopedic implants: Mechanisms, current approaches, and future directions. *Prog. Mater. Sci.* **2019**, *106*, 100588. [CrossRef]
20. Pagel, M.; Hassert, R.; John, T.; Braun, K.; Wiessler, M.; Abel, B.; Beck-Sickinger, A.G. Multifunctional Coating Improves Cell Adhesion on Titanium by using Cooperatively Acting Peptides. *Angew Chem. Int. Ed. Engl.* **2016**, *55*, 4826–4830. [CrossRef]
21. Choi, J.Y.; Kang, S.H.; Kim, H.Y.; Yeo, I.L. Control Variable Implants Improve Interpretation of Surface Modification and Implant Design Effects on Early Bone Responses: An In Vivo Study. *Int J. Oral Maxillofac Implant.* **2018**, *33*, 1033–1040. [CrossRef]
22. Wennerberg, A.; Albrektsson, T. On implant surfaces: A review of current knowledge and opinions. *Int. J. Oral Maxillofac. Implant.* **2010**, *25*, 63–74.
23. Kim, S.; Choi, J.Y.; Jung, S.Y.; Kang, H.K.; Min, B.M.; Yeo, I.L. A laminin-derived functional peptide, PPFEGCIWN, promotes bone formation on sandblasted, large-grit, acid-etched titanium implant surfaces. *Int. J. Oral Maxillofac. Implant.* **2019**, *34*, 836–844. [CrossRef] [PubMed]
24. Kim, J.M.; Min, S.K.; Kim, H.; Kang, H.K.; Jung, S.Y.; Lee, S.H.; Choi, Y.; Roh, S.; Jeong, D.; Min, B.M. Vacuolar-type H+-ATPase-mediated acidosis promotes in vitro osteoclastogenesis via modulation of cell migration. *Int. J. Mol. Med.* **2007**, *19*, 393–400. [CrossRef] [PubMed]
25. Kilkenny, C.; Browne, W.J.; Cuthill, I.C.; Emerson, M.; Altman, D.G. Improving bioscience research reporting: The ARRIVE guidelines for reporting animal research. *Osteoarthr. Cartil.* **2012**, *20*, 256–260. [CrossRef] [PubMed]
26. Donath, K.; Breuner, G. A method for the study of undecalcified bones and teeth with attached soft tissues. The Sage-Schliff (sawing and grinding) technique. *J. Oral Pathol.* **1982**, *11*, 318–326. [CrossRef]
27. Gruber, H.E. Adaptations of Goldner's Masson trichrome stain for the study of undecalcified plastic embedded bone. *Biotech. Histochem.* **1992**, *67*, 30–34. [CrossRef]
28. Buser, D.; Janner, S.F.; Wittneben, J.G.; Bragger, U.; Ramseier, C.A.; Salvi, G.E. 10-year survival and success rates of 511 titanium implants with a sandblasted and acid-etched surface: A retrospective study in 303 partially edentulous patients. *Clin. Implant. Dent. Relat Res.* **2012**, *14*, 839–851. [CrossRef]
29. Van Velzen, F.J.; Ofec, R.; Schulten, E.A.; Ten Bruggenkate, C.M. 10-year survival rate and the incidence of peri-implant disease of 374 titanium dental implants with a SLA surface: A prospective cohort study in 177 fully and partially edentulous patients. *Clin. Oral Implant. Res.* **2015**, *26*, 1121–1128. [CrossRef]
30. Tsolaki, I.N.; Madianos, P.N.; Vrotsos, J.A. Outcomes of dental implants in osteoporotic patients. A literature review. *J. Prosthodont.* **2009**, *18*, 309–323. [CrossRef]
31. Choi, S.H.; Jeong, W.S.; Cha, J.Y.; Lee, J.H.; Lee, K.J.; Yu, H.S.; Choi, E.H.; Kim, K.M.; Hwang, C.J. Overcoming the biological aging of titanium using a wet storage method after ultraviolet treatment. *Sci. Rep.* **2017**, *7*, 3833. [CrossRef]
32. Lee, J.B.; Jo, Y.H.; Choi, J.Y.; Seol, Y.J.; Lee, Y.M.; Ku, Y.; Rhyu, I.C.; Yeo, I.L. The Effect of Ultraviolet Photofunctionalization on a Titanium Dental Implant with Machined Surface: An In Vitro and In Vivo Study. *Materials* **2019**, *12*, 2078. [CrossRef]
33. Choi, J.Y.; Park, J.I.; Chae, J.S.; Yeo, I.L. Comparison of micro-computed tomography and histomorphometry in the measurement of bone-implant contact ratios. *Oral Surg. Oral Med. Oral Pathol. Oral Radiol.* **2019**, *128*, 87–95. [CrossRef]
34. Bernhardt, R.; Kuhlisch, E.; Schulz, M.C.; Eckelt, U.; Stadlinger, B. Comparison of bone-implant contact and bone-implant volume between 2D-histological sections and 3D-SRmicroCT slices. *Eur. Cell Mater.* **2012**, *23*, 237–247, discussion 247–248. [CrossRef]

9

Prediction of Titanium Implant Success by Analysis of microRNA Expression in Peri-Implant Tissue. A 5-Year Follow-Up Study

Maria Menini [1], Paolo Pesce [1,*], Domenico Baldi [1], Gabriela Coronel Vargas [2], Paolo Pera [1] and Alberto Izzotti [2,3]

1 Division of Implant Prosthodontics, Department of Surgical Sciences, University of Genoa, 16132 Genoa, Italy; maria.menini@unige.it (M.M.); baldi.domenico@unige.it (D.B.); paolopera@unige.it (P.P.)
2 Department of Health Sciences, University of Genoa, 16126 Genoa, Italy; gabrielafernanda.coronelvargas@edu.unige.it (G.C.V.); izzotti@unige.it (A.I.)
3 IRCCS Ospedale Policlinico San Martino, 16132 Genoa, Italy
* Correspondence: paolo.pesce@unige.it

Abstract: The aim of the present study is to evaluate the expression of microRNA (miRNA) in peri-implant soft tissue and to correlate epigenetic information with the clinical outcomes of the implants up to the five-year follow-up. Seven patients have been rehabilitated with fixed screw-retained bridges each supported by implants. Peri-implant bone resorption and soft tissue health parameters have been recorded over time with a five-year follow-up. Mini-invasive samples of soft peri-implant tissue have been taken three months after implant insertion. miRNA have been extracted from cells of the soft tissue samples to evaluate gene-expression at the implant sites by microarray analysis. The epigenomic data obtained by microarray technology has been statistically analyzed by dedicated software and compared with measured clinical parameters. Specific miRNA expression profiles predictive of specific clinical outcomes were found. In particular, some specific miRNA signatures appeared to be "protective" from bone resorption despite the presence of plaque accumulation. miRNA may be predictors of dental implant clinical outcomes and may be used as biomarkers for diagnostic and prognostic purposes in the field of implant dentistry.

Keywords: dental implants; micro-RNA; microarray; predictive biomarker; epigenomics

1. Introduction

Currently dental implants are widely used for fixed rehabilitation of partially or completely edentulous patients and demonstrate predictable outcomes. However, the biological mechanisms of possible complications and implant failure are not clear and are debated in the dental scientific community.

In particular, the specific endogenous characteristic of the host (i.e., individual susceptibility) may strongly affect the success of the rehabilitation. Modern innovative technologies using molecular biomarkers may help in identifying individual susceptibility.

In a previous paper [1] we provided evidence that microRNA (miRNA) expression in peri-implant tissue reflects the pathological processes occurring in peri-implant tissues.

miRNAs are small noncoding RNAs (ncRNAs) of approximately 22 nucleotides responsible for specific regulation of gene expression in a post-transcriptional manner. They are the main regulator of gene transcription and bear relevance in predicting clinical outcomes. Indeed, only less than 5% of expressed genes producing messenger RNA is really translated into proteins while microRNAs are fully functionally active in cell cytoplasm [2]. They have an important role in several biological processes, such as development, cell proliferation, apoptosis and carcinogenesis [3,4].

A major problem is currently represented by the lack of a predictive marker to personalize risk after peri-implant surgery. Indeed, some authors have suggested peri-implant soft tissue biotype as a risk indicator of peri-implants tissue disease [5,6]. However, this biomarker is rough and does not reflect the multiple pathogenic mechanisms occurring in the peri-implant tissue hampering or favoring the outcome of implant surgery. Conversely the accurate classification of patients in high or low-risk categories is fundamental to set up follow-up procedures and therapies according to the real risk of each subject. This is a pivotal step in the era of personalized medicine.

Molecular biomarkers are already extensively used in medicine to accurately classify each patient according to their real risk of developing complications. This approach, referred to as personalized or "theranostic" medicine, has been already well developed in oncology but is still under development in dental science.

Molecular predictive biomarkers should reflect the pathogenic process modulating clinical outcome in the target tissue of the diseases. Furthermore, the molecular alteration investigated may occur years before the appearance of the related clinical consequence thus opening the possibility of preventing adverse clinical outcomes before their onset.

At this regard, miRNAs are currently identified as predictive biomarkers for degenerative diseases, because they do not undergo a post-transcriptional selection, being themselves the controllers of gene transcription. Consequently, compared to genomic or transcriptomic biomarkers, miRNA expression has by far a higher probability of being related with clinical variables representing a new tool for predictive medicine.

On the other side, several factors, including the implant surface [7], might affect dental implant success possibly through miRNA expression. Our research group demonstrated in vitro that osteoblasts change their gene expression profile according to the type of implant surface in contact with them [8].

The role of miRNA in implant dentistry has been established. In a clinical trial, we demonstrated that miRNA expressed by peri-implant tissues are related with the clinical outcome [2]. However, it remains to be established the long-term predictivity of miRNA analysis in a long-term follow-up study.

The aim of the present study is to examine the predictivity of miRNA profiling to categorize patients according to risk categories of developing more or less probably adverse consequences of oral implants on a long-term basis.

In particular, the expression of micro-RNA (miRNA) in peri-implant soft tissue will be correlated with the clinical outcomes of dental implants recorded up to the five-year follow-up.

2. Experimental Section

Between January 2013 and July 2014, 7 patients (4 women, 3 men; mean age: 64.6, range: 52–76) who were referred to the Division of Implant and Prosthetic Dentistry of the Surgical Sciences Department (DISC) of the University of Genoa (Genoa, Italy) and that required the insertion of two implants into an edentulous area were recruited if they met the following criteria: desire to be treated with fixed prostheses supported by dental implants and good general health without any contraindications for undergoing oral surgery and the related prosthodontic protocols.

Exclusion criteria included: an uncontrolled medical condition such as diabetes mellitus, immune suppression, intravenous bisphosphonate medication, oro-facial cancer, chemotherapy or head and neck radiotherapy, infarct during the preceding 6 months, heavy smokers (≥20 cigarettes/day).

Healing time since tooth extraction in the intended implant sites had to be longer than 1 year. Post-extractive implants and implant sites that required a bone graft were excluded.

The present report was conducted in accordance with the Helsinki Declaration and was approved by the local Scientific Ethical Committee of the University of Genoa.

Patients were instructed in detail on the planned clinical procedure and signed an informed consent before being scheduled in the experimental protocol.

Each patient of the sample received two adjacent implants: Osseotite implants (Biomet 3i, Palmbeach Gardens, FL) with a dual acid-etched (DAE) surface in the apical portion and a machined coronal part (hybrid implants), and Full Osseotite implants (Biomet 3i) completely DAE (DAE implants).

All the implants had identical macro- and micro-structure, external hexagon connection, a 4 mm diameter, a 10–13 mm length (depending on available bone).

Implants were placed with a single-stage delayed loading approach and were assigned specific codes for blinding.

The healing abutments remained in situ up to the 4-month follow-up appointment when impressions of the implants were taken to fabricate the fixed prostheses. No bone nor soft tissue grafting procedures were performed at the implant sites.

Patients were accurately instructed on the hygienic procedures to be followed and were prescribed adequate dietary guidelines in order to ensure optimal recovery.

Screw-retained prostheses, provided with a metal framework and composite resin veneering material, were delivered 5–6 months (mean 24 weeks) after surgery (Figure 1).

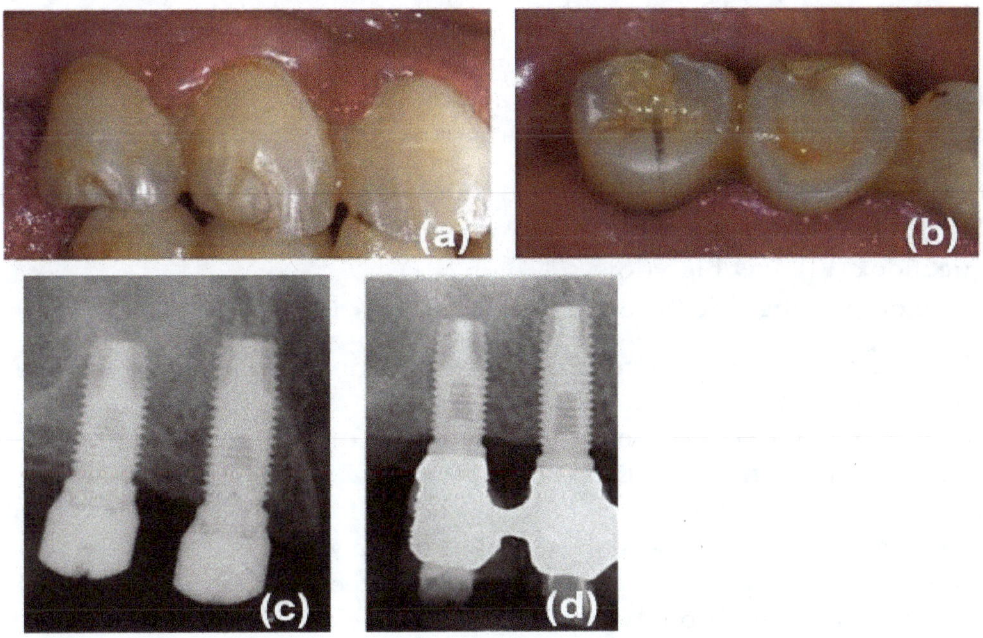

Figure 1. One of the patients included in the present research: (**a**) intraoral view of the bridge at the five-year follow-up appointment; (**b**) occlusal view of the bridge at the five-year follow-up appointment; (**c**) endoral radiograph three months after implant insertion; (**d**) endoral radiograph taken at the five-year follow-up appointment.

Spontaneous bleeding, probing depth (PD), bleeding on probing (BoP), plaque index (PI), and suppuration were recorded at 3 and 6 weeks and at 3-, 6- and 12-months post-surgery and then at the five-year follow-up appointment. At the five-year appointment the fixed prostheses were unscrewed in order to record the parodontal parameters. PD was recorded in four points for each implant (mesial, distal, buccal and lingual) using a non-metallic probe. BoP was simultaneously evaluated in four points for each implant (values from 0 to 4 for each implant). PI was measured at four points for each implant using an erythrosine gel (values from 0 to 4 for each implant).

Technical and biological complications were also recorded.

Intraoral radiographs were taken at the time of implant placement and at 3-, 6- and 12-months post-surgery and then at the five-year follow-up appointment. The implant–abutment interface was used as the reference point for interproximal bone level measurements over time. Bone resorption (BR) over the duration of the study was assessed from these reference points to the most coronal bone at the mesial and distal aspects of each implant.

The above-mentioned clinical parameters recorded at the five-year follow-up appointment were statistically analyzed and differences between DAE and hybrid implants were evaluated by Student's *t*-test.

After 3 months from surgery, a sample of soft tissue containing both epithelium and connective tissue was collected: a mini-invasive sample of soft tissue (diameter < 3 mm) surrounding each implant was taken using a surgical blade to be histologically analyzed by miRNA microarray at the Department of Health Sciences (DISSAL) of Genoa University.

MicroRNA microarray analysis is an innovative technology, which allows the evaluations of thousands of genes in a single experiment. MicroRNAs (miRNA) have been extracted from cells of the soft tissue samples to evaluate gene-expression at the implant sites by microarray analysis.

miRNA expression data was evaluated in the peri-implant tissue as previously reported [1]. The expression of 1928 human miRNA was determined by using a commercially available microarray (miRCURY LNATM, Exiqon, Vedbaek, Denmark).

The results of miRNA microarray have been compared with clinical parameters measured over time for five years since miRNA analysis. The previously published paper reported correlation between miRNA data and one-year outcomes (T0). The present paper reports the correlation between miRNA data and clinical outcomes recorded at the five-year follow-up appointment (T1).

All clinical continuous variables recorded at the five-year follow-up have been turned into categorical ones depending on the following criteria arbitrarily chosen by the authors:

- mean bone resorption (BR): normal/increased (normal ≤ 1 mm, increased > 1 mm)
- mean probing depth (PD): normal/increased (normal ≤ 3 mm, increased > 3 mm)
- mean plaque index (PI): low/high (low ≤ 1, high > 1)
- mean bleeding on probing (BOP): yes/no (yes ≥ 0.5, no < 0.5)

On the base of these parameters, several categories of implants (i.e., implants with normal BR vs. implants with increased BR) have been determined.

In addition, implants with the contemporary presence of BOP, altered PD and bone resorption were considered affected by peri-implantitis (PITI).

Implant sites were also divided in two categories according to the periodontal biotype: thin (TH) and thick (TK). To evaluate the biotype, a periodontal probe was placed into the facial aspect of the peri-implant mucosa. The peri-implant biotype was categorized as thin if the outline of the underlying periodontal probe could be seen through the gingiva and thick if the probe could not be seen [9].

Relationship between miRNA and clinical events were tested by Genespring software (Agilent technologies, Palo Alto, CA, USA).

3. Results

During the five-year follow-up, there were no dropouts and all the patients attended the five-year recall appointment. No implant failure occurred resulting in an implant cumulative survival rate (CSR) of 100%. No technical complications were detected, resulting in a prosthodontic CSR of 100%. All the patients anecdotally reported to be satisfied with their implant rehabilitation.

Five patients presented a thin periodontal biotype and two a thick periodontal biotype.

Mean bone resorption at the five-year follow-up appointment was 1.98 mm (min: 0.7, max: 4 mm): 1.8 mm and 2.2 mm for implants with a machined coronal portion and DAE implants respectively.

No patient presented spontaneous bleeding or suppuration.

No statistically significant differences were found between hybrid implants and DAE implants for the clinical variables recorded at the five-year follow-up.

Mean and median values of the other soft tissue health parameters are reported in Table 1.

Table 1. Bone level and peri-implant health parameters recorded at the five-year follow-up appointment.

	Interproximal Bone Resorption (mm)	Plaque Index	Bleeding on Probing	Probing Depth (mm)
Mean	1.98	2.9	2.1	3.7
Median	2	3	2	4
Min	0.7	0	0	1
Max	4	4	4	6.5
P for DAE vs. hybrid implants	0.1466	0.8641	0.5817	0.6215

An overall view of the miRNA alterations as related to clinical outcomes occurring in the five years after surgery was performed using scatter plot (Figure 2) and volcano plot analyses (Figure 3).

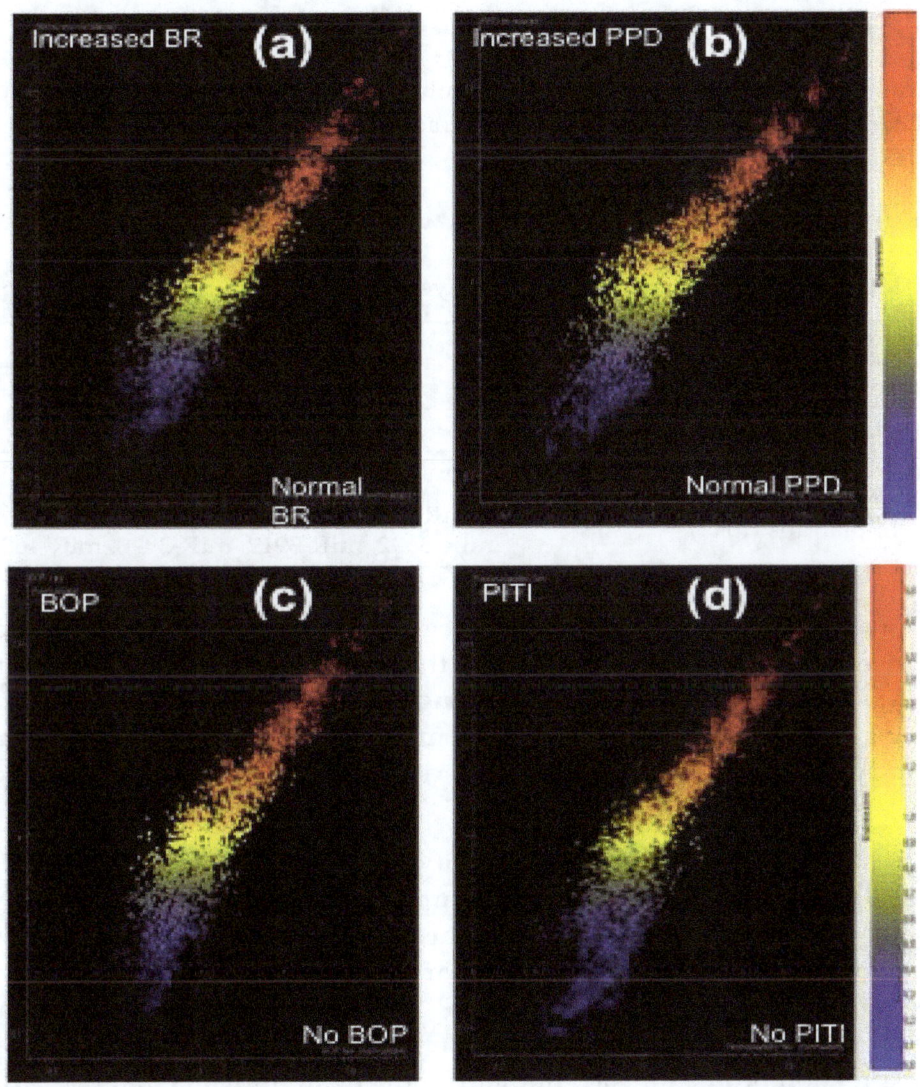

Figure 2. Scatter plot analyses reporting the alteration of microRNA (miRNA) profile as related to the outcome of the following clinical variables recorded at the five-year follow-up appointment: (**a**) bone resorption (BR), (**b**) peri-implant probing depth (PPD), (**c**) bleeding on probing (BOP), (**d**) peri-implantitis (PITI).

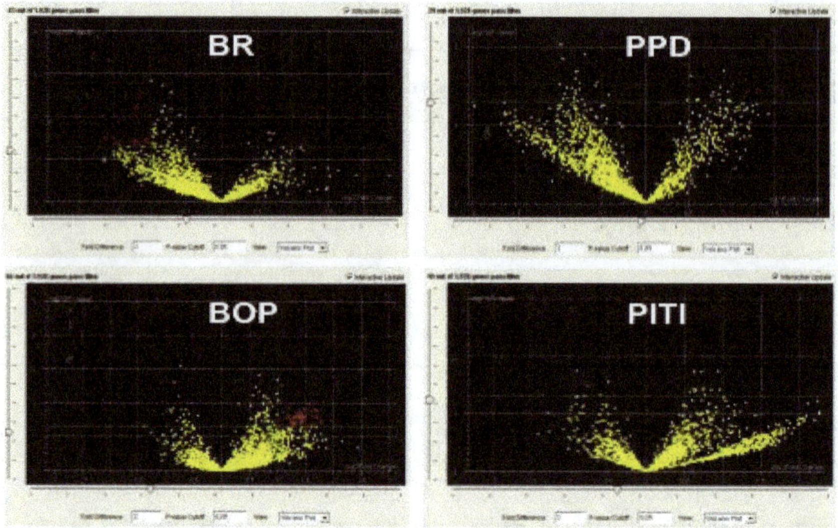

Figure 3. Volcano plot analyses reporting the number of significantly (<2-fold, $p < 0.05$) altered miRNAs as related to the outcome of the following clinical variables recorded at the five-year follow-up appointment: BR, PPD, BOP, PITI.

For each clinical variable, the predictor miRNAs were identified by volcano plot analysis (Table 2).

Table 2. Identity of miRNAs predictor of five-year clinical outcomes of dental implants.

Clinical Variable Predicted	miRNA
Bone Resorption (BR)	miR-33, miR-134, miR-200, miR-378
Bleeding on probing (BOP)	let-7f miR-425, miR-548
Peri-implant pocket depth (PPD)	miR-30, miR-197, miR-218, miR-548, miR-613
Perimplantitis (PITI)	miR-517, miR-525, miR-624, miR-3128, miR-3658, miR-3692, miR-3912, miR-3920, miR-4683, miR-4690

BR: 48 miRNA were significantly (Figure 3) dysregulated at T0 in patients with altered BR (altered) as compared to those with normal BR (normal) in the five years following implant surgery. Venn diagram analyses indicated that in these patients among the miRNAs altered at T0, four were predictors of BR in the following five years. These miRNAs are miR-33, miR-134, miR-200 and miR-378 (Table 2). They play a regulatory role in cell proliferation, stem cell recruitment and differentiation, osteogenesis and inflammation.

Hierarchical cluster analyses were used to classify patients according to their miRNA expression profile as related to BR in the five years following implant surgery. Implants with a normal miRNA expression level (yellow, red) are located in the left part of the cluster, while implants with a decreased miRNA expression (blue) are located in the right part of the cluster. A severe alteration of miRNA expression at three months occurs in patients with BR $\geq$ 2 mm at the five-year follow-up appointment (Figure 4a). These findings were confirmed by unsupervised principal component analysis of variance (PCA) of miRNA expression profile for each implant. Indeed, all implants that had a BR $\geq$ 2 mm in the five years after surgery were located in a different quadrant as compared to other implants (Figure 4b).

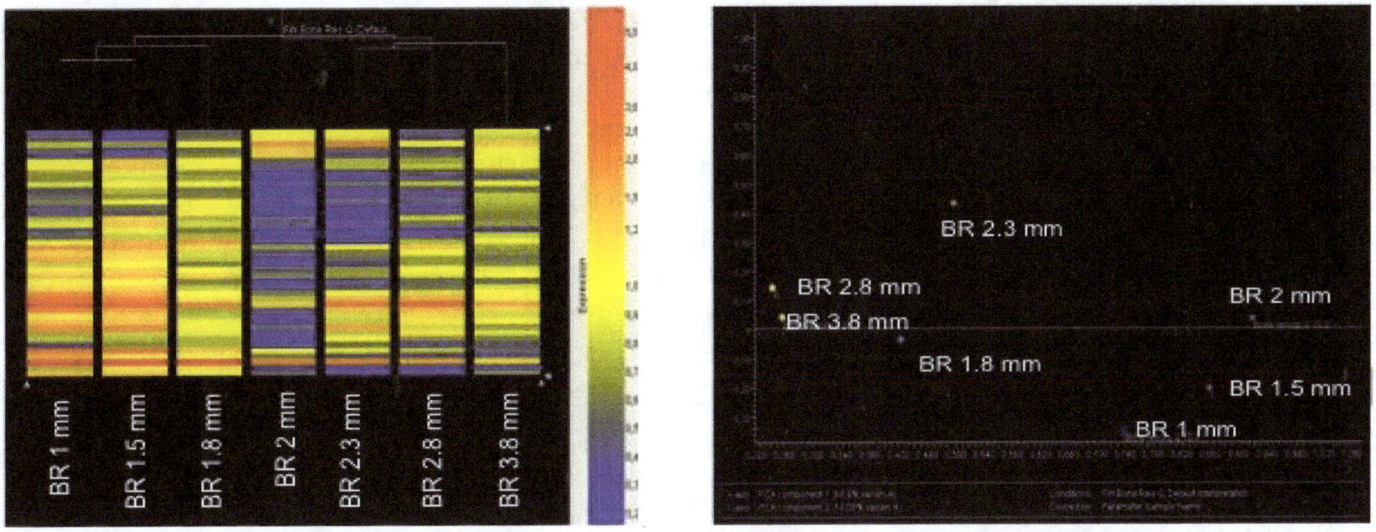

(a) (b)

Figure 4. Hierarchical cluster (**a**) and principal component analysis of variance (**b**) analyses showing the occurrence of miRNA alteration in implants with BR > 2 mm.

PD: 29 miRNA were significantly (Figure 3, volcano plot) altered at T0 in patients with PD increase (increased) as compared to those having normal PD (normal) in the five years following implant surgery. Venn diagram analyses indicated that among the 10 miRNA altered in these implants at T0 (see data reported in Menini et al. [1] first year after surgery) five were predictors of PD increase in the following five years. These miRNAs are miR-30, miR-197, miR-218, miR-548 and miR-613 (Table 2). They play a regulatory role in the following biological functions: osteogenesis and cartilage homeostasis.

BOP: 66 miRNA were significantly (Figure 3, volcano plot) altered at T0 in patients with BOP (yes) as compared to those without BOP (no) at five years following implant surgery. Venn diagram analyses indicated that among the six miRNA altered in these patients at T0 (see data reported in Menini et al. [1] first year after surgery) three were predictors of BOP increase in the following five years. These miRNAs are let-7f, miR-425 and miR-548 (Table 2). They play a regulatory role in the following biological function: inflammation.

PITI: 10 miRNA were significantly (Figure 3, volcano plot) altered at T0 in patients having PITI (yes) as compared to those not having PITI (no) at five years following implant surgery. This condition was not evaluated at T0 (at the one-year follow-up appointment only two implants in one single patient presented PITI). These miRNAs are miR-517, miR-525, miR-624, miR-3128, miR-3658, miR-3692, miR-3912, miR-3920, miR-4683 and miR-4690 (Table 2). They play a regulatory role in the following biological functions: inflammation, cellular proliferation and cartilage homeostasis.

The number of altered miRNAs as related to BR, peri-implant probing depth (PD) and BOP recorded at the five-year follow-up was dramatically increased (T1) as compared to T0 (Table 3). These findings reflect the progressive recruitment of new pathogenic mechanisms during the progression of the diseases.

Table 3. Number of altered miRNAs as related to BR, PD and BOP recorded at the one-year (T0) and at the five-year follow-up (T1).

	BR	PD	BOP
T0	7	10	6
T1	48	29	66

The efficacy of miRNA as biomarkers predicting clinical outcome was compared with those of periodontal biotype classified for each patient as thick (low-risk) or thin (high-risk). The ability of periodontal biotype to predict the clinical outcome of dental implants in the following five years was tested by chi square analysis (Figure 5). Of the patients with a thick biotype 33% underwent PITI, while none of the patients with a thin biotype underwent PITI. These differences were not significantly different (chi square = 2.727; chi square p-value = 0.0986; Fischer's exact p-value = 0.2308). Conversely, miRNA expression as focused on the cluster of PITI miRNA predictors (see Table 2 and Figure 6) was able to predict PITI occurrence in all (100%) patients.

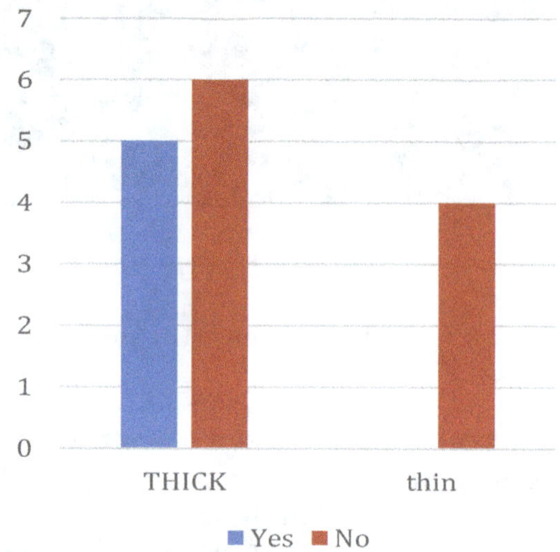

Summary table for PITI, Biotype	
Num. missing	0
DF	1
Chi Square	2.727
Chi Square p-Value	0.0986
G-Squared	*
G-Squared p-Value	*
Contingency Coef.	0.392
Phi	0.426
Cty. Cor. Chi Square	1.152
Cty. Cor. p-Value	0.2831
Fisher's exact p-Value	0.2308

Observed Frequencies for PITI, Biotype			
	THICK	Thin	Totals
PITI	5	0	**5**
No PITI	6	4	**10**
Totals	11	4	**15**

Figure 5. PITI occurrence as related to parodontal biotype.

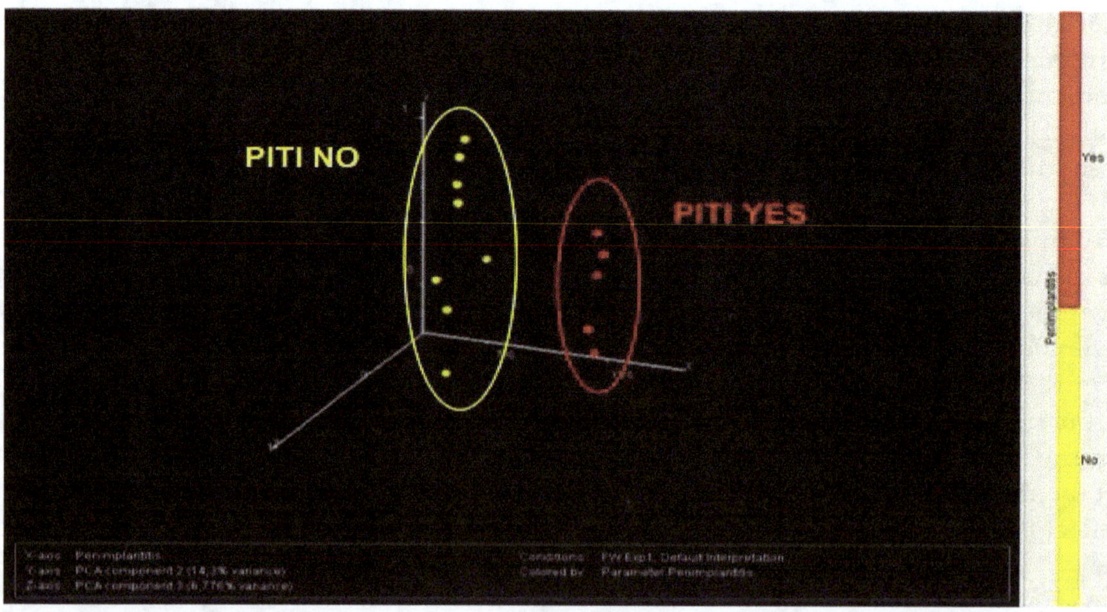

Figure 6. Principal component analysis of variance showing differences in miRNA expression in implants with or without PITI.

In fact, PCA of miRNA expression at T0 (Figure 6) distinguished between patients that would develop PITI in the following five years (red dots) from those who would not develop PITI (yellow dots) in a clear-cut manner, as highlighted by the lack of any overlap between the grouping circles. The ability of miRNA profiling in predicting PITI was also statistically evaluated by k-nearest neighbors and support vector machine algorithms. The sensitivity (percentage of patients with prediction) was 80%

and 93% respectively; the specificity (percentage of patients with true prediction) was 100% and 93% respectively. Accordingly, the accuracy of this test was >90% independently of the algorithm adopted.

The miRNA pattern was compared in patients undergoing plaque accumulation (high PI) between those with or without BR. The aim of this approach was to identify miRNA protecting peri-implant tissue from the adverse effect of plaque accumulation. Obtained results are reported in Figure 7.

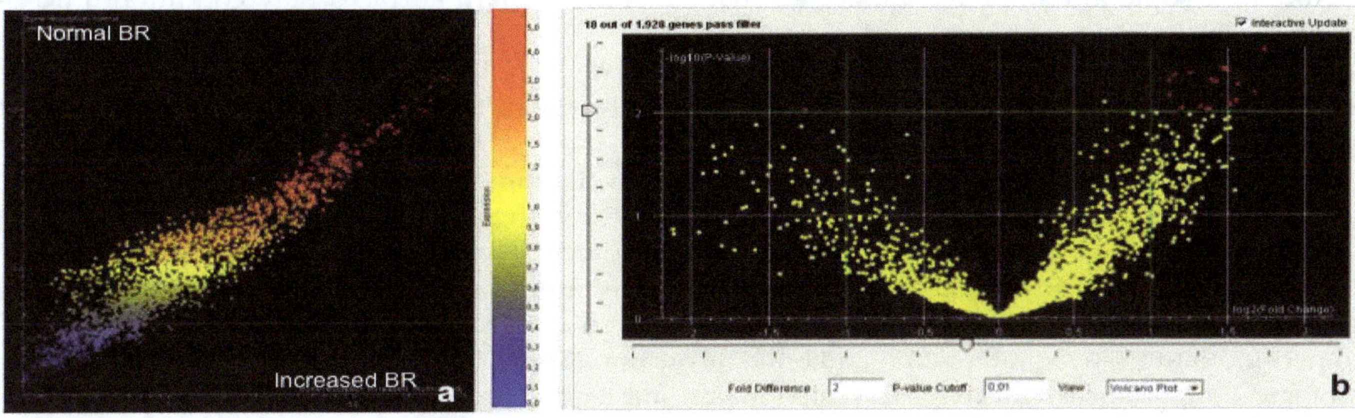

Figure 7. Scatter plot (**a**) and volcano plot (**b**) analyses reporting the alteration of miRNA profile as related to BR at the level of implants with high plaque index (PI).

Both scatter plot and volcano plot identified differences between these two groups of patients. The miRNAs that protected peri-implant tissue from BR despite the presence of plaque deposits are reported in Table 4.

Table 4. miRNA that were found to be "protective" from bone resorption despite the presence of plaque deposits (high PI) and their fold variation. The fold change indicates the ratio of miRNA expression intensity between the two categories of implants stratified according to differences in bone resorption (increased vs. normal) next to implants with high PI.

Gene Name	Fold Change
hsa-miR-4677-5p	3.328
hsa-miR-3914	3.189
hsa-miR-4679	2.948
hsa-miR-378b	2.929
hsa-miR-4434	2.858
hsa-miR-32-3p/mmu-miR-32-3p/rno-miR-32-3p	2.804
hsa-miR-1/mmu-miR-1a-3p	2.769
hsa-miR-4778-5p	2.681
hsa-miR-99b-3p/mmu-miR-99b-3p/rno-miR-99b-3p	2.615
hsa-miR-7-5p/mmu-miR-7a-5p/rno-miR-7a-5p	2.496
hsa-miR-3146	2.389
hsa-miR-4439	2.296
hsa-miR-539-3p	2.247
hsa-miR-222-3p/mmu-miR-222-3p/rno-miR-222-3p	2.225
hsa-miR-124-5p/mmu-miR-124-5p/rno-miR-124-5p	2.169
hsa-miR-4689	2.167

4. Discussion

miRNA are biomarkers of several diseases and in recent years, some studies have begun to focus on the regulatory role of miRNAs in the inflammatory response [10,11].

miRNA are fundamental in controlling cell function and also influence osteoinductive pathways and inflammation in several ways. On the other side, miRNA expression is influenced by many factors and some authors have suggested that different implant surfaces may condition miRNA expression [12,13].

However, studies investigating the role of miRNA in implant dentistry are still scarce. Some in vitro studies are present [12,14] and studies focused on the differences of miRNA profiles between periimplantitis and periodontitis [15].

A recent review [16] found only one clinical trial evaluating the role of miRNA expression in the osseointegration of dental implants. This study was the investigation conducted by the present team of authors [1] and the present paper reports follow-up data for the same patients' samples.

Our previous study suggested that miRNAs play an important role in conditioning clinical outcomes after implant insertion [1]. Specific miRNA profiles appeared to indicate lower susceptibility to peri-implant tissue inflammation and bone resorption. These findings highlighted the remarkable biological importance of miRNA expression in peri-implant tissue in determining the clinical outcome of dental implant rehabilitations.

The present study with a five-year follow-up confirmed the potential role of miRNA in patients' susceptibility to peri-implant disease and the potential role of miRNAs as predictors of clinical outcomes of dental implants. In fact, miRNA expression at three months of healing was predictive of the clinical variables recorded at five years of follow-up.

The miRNA mostly involved in the prediction of clinical outcomes was miR-548. Indeed, this miRNA predicted PD and BOP (Table 2). This miRNA is an established regulator of the balance between cell proliferation and apoptosis. This miRNA was found to be upregulated in patients undergoing these adverse events; indeed this upregulation results in cell proliferation arrest and apoptosis activation, two conditions fundamental in triggering degenerative diseases of the peri-implant tissue and to hamper wound healing.

The definition and etiology of peri-implant disease are controversial [17]. In particular, a clear link between plaque accumulation and bone loss has yet to be demonstrated [18,19]. The possible etiological effect of plaque accumulation on peri-implant disease may be decreased or enhanced by specific miRNAs.

Indeed, a specific miRNA expression profile was found in patients with normal BR at five years, despite the presence of plaque accumulation (6,7), and miRNA expression analysis was far more accurate than periodontal biotype in predicting PITI occurrence in the five years after implant surgery (5,6).

The present investigation shed light on possible biomarkers that may be predictable of dental implants clinical outcomes. The variables that can compromise implant therapy are numerous (systematic diseases, residual bone density and 3-D morphology, smoking, bruxism, regularity and effectiveness of the follow-up etc.) and the miRNA can be considered a useful tool for only evaluating the "predisposition" of the peri-implant tissues to a stable osseointegration process.

The integrated findings derived from clinical and laboratory analysis helped with understanding the biological mechanisms affecting peri-implant tissue healing and maintenance. This will help clinicians in the choice of a better treatment plan for a predictable success of dental implant rehabilitations. In fact, specific miRNA expression profiles are predictive of specific clinical outcomes in implant dentistry and may be used as diagnostic and prognostic tools, thus affecting therapeutic strategies. These findings can be tools for a more personalized medicine approach in the treatment of edentulous patients using dental implants.

Moreover, the possible identification of "protective" miRNA also discloses the possibility of using miRNAs in future studies as therapeutic agents in implant dentistry. miRNAs might be used as possible drugs or coatings for implant surfaces, in order to improve healing and maintenance of peri-implant tissues.

5. Conclusions

The results of the present clinical trial suggest that miRNA may be predictors of dental implants clinical outcomes and may be used as biomarkers for diagnostic and prognostic purposes in the field of implant dentistry.

Author Contributions: Conceptualization, M.M., P.P. (Paolo Pera)Paolo Pera, D.B. and A.I.; methodology, M.M., D.B. and A.I.; software, A.I. and G.C.V.; validation, M.M., P.P.(Paolo Pesce), D.B. and A.I.; formal analysis, M.M., P.P. (Paolo Pesce) and A.I.; investigation, M.M., P.P. (Paolo Pesce), D.B., G.C.V. and A.I.; resources, P.P.(Paolo Pera) and A.I.; data curation, P.P. (Paolo Pesce) and M.M.; writing—original draft preparation, M.M. and A.I.; writing—review and editing, M.M., A.I. and P.P. (Paolo Pesce); visualization, M.M., A.I. and P.P. (Paolo Pesce); supervision, P.P. (Paolo Pera); project administration, M.M.; funding acquisition, M.M. and P.P. (Paolo Pera).

References

1. Menini, M.; Dellepiane, E.; Baldi, D.; Longobardi, M.G.; Pera, P.; Izzotti, A. Microarray expression in peri-implant tissue next to different titanium implant surfaces predicts clinical outcomes: A split-mouth study. *Clin. Oral. Implant. Res.* **2017**, *28*, e121–e134. [CrossRef] [PubMed]
2. Izzotti, A. Molecular medicine and development of cancer chemopreventive agents. *Ann. N. Y. Acad. Sci.* **2012**, *1259*, 26–32. [CrossRef] [PubMed]
3. Osada, H.; Takahashi, T. MicroRNAs in biological processes and carcinogenesis. *Carcinogenesis* **2007**, *28*, 2–12. [CrossRef] [PubMed]
4. Pasquinelli, A.E.; Reinhart, B.J.; Slack, F.; Martindale, M.Q.; Kuroda, M.I.; Maller, B.; Hayward, D.C.; Ball, E.E.; Degnan, B.; M€uller, P.; et al. Conservation of the sequence and temporal expression of let-7 heterochronic regulatory RNA. *Nature* **2000**, *408*, 86–89. [CrossRef] [PubMed]
5. Isler, S.C.; Uraz, A.; Kaymaz, O.; Cetiner, D. An Evaluation of the Relationship between Peri-implant Soft Tissue Biotype and the Severity of Peri-implantitis: A Cross-Sectional Study. *Int. J. Oral. Maxillofac. Implant* **2019**, *34*, 187–196. [CrossRef] [PubMed]
6. Mailoa, J.; Miron, R.J.; Wang, H.L. Risk Indicators and Prevention of Implant Soft-Tissue Complications: Interproximal Papillae Loss and Midfacial Implant Mucosal Recessions. *Compend. Contin. Educ. Dent.* **2017**, *38*, 436–443. [PubMed]
7. Menini, M.; Dellepiane, E.; Chvartszaid, D.; Baldi, D.; Schiavetti, I.; Pera, P. Influence of Different Surface Characteristics on Peri-implant Tissue Behavior: A Six-Year Prospective Report. *Int. J. Prosthodont.* **2015**, *28*, 389–395. [CrossRef] [PubMed]
8. Baldi, D.; Longobardi, M.G.; Cartiglia, C.; La Maestra, S.; Pulliero, A.; Bonica, P.; Micale, R.; Menini, M.; Pera, P.; Izzotti, A. Dental Implants Osteogenic Properties Evaluated by cDNA Microarrays. *Implant Dent.* **2011**, *20*, 299–304. [CrossRef] [PubMed]
9. Kan, J.Y.; Rungcharassaeng, K.; Umezu, K.; Kois, J.C. Dimensions of peri-implant mucosa: An evaluation of maxillary anterior single implants in humans. *J. Periodontol.* **2003**, *74*, 557–562. [CrossRef] [PubMed]
10. Lindsay, M.A. MicroRNAs and the immune response. *Trends Immunol.* **2008**, *29*, 343–351. [CrossRef] [PubMed]
11. O'Connell, R.M.; Taganov, K.D.; Boldin, M.P.; Cheng, G.; Baltimore, D. MicroRNA-155 is induced during the macrophage inflammatory response. *Proc. Natl. Acad. Sci. USA* **2007**, *104*, 1604–1609. [CrossRef] [PubMed]
12. Iaculli, F.; Di Filippo, E.S.; Piattelli, A.; Mancinelli, R.; Fulle, S. Dental pulp stem cells grown on dental implant titanium surfaces: An in vitro evaluation of differentiation and micro-RNAs expression. *J. Biomed. Mater. Res. Part B. Appl. Biomater.* **2017**, *105*, 953–965. [CrossRef] [PubMed]
13. Sartori, E.M.; Magro-Filho, O.; Silveira Mendonça, D.B.; Li, X.; Fu, J.; Mendonça, G. Modulation of Micro RNA Expression and Osteoblast Differentiation by Nanotopography. *Int. J. Oral. Maxillofac. Implant* **2018**, *33*, 269–280. [CrossRef] [PubMed]

14. Chakravorty, N.; Ivanovski, S.; Prasadam, I.; Crawford, R.; Oloyede, A.; Xiao, Y. The micro-RNA expression signature on modified titanium implant surfaces influences genetic mechanisms leading to osteogenic differentiation. *Acta. Biomater.* **2012**, *8*, 3516–3523. [CrossRef] [PubMed]
15. Xie, F.; Shu, R.; Jiang, S.; Liu, D.; Zhang, X. Comparison of microRNA profiles of human periodontal diseased and healthy gingival tissues. *Int. J. Oral. Sci.* **2011**, *3*, 125–134. [CrossRef] [PubMed]
16. Sartori, E.M.; das Neves, A.M.; Magro-Filho, O.; Mendonça, D.B.S.; Krebsbach, P.H.; Cooper, L.F.; Mendonça, G. The Role of MicroRNAs in the Osseointegration Process. *Int. J. Oral. Maxillofac. Implant.* **2019**, *34*, 397–410. [CrossRef] [PubMed]
17. Albrektsson, T.; Canullo, L.; Cochran, D.; De Bruyn, H. "Peri-Implantitis": A Complication of a Foreign Body or a Man-Made "Disease". Facts and Fiction. *Clin. Implant Dent. Relat. Res.* **2016**, *18*, 840–849. [CrossRef] [PubMed]
18. Pesce, P.; Menini, M.; Tealdo, T.; Bevilacqua, M.; Pera, F.; Pera, P. Peri-implantitis: A systematic review of recently published papers. *Int. J. Prosthodont.* **2014**, *27*, 15–25. [CrossRef] [PubMed]
19. Menini, M.; Setti, P.; Pera, P.; Pera, F.; Pesce, P. Peri-implant tissue health and bone resorption in immediately loaded, implant-supported full-arch prostheses. *Int. J. Prosthodont.* **2018**, *31*, 327–333. [CrossRef] [PubMed]

10

Aseptic Ligatures Induce Marginal Peri-Implant Bone Loss—An 8-Week Trial in Rabbits

David Reinedahl [1,*], Silvia Galli [2], Tomas Albrektsson [2,3], Pentti Tengvall [3], Carina B. Johansson [1], Petra Hammarström Johansson [1] and Ann Wennerberg [1]

1 Department of Prosthodontics, Institute of Odontology, Sahlgrenska Academy, University of Gothenburg, Gothenburg 405 30, Sweden
2 Department of Prosthodontics, Faculty of Odontology, Malmö University, Malmö 205 06, Sweden
3 Department of Biomaterials, Institute of Clinical Sciences, Sahlgrenska Academy, University of Gothenburg, Gothenburg 405 30, Sweden
* Correspondence: d.reinedahl@gmail.com

Abstract: The clinical value of ligature-induced experimental peri-implantitis studies has been questioned due to the artificial nature of the model. Despite repeated claims that ligatures of silk, cotton and other materials may not induce bone resorption by themselves; a recent review showed that the tissue reaction toward them has not been investigated. Hence, the current study aimed to explore the hard and soft tissue reactions toward commonly used ligature materials. A total of 60 dental implants were inserted into the femur (n = 20) and tibia (n = 40) of 10 rabbits. The femoral implants were ligated with sterile 3-0 braided silk in one leg and sterile cotton retraction chord in the other leg. The tibial implants were ligated with silk or left as non-ligated controls. All wounds were closed in layers. After a healing time of 8 weeks, femoral (silk versus cotton) and proximal tibial (silk versus non-ligated control) implants were investigated histologically. Distal tibial (silk versus non-ligated control) implants were investigated with real time polymerase chain reaction (qPCR). The distance from the implant-top to first bone contact point was longer for silk ligated implants compared to non ligated controls (p = 0.007), but did not vary between cotton and silk. The ligatures triggered an immunological reaction with cell infiltrates in close contact with the ligature materials, adjacent soft tissue encapsulation and bone resorption. qPCR further demonstrated an upregulated immune response toward the silk ligatures compared to non-ligated controls. Silk and cotton ligatures provoke foreign body reactions of soft tissue encapsulation type and bone resorption around implants in the absence of plaque.

Keywords: ligature induced peri-implantitis; dental implant; marginal bone loss; osseointegration; aseptic loosening

1. Introduction

Dental implant therapy is a well-documented treatment for edentulism with an overall success rate of approximately 95% after 10 years [1]. A small degree of marginal bone resorption can often be observed during the first year of implant loading, probably due to tissue adaptation to the foreign material. Even though it is self-limiting in most cases, the marginal bone resorption sometimes progresses to the extent that the osseointegration becomes threatened. In a systematic review on implants with different surface types, Doornewaard et al., reported a 5% overall rate of implants with ≥3 mm of marginal bone loss after at least 5 years of function. They further indicated that smoking and a history of periodontitis yielded more bone loss [2]. With regards to treatment need, Albrektsson et al. reported that 2.7% of modern, moderately rough implants were either removed or subjected to other surgical procedures due to progressive marginal bone resorption during 7 to 16 years of follow up. [3].

In severe cases, continuous marginal bone loss may be locally detrimental to patients due to significant peri-implant bone defects that may impede future implant revision. Hence, animal models have been developed to study the onset and progression of marginal bone loss [4]. Such models have generally been based on the theory of peri-implantitis, which defines all marginal bone loss after osseointegration as solely a bacterial infection if coupled with bleeding from the peri-implant pocket in response to pocket probing [5].

The infectious peri-implantitis theory has been criticized for being narrow and exclusive of other potential causes for marginal bone resorption, such as poor implants, traumatic implantation or change of marginal conditions over time in response to wear products [6–8]. Furthermore, the marginal bone level has been shown to both increase and decrease around some implants over time, indicating a dynamic foreign body response to implants that may not require treatment, rather than a progressive infectious condition that demands intervention [9]. It has also been well-established that other types of endosseous implants that function in presumably sterile environments, such as hip and knee arthroplasties are equally susceptible to progressive bone loss and long-term failure (>10 years), as are transmucosal dental implants [10,11]. Aseptic loosening, caused by an immunological response to increasing amounts of wear debris at the bone-implant interface over time is believed to be the main cause of such late prosthetic joint failures [12,13].

In animal studies, undisturbed peri-implant plaque accumulation has resulted in negligible or absent marginal bone loss [14–16]. In order to speed up the process, a large majority of previous experimental peri-implantitis studies have therefore utilized sub-marginal ligatures of cotton, silk or other materials. Sub-marginal ligation has commonly resulted in significant bone loss after a few months, especially when the ligatures were replaced or added to in number every few weeks [17]. The ligature method aims to mimic infectious, clinical peri-implantitis and several authors have claimed that the utilized ligatures merely act as carriers of bacteria, without capacity to induce bone resorption by themselves [4,18,19]. In one of the very first ligature studies on implants, Lindhe et al. referred to a study that used silk ligatures in the periodontal tissues (natural teeth not implants) of germ free and conventional rats from 1966 to support this claim; however, none of the rats in either group lost any bone in that study [20]. The validity of the claim was further questioned in a recent systematic review by our group, in which we failed to identify any attempts to prove that ligatures cannot induce peri-implant bone resorption by themselves. Along with previous reviews on the method, we concluded that it remains unknown whether bone resorption can be induced by a foreign body reaction to the ligature materials themselves or the tissue trauma that results from their insertion [17,21,22]. An eventual capacity for ligatures to induce bone resorption in absence of bacteria would cast serious doubt on the clinical value of the method, especially when considering that ligation is an artificial manipulation that does not mimic any clinical condition, with the possible exception if someone unintentionally leaves a retraction chord in a peri-implant pocket, which, however, must be regarded a most unusual clinical error. Hence, a validation of the infectious model of explanation provided for the ligature method is warranted.

The aim of the current study was to evaluate the capacity of aseptic ligatures to induce peri-implant bone resorption in rabbits. We chose silk ligatures due to their common use in other small animals, i.e., rodents, as well as existing, relevant real time polymerase chain reaction (qPCR) data from one of these studies [23] and an ongoing aseptic silk ligature trial on rats, by another group at our faculty. The hard and soft tissue reactions against the silk ligatures were evaluated for tibial implants, with histological methods and also selected qPCR markers in order investigate the immunological activity of adjacent cells, as well as the local bone reactions. Furthermore, since no comparisons of different ligature materials have been published previously according to our knowledge, a histological comparison of silk and cotton ligatures was also performed on femoral implants. Our null hypothesis was that marginal ligatures should not be able to induce marginal bone loss in the absence of a bacterial plaque, as repeatedly claimed in previous ligature induced peri-implantitis studies [4,18,19].

2. Experimental Section

2.1. Implants

The implants used (Ospol Regular, Malmö, Sweden) were turned/machined (diameter 4 mm and length 8 mm) from rods of commercially pure titanium (grade 4) followed by an anodising process.

Surface Roughness

The implant surface roughness was characterized by white light interferometry, GBS, mbH, Ilmenau, Germany and MountainsMap Imaging Topography software (version 7.0, Digital Surf, Besancon, France). Three implants were measured on nine sites each: three tops, three valleys and three flanks. Each measurement had a size of 350 × 224 μm. Errors of form and waviness were removed with a Gaussian filter size of 50 × 50μm. Three parameters were selected to describe the surface, one height descriptive parameter (Sa), one spatial parameter (Sds) and one hybrid parameter (Sdr).

Sa is the average height deviation over the surface calculated from a mean plane. Calculated in μm.

Sds is the density of summits, expressed in number/mm^2.

Sdr is the increase in surface area compared to a completely flat area reference. Expressed in %.

2.2. Animal Model and Surgical Procedure

Ten male Swedish lop-eared rabbits with weight between 3.65 to 4.95 Kg were used in this experiment, with ethical approval (number 188-15) from the Regional Ethics Committee for Animal Research of Malmö/Lund, Sweden. All experiments were carried out in accordance with the rules and regulations of the Swedish Board of Agriculture. The number of the animals included in the study was selected after power analysis performed with G*Power software (version 3.1.9.4, Department of Psychology, University of Düsseldorf, Düsseldorf, Germany) to achieved a statistical power of 80%, given an α-error of 0.05 and an effect size of 0.8.

General anesthesia was induced by intramuscular injection of ketamin (Ketaminol; Intervet, Stockholm, Sweden) and dexmedetomidine (Dexdomitor; Orion Pharma Animal Health, Danderyd, Sweden) followed by subcutaneous injection of buprenorfin (Temgesic; Indivior, Berkshire, Great Britain).

The surgical site was shaved and cleaned with chlorhexidine ethanol solution 0.5 mg/mL (Klorhexidinsprit; Fresenius Kabi, Uppsala, Sweden) and covered with a sterile surgical drape. After injection of lidokain 10 mg/mL (Xylocain; Aspen Nordic, Ballerup, Denmark) at the surgical sites, the femoral and tibial metaphyseal plates were exposed by incision and dissection of covering tissue layers, including skin, muscle and periosteum on the medial side. A total of 60 implants ($n = 60$) were inserted according to Figure 1; one in each condylar metaphyseal plate and two in each tibial metaphyseal plate, with a center to center implant distance of 10 mm.

The implant insertion and ligature application technique are depicted in Figure 2. Osteotomies were performed with burrs of increasing diameter up to 3.5 mm under constant irrigation with physiological saline solution. After inserting the implants halfway, a single ligature loop of sterile 3-0 braided silk (Ethicon, Cincinnati, OH, USA) were tied with a surgical knot around the neck of the (i) right femoral, (ii) right proximal and (iii) left distal tibia implants of all rabbits. The ligature was then compressed between the implant neck and marginal bone, by finishing the fixture insertion. With an identical procedure, the left femoral implants were ligated with non-impregnated cotton gingival retraction cord (GingiKNIT non-impregnated; Kerr Dental, Bioggio, Switzerland). The right distal and left proximal implants were inserted without ligatures and used as controls. Multi-layered wound closure was performed with resorbable sutures in fascia and skin (Vicryl 3-0, Ethicon, Cincinatti, OH, USA) at all sites in order to ensure a submerged and non-contaminated healing environment for all implants.

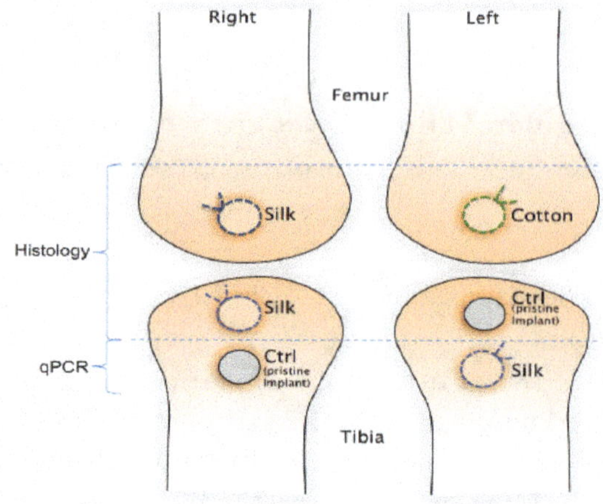

Figure 1. Schematic drawing of implant and ligature placement.

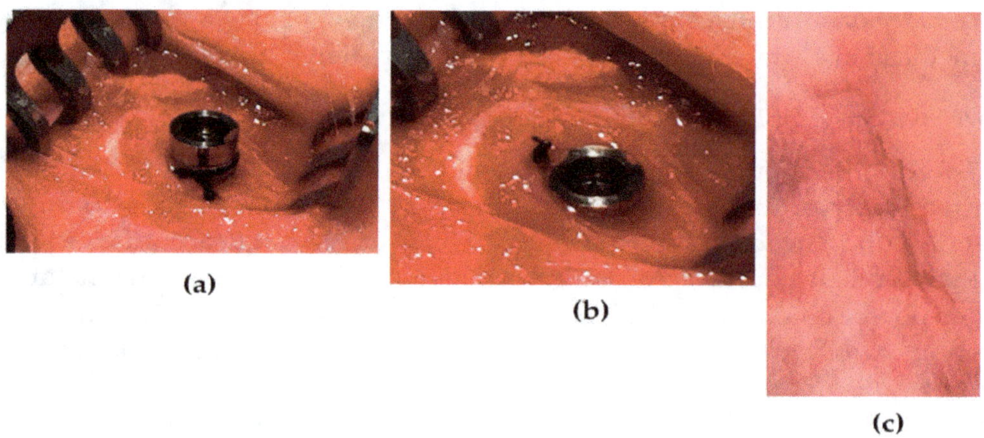

Figure 2. (**a**) Ligature tied around the implant neck after half-way insertion of the implant. (**b**) Ligature compressed against the bone by finishing the implant insertion. (**c**) Wound closure with interrupted resorbable sutures in a layered fashion.

At 8 weeks, the rabbits were sacrificed with a lethal injection of intra peritoneal pentobarbital (Euthasol; Virbac, Kolding, Denmark). Femoral- ($n = 20$) and proximal tibial ($n = 20$) implants were resected en bloc and directly immersed in 4% buffered formaldehyde (Merck, Darmstadt, Germany) for three days.

The distal tibia samples (tissues and implants) were harvested for gene expression analysis in the following way:

(i) The soft tissue that adhered to the implant margin was removed by a 6 mm punch after removing the cutis.
(ii) The implants were then unscrewed and the marginal bone trephined out using a 6 mm trephine.

These respective tissues were placed in RNA-later store in +4 °C overnight and then −20 °C until processing.

2.3. Histology

2.3.1. Histological Sample Preparation

Following the formalin fixation, the femoral ($n = 20$) and distal tibia ($n = 20$) samples were rinsed in tap water and then dehydrated in increasing concentrations of ethanol from 70% up to 99.9% (Solveco, Rosersberg, Sweden). The next steps involved pre-infiltration in diluted resin and pure resin followed by embedment in light-curing resin (Technovit 7200 VLC; Heraeus Kultzer, Wehrheim, Germany). All samples were divided in a similar direction i.e., in the center of the implant (in a longitudinal manner of the implant) using the cutting and grinding system, i.e., the ExaktR equipment (Exakt Apparatebau, Norderstedt, Germany). A central section of about 150–200 μm were cut. The samples were ground with Silicon carbide wet grinding papers of 800–1200 grit (Struers ApS, Ballerup, Denmark) to a final thickness of about 15 μm. The section surfaces were cleaned and dried prior to histological staining in toluidine blue mixed with pyronin G.

Finally, the sections were glass cover-slipped using a routine glue (Pertex, Histolab Products AB, Göteborg). The sample preparation related to the cutting and grinding procedure followed the routine laboratory-guidelines as deduced by Donath et al. [24] and Johansson and Morberg [25,26]

2.3.2. Histological Analysis: Qualitative and Quantitative

The histological sections were qualitatively and quantitatively investigated in a light microscope (L.M., Eclipse Nikon ME600, Nikon, Tokyo, Japan) by two of the authors: C.J. and D.R. Measurements were performed with the NIS-Elements D 64-bit software (version 3.2, Nikon Metrology, SARL, Lisses, France) using a 10× objective. Light microscopic (LM) images of the histological features were obtained with a Nikon DS-Ri1 camera (Nikon Instruments Inc. Meville, NY, USA). The first implant-bone contact was ascertained with a 40× objective.

The distance from the implant top to first bone contact was measured on both sides of each implant (anterior and posterior) sides. The difference between the distances for control versus test (silk ligatures) samples in the proximal tibia and for the cotton versus silk samples in the femur, were analyzed using non-parametric Wilcoxon Signed Rank with the pair considered as the control and test samples from the same rabbit. Statistical significance was set for $p < 0.05$. A level of 0.05 was selected for the α-error and the statistical significance was set for $p < 0.025$ after Bonferroni's adjustment for multiple calculations. A qualitative investigation of the marginal hard and soft tissues was also performed.

2.4. Gene Expression Analysis—qPCR

The samples for the gene expression analysis originated from the soft tissues that were in direct contact with the implant heads in the distal tibias and bone tissue that was adherent to the implants in distal tibia and constituted four study groups (soft tissues specimens from implants with and without ligature and bone specimens from implants with and without ligatures). A total of 32 samples (20 soft tissues and 12 bone tissue) were analyzed. The soft tissues were cut with sterile, disposable tissue punches of 6 mm diameter (1 punch per specimen) and dissected from the implant surface with a curette (Miltex, Inc. York, PA, USA).

The specimens were immediately placed in separate sterile plastic tubes containing RNA*later* solution (Ambion, Inc., Austin, TX, USA), for fixation. The samples were then stored at 4 °C overnight and further stored at −20 °C until processing.

2.4.1. mRNA Isolation

(This step is performed to purify the mRNA from the samples.)

mRNA isolation and qPCR amplification were performed at TATAA Biocenter, Gothenburg, Sweden.

Before mRNA isolation and extraction, the samples were thawed on ice. The samples were extracted using Qiazol (Cat.No 79306) and the RNeasy mini kit (Cat.No 74104) (Qiagen GmbH, Venlo, Netherlands) according to manufacturer's instructions.

Sample concentrations where determined using spectrophotometry (Dropsense, Trinean, Pleasanton, CA, USA) and RNA integrity was analyzed using capillary electrophoresis (Fragment Analyzer, Thermo Fisher Scientific, Waltham, MA, USA).

After extraction, the RNA was cleaned of inhibitory factors using the RNeasy MinElute Clean up kit (Qiagen GmbH, Venlo, Netherlands, Cat no. 74204).

2.4.2. Reverse Transcription (RT)

(This step produces complementary DNA (cDNA) to the mRNA isolated from the respective samples.)

RNA was reverse transcribed in single 20 μL reactions on all 32 samples.

Samples where first normalized to 33.33 ng/μL to reach a quantity of 500 ng RNA per tube that was loaded into the reaction. The RT was performed according to manufacturer's instructions with TATAA Grandscript cDNA synthesis kit Cat.No A103 (TATAA Biocenter AB, Gothenburg, Sweden), with the following concentration: 1 μL RT enzyme, 4 μL reaction mix, 15 μL normalized sample RNA.

2.4.3. Assays Design and Validation

(This step is performed to create short DNA fragments that are later used to determine each specific region of DNA to be copied, in this case the regions that encode the proteins of interest for the study.)

Eleven assays where designed and validated by TATAA (according to SOP 009 ver 1.2 SOP 001 ver1.4) (Validation plan qPCR assay validation). A list of all assays can be found in Table 1. For validation, a control genomic DNA (gDNA) from male rabbit (Zyagen) and a pool of all the cDNA samples was used. Seven-point standard curves in 10-fold dilutions were run for all the assays, in quadruplicates. The annealing temperature was set to 60 °C for all assays. PCR products; gDNA, cDNA, selected standard point and NTC were then run on Fragment Analyzer using the DNF-910-33-DNA 35-1500bp kit (Thermo Fisher Scientific, Waltham, MA, USA) to check the product lengths and primer specificity. The qPCR data for the assay validation was analysed with GenEx software (version 6, MultiD Analyses AB, Göteborg, Sweden) to calculate the efficiencies and performance of the assays with a confidence interval of 95%.

Table 1. Gene sequences and biological entity.

Primer	Forward Sequence	Reverse Sequence	Accession Number	Biological Entity
ACTβ	GAGATGCCATGTGACGGAAG	TTACACAAATGCGATGCTGC	NM_001101683.1	Reference gene
ALPL	ACTGTGGACTACCTCTTG	GGTCAGTGATGTTGTTCC	XM_017346489	Bone mineralization
ARG1	GGATCATTGGAGCCCCTTTCTC	TCAAGCAGACCAGCCTTTCTC	NM_001082108.1	M2 macrophage
C5aR1	ACGTCAACTGCTGCATCAACC	AGGCTGGGGAGAGACTTGC	NM_017338812.1	The complement system
CD11β	TTCAACCTGGAGACTGAGAACAC	TCAAACTGGACCACGCTCTG	XM_008248697.2	M1 macrophage
CD19	GGATGTATGTCTGTCGCCGT	AAGCAAAGCCACAACTGGAA	NM_002711879.3	B lymphocytes
CD4	CAACTGGAAACATGCGAACCA	TTGATGACCAGGGGAAAGA	NM_008254148.2	T lymphocytes
CD8	GGCGTCTACTTCTGCATGACC	GAACCGGCACACTCTCTTCT	NM_008254148.2	T lymphocytes
GAPDH	CCGAGACACGATGGTGAAGG	TGTAGACCATGTAGTGGAGGTCA	NM_001082253.1	Reference gene
IL8	CTTTTTGCCCTGACCATGCC	TCCTTCACAAGCGAGACCAC	NM_001171082.1	Macrophage
LDHA	ACAAGTGCACAAACAAGTGGT	AGAGCCCCTTAAGCATGGTG	NM_001082277	Reference gene
MCP1	GCTCATAGCAGTCGCCTTCA	CATGAAGATCACAGCTTCTTTGGG	NM_001082294	Macrophage fusion
NCF1	TTCATCCGCCACATTGCCC	GTCCTGCCACTTCACCAAGA	XM_001082102.1	Neutrophil
OC	AGAGTCTGGCAGAGGCTCAG	TCGCTTCACCACCTCGCT	XM_002715383	Bone mineralization
CTSK	ACTCTGAAGATGCCTACCCCT	TTCAGGGCTTTCTCATTCCCC	NM_001082641	Bone resorption
FGF2	ATCTACACTGTGGAGCTTGCAG	TCATGCGGTCACACACTTCC	XM_002711077	Fibroblast
IL1β	TCCTTGGTGTTGTCTGGCAC	GGCCACAGGTATCTTGTCGTT	NM_001082201	M1 macrophage
IL6	GAGGAAAGAGATGTGTGACCAT	AGCATCCGTCTTCTTCTATCAG	NM_001082064	M1 macrophage
VEGFα	CTTGGGTGCATTGGAGCCTT	CTTCACCACTTCGTGGGTTTA	XM_017345155	Endothelial cells
TNFα	CTCTTTCCTGCTCGTGGCTG	GGAGGTTGTTTGGGGACTCTT	NM_001082263	M1 Macrophage
TRAP	CTGGGTTTGCAGGAGTTG	TTGAAGAGCAGCGACAGA	NM_001081988	Bone resorption

ACTβ, β-actin (reference gene); ALPL, alkaline phosphatase; ARG1, arginase 1; C5aR1, complement C5a Receptor 1; CD11β, macrophage marker CD11β; CD19, B-lymphocyte surface protein CD19; CD4, T-cell surface glycoprotein CD4; CD8, T-cell transmembrane glycoprotein CD8; GAPDH, glyceraldehyde 3-phosphate dehydrogenase (reference gene); IL8, interleukin 8 receptor alpha; LDHA, lactate dehydrogenase A (reference gene); MCP1, monocyte chemotactic and activating factor; NCF1, neutrophil cytosolic factor; OC, osteocalcin; CTSK, Cathepsin K; FGF2, fibroblast growth factor 2; IL1β, interleukin 1 beta; IL6, interleukin 6; VEGFα, vascular endothelial growth factor alpha; TNFα, tumor necrosis factor alpha; TRAP, Triiodothyronine receptor auxiliary protein.

2.4.4. Real-Time Quantitative Polymerise Chain Reaction (RT-qPCR)

(This final step monitors the amplification of the selected DNA segments in real time and enables the researcher to quantify the amount of each DNA segment at the start of the reaction.)

The cDNA samples were diluted 10× to have enough volume and were then analyzed using TATAA SYBR GrandMaster® Mix Cat. No. TA01-625 (TATAA Biocenter AB, Gothenburg, Sweden). Five μl of TATAA SYBR Green Master Mix, 0.4 μL of Primer (forward & reverse), 2.6 μL of nuclease-free water and 2 μL of cDNA templates were used for each reaction mix. All pipetting was performed by a pipetting robot (EpMotion 5070, Eppendorf, Germany). Duplicate NTCs were included for all the assays and cDNA samples were run in duplicate reactions. Universal ValidPrime assay, Cat No. A107P (TATAA Biocenter AB, Göteborg, Sweden) was used to compensate for possible gDNA contamination.

The quantification was performed using the LightCycler 480 (Roche, Basel, Switzerland) and detection was performed in the SYBR channel. Cq values were based on the second derivative maximum threshold method. Inter-plate calibrator, IPC Cat. No. IPC250 (TATAA Biocenter AB, Göteborg, Sweden) was run on each plate to be able to correct for inter-run differences. qPCR raw data were pre-processed and analyses with GenEx software (version 6, MultiD Analyses AB, Gothenburg, Sweden) and were thereafter imported in Qbase+ software (version 3.1, Biogazelle, Zwijnaarde, Belgium) for calibrated normalized relative quantification of the gene expression. Three assays were used as reference genes (ACTB, GAPDH and LDHA) and their quality as reference genes was assessed with the GeNorm algorithm.

2.4.5. Statistical Analysis

The gene expression results were reported as calibrated normalized relative quantities (CNRQ). Mean and 95% confidence intervals were reported for each assay for each group.

The difference in mean between the test (silk ligated implants) and the control (pristine Ti-implant) groups in the soft tissue samples and between the test and control groups in the bone samples were analyzed using non-parametric Wilcoxon Signed Rank. The test and control samples from the same rabbit were considered as paired. The level of α-error was set to 0.05 and statistical significance was adjusted according to Bonferroni´s method for multiple testing; therefore, it was set to $p < 0.0027$.

3. Results

3.1. Clinical Appearance at Sacrifice

The tissue harvesting procedure is shown in Figure 3. Uneventful healing and primary wound closure were achieved in all cases. Dissection of the tissues revealed no pus or other signs of infection around the implants. Exposure of the bone adjacent to the implants revealed small saucerization-like defects around most ligated implants and sometimes callus formation lateral to the ligatures. Some control implants presented with callus formation lateral to the implants, but no saucerization-like bone defects were noted.

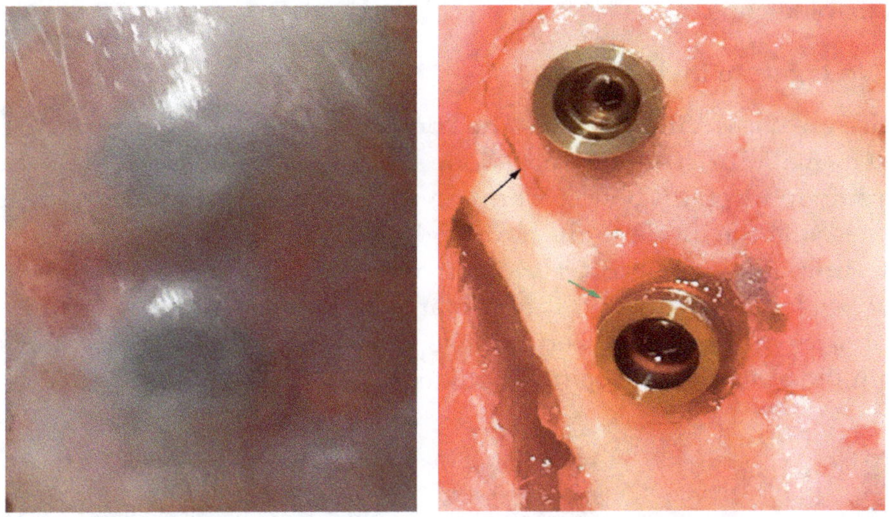

(a) (b)

Figure 3. (**a**) The soft tissue covering a tibial control implant (superior) and test implant (inferior) after removal of skin and subcutaneous tissues. (**b**) A small saucerization-like defect (green arrow) visible after removal of the silk ligature around the inferior implant and callus formation (black arrow) around the superior control implant.

3.2. Histological Results

3.2.1. Histomorphometrical Results

One implant with a cotton ligature was excluded from the histomorphometrical analysis due to a superior displacement of the ligature and unfavorable implant location that engaged the dorsal femoral bone plate and showed non-union of the implant on that side. The distance from the implant top to first bone contact was significantly longer for test implants ligated with silk compared to controls ($p = 0.007$) (Figure 4). This difference was due to the combined effect of bone resorption inferior to the ligatures in the test implants and also bone gain due to callus formation adjacent to protrusive implant tops in some control implants. The difference between implants ligated with silk or cotton was not statistically significant ($p = 0.37$).

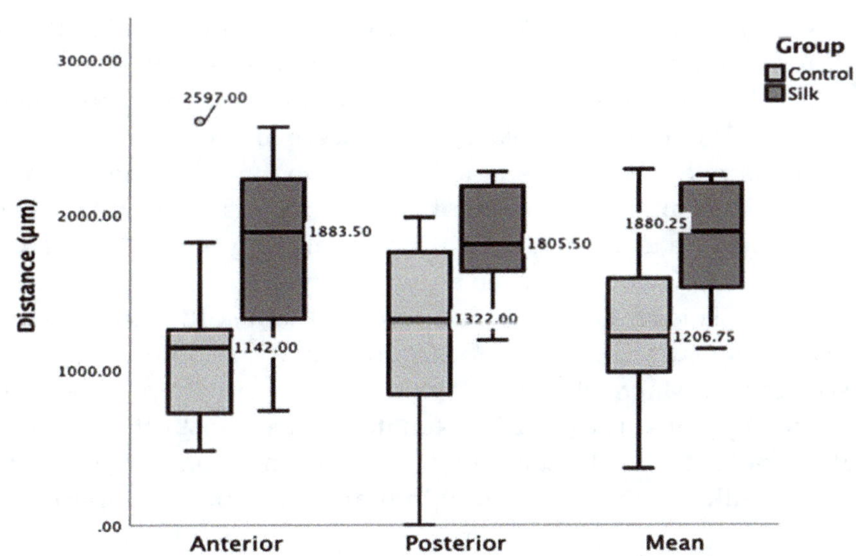

Figure 4. Box-plot showing the distance from implant top to first bone-to-implant contact for implants with silk ligatures (Silk) and pristine implants (Control).

3.2.2. Qualitative Histological Results

Control Implants (No Ligature Involved)

Control samples are shown in Figure 5. The control samples demonstrated both periosteal and endosteal new bone formation. The old cortical bone surfaces, observed in regions close to the implant, were undergoing remodeling with bone forming and bone resorption areas present. Most control sections demonstrated that the implant interface regions consisted of new formed bone with various amounts of bone-to-implant contact (BIC) and active bone forming regions (bone tissue covered by osteoid with osteoblasts visible) close to the implant. In some sections, multinucleated giant cells (MNGCs) of various sizes could be observed in close vicinity to metal oxide debris and particles (most likely detached from the bulk implant being anodized).

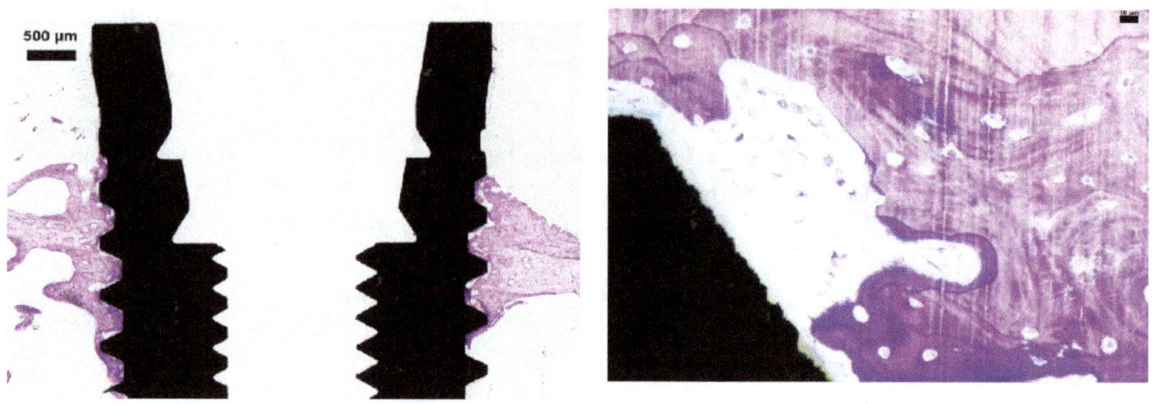

(a) (b)

Figure 5. (**a**) A typical example of a control sample (no ligature involved) with darker stained periosteal and endosteal new bone formation. (**b**) This figure illustrates seemingly an ongoing bone remodeling region with clear demarcation between old bone (lighter stained) and younger bone (larger osteocytes and a bit darker stained bone tissue). Possibly some macrophages can be observed in the region closer to the implant.

Test Implants (Ligated with Silk or Cotton)

Silk samples are shown in Figure 6. The silk samples demonstrated soft tissue encapsulation of the material with capsules of varying thickness and sometimes also distant bony encapsulation. The capsules appeared both as a "loose" and a "tight" formation with macrophages of various sizes as the dominating cell type. Possibly some plasma-cells were also part of the cell population in such regions. One section demonstrated loosened single silk fibers in the soft tissue region appearing as being encapsulated by a rather thick formation of macrophages of various sizes and shapes. The silk material was not in contact with bone and a capsule formation separating bone and silk could sometimes be observed. In five samples, MNGCs could be seen as long elongated rims that captured the silk material (i.e., foreign body reaction). This rim of cells was involved in a soft tissue space that separated the bone from the silk. The bone surfaces, at some distance away, showed signs of resorption but no osteoclasts could be observed. Macrophages of various sizes and shapes were observed in the soft tissue regions close to the implant surface. The silk material was most often located "above" the bone surface, seemingly glued onto the implant, compared to cotton being "spread out". One silk sample demonstrated a shell/dome-like bone formation with marrow tissue at the periosteal side.

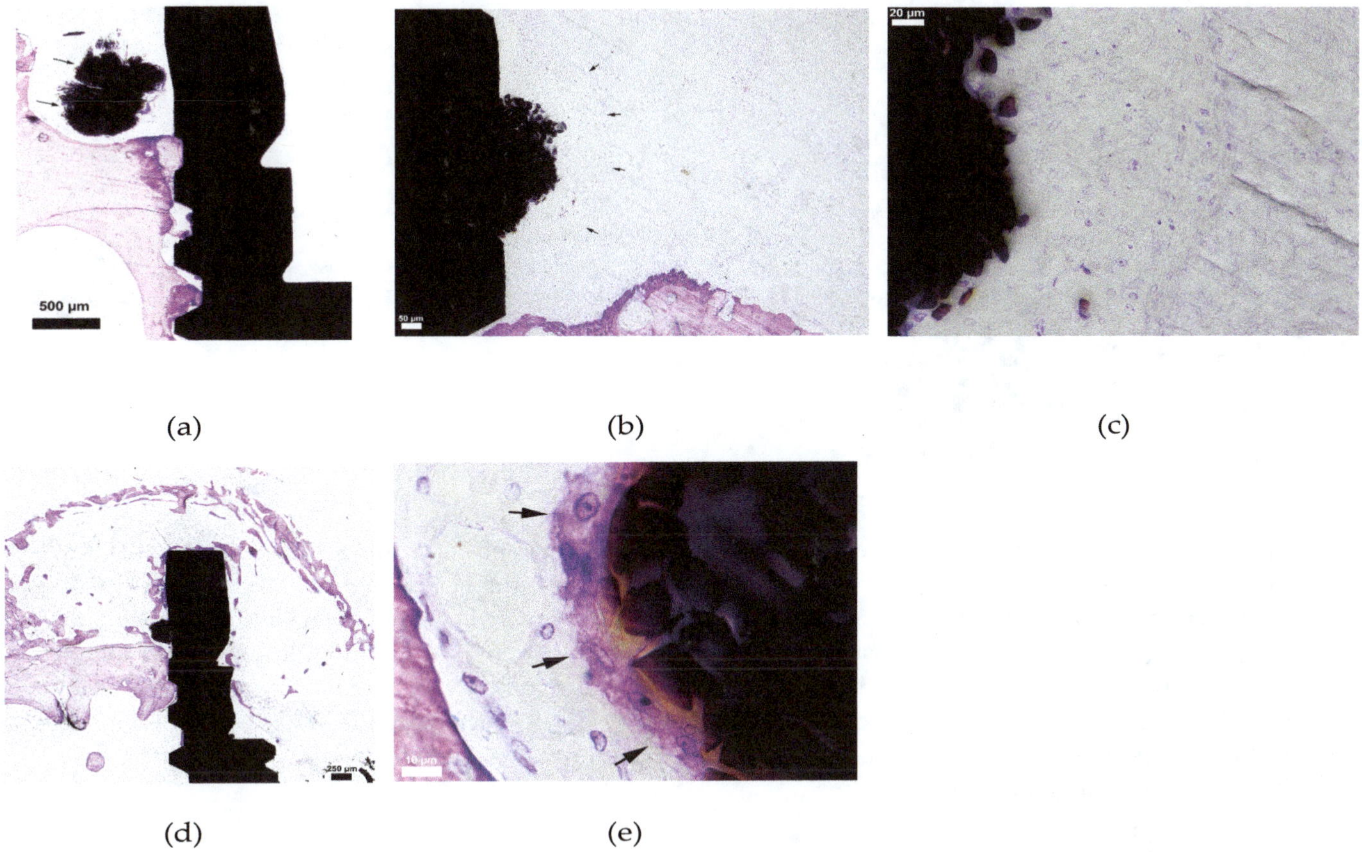

Figure 6. Sample figures from different silk sections. (**a**) Survey figure of a typical section with a silk ligature (arrows) above a partly resorbed cortical bone surface in the periosteal region. (**b**) In some cases, the silk ligatures (in close contact to the implant) were surrounded by a thick cellular infiltrate layer (arrows) dominated by macrophages of various sizes and shapes. Outside this formation, loose connective tissue was formed. (**c**) The same section in higher resolution. (**d**) This figure illustrates a rather large "dome-like" callus formation of the periosteal bone and it seems like the implant part above the silk ligature is almost covered by new formed bone. (**e**) The arrows illustrate a large, elongated multinucleated giant cell (MNGC) in intimate contact with the silk.

Cotton samples are shown in Figure 7. The majority of the sections of the cotton material could be observed as "huge loosened regions" with the material encapsulated by soft tissue situated above the periosteal bone surface. The capsule itself was often surrounded by bone trabecula and the interface between the periosteal bone surface and soft tissue seemed to undergo resorption, with regions of "mouse-eaten" bone; however, no osteoclasts could be observed. Cotton demonstrated a larger diameter of the material than silk, with several separate "cotton rolls" visible both at a distance from the implant and in close contact, compared to the silk. No active bone forming surface (i.e., osteoid rim with osteoblasts) could be observed close to the soft tissue. Although the bone surface, in general, seemed to be resorbed ("mouse-eaten" surface) no osteoclasts were visible, except in one cotton-section. In higher magnification MNGCs could be observed in close vicinity to cotton. Macrophages were also visible but seemingly in less amount (albeit not counted) compared to silk. Cotton seemed to have a greater soft tissue area surrounding the material compared to silk, which possibly indicated a higher degree of encapsulation of cotton compared to silk.

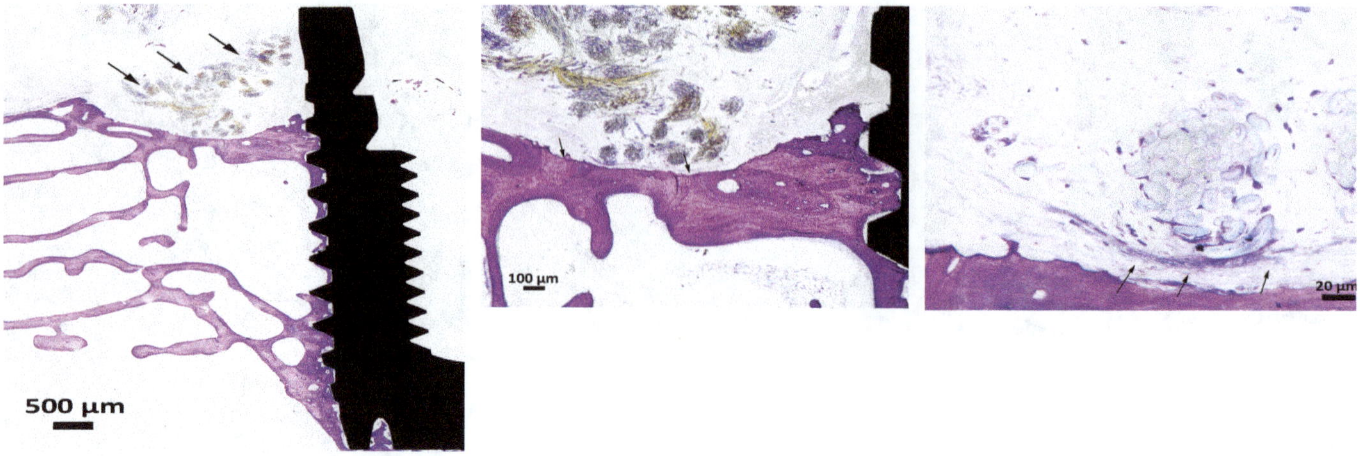

(a) (b) (c)

Figure 7. Three images from one cotton section with arrows showing the cotton ligature. (**a**) An illustration of a typical section with cotton suture situated above the periosteal bone. (**b**) The periosteal bone surface is separated from the cotton ligature by a soft tissue layer and the bone surface appears to be resorbed (arrows), although no osteoclasts could be observed. (**c**) The amount of macrophages in the soft tissue between the bone and the cotton seemed to be less compared to the silk sections. However, macrophages were visible as being more spread out and "darker" compared to silk samples. None of the cotton samples demonstrated a typical MNGC formation and the "encapsulation" of cotton was often loosely arranged (arrows).

3.3. Gene Expression Results

The expression of a panel of genes in the soft tissue around titanium implants either left pristine (control) or treated with a silk ligature placed around the implant neck (test) was evaluated with RT-qPCR. The relative expressions of the selected markers are presented in Table 2 and Figure 8 for soft tissue and in Table 3 and Figure 9 for bone tissue.

Table 2. Relative expression of the selected gene targets in the soft tissues around implants with silk ligature versus the soft tissues around controls (no ligature involved).

Target Gene	Relative Expression in Test versus Control	95% CI Low	95% CI High	*p*-Value
NCF1	4.9	1.9	12.4	0.008
CD11β	2.8	1.5	5.4	0.016
CD4	2.3	1.7	3.1	0.016
VEGFα	1.6	1.0	2.5	0.05
TNFα	1.7	0.9	2.9	0.08
ARG1	2.4	0.9	6.5	0.11
IL8	0.5	0.2	1.2	0.11
FGF2	0.8	0.5	1.2	0.11
CD8	3.9	0.5	27.4	0.22
CD19	2.1	0.5	12.3	0.22
OC	1.7	0.7	4.2	0.25
C5aR1	1.3	0.9	2.0	0.31
TRAP	1.7	0.5	5.4	0.37
IL1β	0.7	0.2	2.5	0.58
IL6	0.8	0.3	2.5	0.58
ALPL	1.2	0.5	3.1	0.64
MCP1	0.9	0.3	2.8	0.84
CTSK	1.0	0.7	1.5	0.84

CI = confidence interval. *p*-value was calculated with Wilcoxon Signed Rank test, significance level was set to $p \leq 0.0027$ after Bonferroni´s adjustment for multiple testing. No gene showed significant difference in expression.

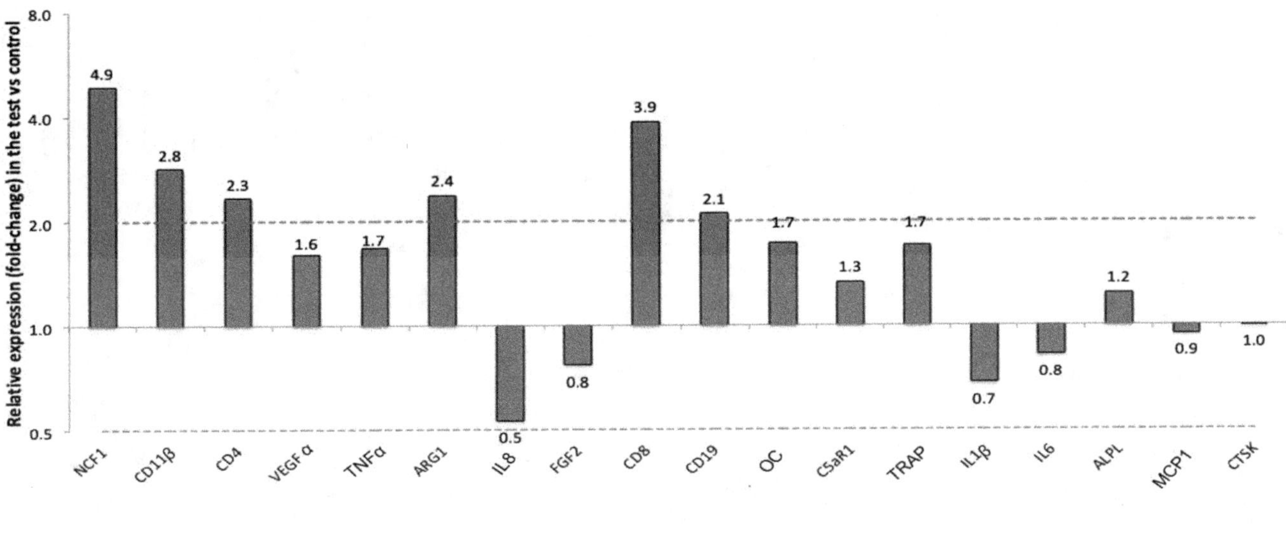

Figure 8. Up and down regulation of the selected markers in the soft tissues around implants with silk ligatures versus controls (no ligature).

Table 3. Relative expression of the selected gene targets in the bone around implants with silk ligature versus the bone around controls (no ligature).

Target Gene	Relative Expression in Test versus Control	95% CI Low	95% CI High	*p*-Value
IL6	0.1	0.0	0.9	0.04
CTSK	0.7	0.5	1.0	0.04
OC	0.6	0.4	1.1	0.07
NCF1	3.5	0.8	15.2	0.07
MCP1	2.2	0.8	5.9	0.08
CD19	2.7	0.6	12.3	0.13
CD11β	2.6	0.6	12.2	0.14
TNFα	0.4	0.1	2.3	0.19
FGF2	0.6	0.2	1.6	0.19
IL1β	2.1	0.5	8.8	0.19
IL8	0.5	0.1	2.4	0.26
C5aR1	1.9	0.4	9.3	0.28
CD4	2.6	0.3	25.0	0.28
CD8	1.4	0.4	5.2	0.42
TRAP	2.2	0.1	40.0	0.46
VEGFα	1.8	0.2	20.4	0.49
ALPL	0.8	0.2	4.4	0.76

CI = confidence interval. *p*-value calculated with Wilcoxon Signed Rank test, significance level was set to $p \leq 0.0027$ after Bonferroni´s adjustment for multiple testing. No gene showed significant difference in expression.

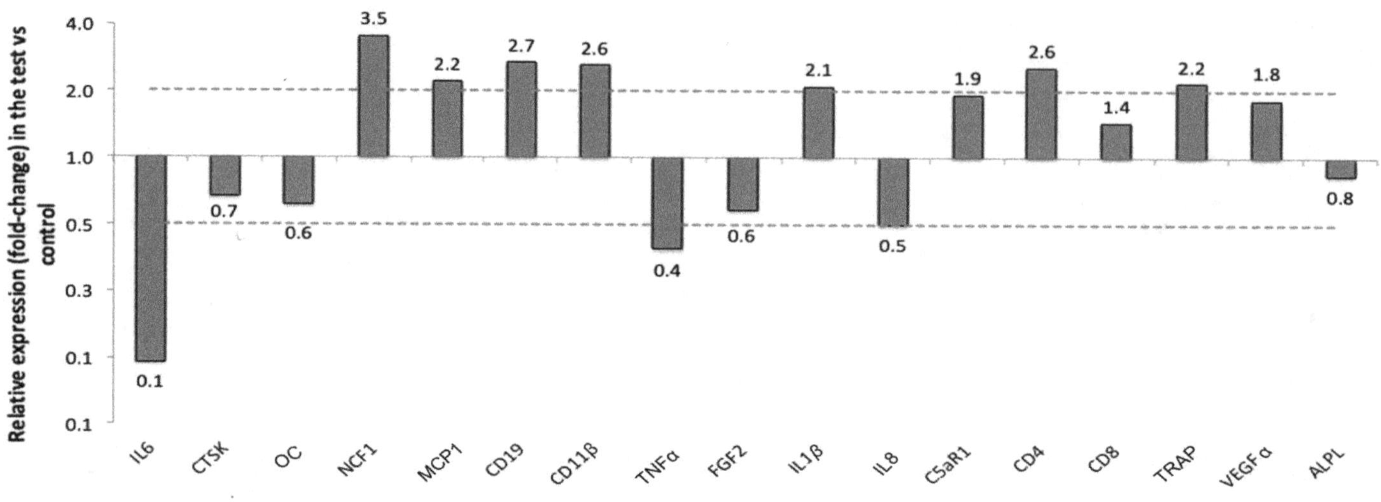

Figure 9. Up and down regulation of the selected markers in the bone around implants with silk ligatures versus controls (no ligature).

In the soft tissues near the silk ligature, several genes mediating reactions of immune cells were more than two-folds up-regulated compared to the controls. Those were NCF1 (CNRQ 4.9), which is specific for neutrophils, CD8 (CNRQ 3.9), which is a marker for T-lymphocytes, CD11β (CNRQ 2.8), a M1 macrophages marker, ARG1 (CNRQ 2.4), a marker for M2 macrophages, CD4 (CNRQ 2.3), which is another gene specific for T-lymphocytes, and CD19 (CNRQ 2.1), which is associated with B-lymphocytes. One gene, IL8, related to macrophages was two-folds down-regulated in the tests versus the controls. None of the markers reached a level of significance of $p \leq 0.0025$ in expression between the tests and the controls, which was the adjusted p-value (Table 2, Figure 8).

In the bone surrounding the implants ligated with silk, six genes related to the immune response were expressed more than two-folds compared to the bone surrounding pristine implants. Of those, four were the same that were overexpressed in the soft tissues near the ligatures: NCF1 (CNRQ 3.5), CD19 (CNRQ 2.7), CD11β (CNRQ 2.6) and CD4 (CNRQ 2.6). Other genes up-regulated in the bone of the test samples were MCP1 (CNRQ 2.2), which is related to macrophage fusion, ILβ1 (CNRQ 2.1) which is another gene related to M1 macrophages, and Triiodothyronine receptor auxiliary protein (TRAP) (CNRQ 2.2), which is an osteoclast marker for bone resorption.

Three genes were instead two-folds or more down-regulated in the bone around the test implants compared to the controls. They were IL6 (CNRQ 0.1), which is a cytokine related to inflammation, but also to bone formation [1], TNFα (CNRQ 0.4), another cytokine related to inflammation, and IL8 (CNRQ 0.5), which is related to macrophages and that was down-regulated also in the soft tissues of the test implants. None of these investigated genes in the bone reached a level of significant difference in expression for $p \leq 0.0025$ (Table 3, Figure 9).

4. Discussion

The current study described marginal peri-implant bone and soft tissue reactions to marginal silk and cotton ligatures without plaque accumulation. Our findings present clear criticism to the present interpretation of ligature models that they verify bacteria to be the initiating problem behind marginal bone loss. In reality, previous claims that ligatures induce bone loss solely by plaque accumulation and not by themselves are incorrect [4,18,26]. The present findings also raise questions as to what extent potential clinical provocations may also induce bone loss. Consider for example apically displaced cementum residues, unsuitable, lose or ill-fitting abutments or increasing amounts of wear debris in peri-implant tissues over time. Indeed, wear particles of both cementum and titanium has been found in abundance in human biopsies of peri-implantitis lesions [27]. Furthermore, the possible role of sterile Ti debris in the development of soft tissue inflammation and marginal bone resorption was recently demonstrated by Wang et al., who showed marginal bone resorption around submerged titanium implants in Sprauge Dawley rats and also demonstrated a role of M1 macrophages in that process. [28]. Future studies may strive to provide more knowledge about potential aseptic causes for marginal bone resorption, with the ultimate goal to prevent and treat such conditions.

As described by Donath et al., the body will always strive to alienate an implanted material by rejection, dissolution, resorption, demarcation (i.e., fibrous or bony encapsulation) or a combination of these reactions [29]. The type and extent of the immunological response has been shown to depend on multiple factors, such as material type, surface characteristics, type of receiving tissue, degree of surgical trauma, micromovement between material and host and other factors [7,29]. From studies on osteoimmunology we know that focal bone loss is achieved by osteoclasts when activated by adjacent inflammation, and that TNFα is likely the most significant inflammatory cytokine necessary to activate the osteoclasts [30]. TNFα is expressed in the acute inflammatory response against many types of provocations, such as surgical trauma or presence of infectious microorganisms, necrotic tissue or certain foreign materials. Hence, bone resorption can be expected to occur from almost any type of adjacent, pro-inflammatory provocation of a certain magnitude and may also be continuous if the provocation is sustained or repeated. In experimental peri-implantitis, this is well-exemplified by the rapid marginal bone loss that often occurs when ligatures are frequently exchanged and new ligatures are pushed apically towards the bone, as compared to the frequent self-containing resorption that often occurs from non-exchanged ligatures [17].

The extensive, macrophage-dominated infiltrates adjacent to the silk and cotton ligatures in the present study demonstrates a stronger inflammatory reaction to the ligatures compared to non-ligated control implants, which may likely explain the resorbed bone defects frequently found adjacent to the ligatures. Macrophages can initiate bone resorption in different ways: indirectly by secretion of pro-inflammatory cytokines that stimulate osteoclast generation and activation as described above [30] or directly by the secretion of certain matrix metalloproteinases that can degrade bone matrix [31]. However, the present study demonstrated a late stage foreign body reaction, with fibrous encapsulation of the ligatures, lack of up-regulation of the pro-inflammatory cytokine markers for TNFα, IL1β and IL6 in the soft tissues around them and seemingly arrested bone resorption as evident by the lack of osteoclasts in the resorbed bone defects adjacent to them. This late stage reaction was likely due to the long healing time of 8 weeks and is consistent with the previous findings of Setzen et al., who reported a quite extensive inflammatory response to black braided silk sutures during the first few weeks, followed by the thickest fibrous capsule formation compared to 10 other suture types inserted subcutaneously in rabbits [32]. Recent findings by Nguyen et al. suggested that active bone resorption occurs much earlier, even when plaque accumulation is allowed. In their recent experimental peri-implantitis study in mice, high expression levels of TNFα and IL1 were observed during the first 2 weeks after application of plaque accumulating 5-0 silk-ligatures, followed by a subsequent decrease back to baseline levels after 4 weeks. Simultaneously, the number of osteoclasts and rate of marginal bone resorption both decreased towards the end of the study at 4 weeks [23]. The tissue reactions to strictly bacterial assaults also share many similarities, and is perhaps best exemplified by the closed confines of the periapical bone, when provoked by endodontic pathogens. As explained by Nair et al., the endodontic pathogens typically trigger an acute inflammatory reaction with simultaneous active bone resorption, followed by a chronic stage, or equilibrium, with arrested bone resorption and a dense fibrous capsule that shields off the inflammatory infiltrate from the bone while it continues to hold back the infection [33]. New acute episodes may then be triggered years later, in response to changed local or systemic circumstances.

In contrast to the complex combined assault of repeated mechanic tissue trauma, hostile ligatures and hostile bacteria provided by classical experimental peri-implantitis, the present study demonstrated the isolated capacity of silk and cotton ligature to initiate bone loss. While the distance from the implant top to the first bone contact point varied significantly between silk and controls, the difference between silk and cotton was not significant. However, the fact that the soft tissue capsules that separated the ligatures from the bone were thicker around cotton than silk, may indicate a more consistent bone resorption against cotton. Future studies could benefit from a histomorphometrical method, which unfortunately cannot be performed successfully on non-decalcified, resin-embedded, cut-and-ground sections. The difference in bone loss between similar study subjects (the rabbits in our study) conforms to the findings of traditional ligature induced peri-implantitis studies, where the time to achieve a certain amount of bone loss has also varied greatly [34,35]. These differences are likely due to both immunological differences between animals, as indicated by recent knock out models [36], as well as methodological aspects such as possible variations in the distance between ligature and bone at the time of ligation. The choice of a rabbit model in the present study makes it difficult to compare the present results to those of previous studies that used different mammals as experimental models, considering the great differences in the resulting bone loss for different animal species [17]. For example, Beagle dogs have shown >3 mm of bone loss after 10-weeks with ligatures [37], while monkeys have sometimes required a year of regularly exchanged ligatures to induce 1 mm of bone loss [15].

Another important difference between the present and previous studies was the simultaneous implant and ligature insertion, as opposed to the few months of implant healing before ligation utilized in the majority of previous studies. Jovanovic et al. demonstrated that the amount of marginal bone loss and configuration of peri-implant pockets did not differ from ligation at implant placement compared to a preceding 3 months implant healing time [38].

Although the impact of the ligature has often been overlooked in ligature induced peri-implantitis studies, as evident from the fact that some authors have not specified any details about the type of material used [39,40], information about the ligature materials can be found from other research fields. The most commonly used ones are the organic materials cotton and silk. In surgery, cotton gauze sponges are used to soak up fluids and maintain the surgical field, but are then carefully removed from the tissues due to their capacity to provoke extensive foreign body reactions. When extensive, these foreign body reactions can manifest themselves as tumor-like lesions referred to as cotton-ballomas or gossypibomas. In some cases, these lesions have induced significant bone resorption and may then mimic an osteolytic tumour such as a sarcoma [41,42]. A study on mice also showed that even microscopic remnants of sterile cotton may induce foreign body reactions when left in a surgical wound [43].

Silk, on the other hand, has been used as a suture material for over a century, and the black, braided silk sutures used in the present study are made from fibroin, extracted from virgin Bombyx mori silk in a process that separates the fibroin from a second, glue-like protein called sericin [44]. In addition to fibroin, the utilized suture type also contains a beeswax coating. It is unknown to what extent this particular coating affects the immunological response, but it should be noted that beeswax is the main ingredient of bone wax, a product used to stop osseous bleeding during surgery and well known to arrest bone healing and induce significant foreign body reactions [45]. Older pre-1980s silk sutures contained both fibroin and sericin and were known to induce considerable acute and chronic inflammatory responses, as well as frequent late allergic reactions. Modern fibroin type silk sutures very rarely induce allergy, but still elicit a relatively strong acute inflammatory reaction in the early healing phase. Silk also undergoes slow proteolytic degradation, even though the sutures are defined as non-resorbable [44,46]. Spelzini et al., compared two types of fibroin silk implants with a polypropylene implant for fascial repair in mice and reported a somewhat stronger acute inflammatory reaction to the silk implants, followed by a much stronger chronic inflammatory response with progressive accumulation of chronic inflammatory cells up until 30 days that remained virtually unchanged after 90 days. They also reported a high initial presence of polymorphnuclear neutrophil (PMN) cells, which subsequently dropped in numbers with time but still remained in smaller numbers after 90 days [46].

The clinical significance of the PCR results of the present study must be considered in light of the histological sections and the evident late healing stage and arrested bone resorption described above. It must also be kept in mind that the PCR results only demonstrate the difference between test (silk ligature) and control (no ligature) implants, and hence do not show the immunological reaction to the Ti-implants that were identical for tests and controls. For example, CD11β was 2.8 times upregulated in the present study but 13 times upregulated in response to Ti compared to sham after 28 days in a previous rabbit study, which suggests a pronounced immunological reaction dominated by macrophages to Ti that was masked in the present study design [47]. Additional biopsies at baseline or from untouched distant tissues at sacrifice may facilitate the interpretation in future studies. Regarding the bone specimens, the small differences between tests and controls may in part be due to the harvesting technique, considering that the entire implants + surrounding bone were harvested and analyzed, while only a very small marginal portion of them was ever in contact with the ligatures.

With the above factors in mind, the more than two-fold upregulation of the soft tissue markers NCF1, CD11β, and CD4, ARG1, CD8 and CD19 for silk ligated test implants compared to pristine implants demonstrated a greater activation of the immune response in the test compared to the controls that corresponded to the chronic inflammatory cell infiltrates present around the ligatures. The upregulation of CD11β and ARG1 indicate a mixed M1/M2 phenotype of the macrophages in this tissue. CD4 and CD8 upregulation indicate T-cell presence. T-cells play a key role in antigen specific defense, but are also involved in foreign body reactions in absence of known antigens [48]. Their increased presence in the present study may correspond to the larger number of adherent macrophages and MNGCs on the silk ligatures as compared to controls (Ti), as demonstrated by Brodbeck et al., who described that lymphocytes (mainly CD8+ T-cells and CD4+ T-cells) "rosetted around" biomaterial-adherent macrophages and MNGCs in a co-cell culture study [48]. The authors further demonstrated that the presence of lymphocytes augmented macrophage adherence to biomaterials as well as MNGC-fusion, when both cell types were present from the start of the in vitro experiment [48]. However, a later study on T-cell deficient mice demonstrated a seemingly normal foreign body response with adhesion and fusion of macrophages to an implanted material even in absence of T-cells, which indicates that, while present, T-cells are probably not necessary for a normal foreign body reaction to occur [49]. The prolonged neutrophil presence in soft tissue indicated by upregulation of NCF1 further indicates a more pronounced foreign body reaction to the silk ligatures than controls (no ligature involved). Recent studies demonstrate a long-term role of neutrophils in foreign body reactions, as well as a capacity for them to regulate the long term reaction toward an implant [50]. Jhunjhunwala et al., recently demonstrated a 30-500-fold increased neutrophil presence in the peritoneal lavage of mice in response to sterile implanted microcapsules after 2 weeks, which is much longer than the hours or few days they have previously been thought to survive at a wound site. Jhunjhunwala et al. further demonstrated that the neutrophils became activated in response to the implant, resulting in the secretion of different immunomodulatory cytokines and chemokines and formation of extracellular traps (NETs) on the material surface [51]. The increasing knowledge about the pivotal role of neutrophils in the regulation of foreign body reactions suggests that a strong acute inflammation, associated with the implantation, can predispose an equally strong chronic inflammation orchestrated by neutrophils and characterized by prolonged neutrophil presence and frustrated phagocytosis in the very long run [50]. Beside the impact of material properties on the long-term neutrophil response indicated in the present study, the eventual influence of other factors, such as traumatic surgery and pre-existing disorders that influence the inflammatory response, such as diabetes, may be considered in future studies [52–54].

The immunological reactions to aseptic provocations of dental implants remains largely unexplored and future studies may focus on investigating the details in the immune response to different provocations at different time points throughout the healing phase, as well as refining the methods for such investigation.

5. Conclusions

Within the limitations of the present study, it was demonstrated that aseptic marginal ligatures made of silk and cotton triggered an immunological reaction in the peri-implant tissue of rabbits, with abundant numbers of inflammatory cells in contact with the ligatures. Marginal bone resorption was also evident adjacent to the ligatures, which rejected our null-hypothesis that ligatures cannot induce bone resorption in the absence of a bacterial plaque. Future studies may aim to describe the tissue reactions at both earlier and later time points, as well as further elucidate the details of the immunological events responsible for bone resorption adjacent to aseptic marginal ligatures.

Author Contributions: Conceptualization, D.R., S.G., T.A., P.T. and A.W.; Data curation, S.G., P.H.J. and A.W.; Formal analysis, D.R., P.H.J. and A.W.; Funding acquisition, A.W.; Investigation, D.R., S.G., T.A., P.H.J. and A.W.; Methodology, D.R., S.G., T.A., P.T., C.B.J. and P.H.J.; Project administration, T.A., and A.W.; Supervision, T.A., P.T., C.B.J. and A.W.; Validation, C.B.J.; Visualization, D.R., S.G., C.B.J. and P.H.J.; Writing—Original Draft, D.R., S.G., C.B.J. and P.H.J.; Writing—Review & Editing, D.R., S.G., T.A., P.T., C.B.J. and A.W.

References

1. Moraschini, V.; Poubel, L.A.; Ferreira, V.F.; Barboza Edos, S. Evaluation of survival and success rates of dental implants reported in longitudinal studies with a follow-up period of at least 10 years: A systematic review. *Int. J. Oral Maxillofac Surg.* **2015**, *44*, 377–388. [CrossRef] [PubMed]
2. Doornewaard, R.; Christiaens, V.; De Bruyn, H.; Jacobsson, M.; Cosyn, J.; Vervaeke, S.; Jacquet, W. Long-Term Effect of Surface Roughness and Patients' Factors on Crestal Bone Loss at Dental Implants. A Systematic Review and Meta-Analysis. *Clin. Implant. Dent. Relat. Res.* **2017**, *19*, 372–399. [CrossRef] [PubMed]
3. Albrektsson, T.; Buser, D.; Sennerby, L. Crestal bone loss and oral implants. *Clin. Implant. Dent. Relat Res.* **2012**, *14*, 783–791. [CrossRef] [PubMed]
4. Lindhe, J.; Berglundh, T.; Ericsson, I.; Liljenberg, B.; Marinello, C. Experimental breakdown of peri-implant and periodontal tissues. A study in the beagle dog. *Clin. oral implant res.* **1992**, *3*, 9–16. [CrossRef]
5. Zitzmann, N.U.; Berglundh, T. Definition and prevalence of peri-implant diseases. *J. Clin. Periodontol.* **2008**, *35*, 286–291. [CrossRef] [PubMed]
6. Albrektsson, T.; Dahlin, C.; Jemt, T.; Sennerby, L.; Turri, A.; Wennerberg, A. Is marginal bone loss around oral implants the result of a provoked foreign body reaction? *Clin. Implant Dent. Relat. Res.* **2014**, *16*, 155–165. [CrossRef]
7. Albrektsson, T.; Chrcanovic, B.; Ostman, P.O.; Sennerby, L. Initial and long-term crestal bone responses to modern dental implants. *Periodontology 2000* **2017**, *73*, 41–50. [CrossRef]
8. Frydman, A.; Simonian, K. Review of models for titanium as a foreign body. *C.D.A. J.* **2014**, *42*, 829–833.
9. Jemt, T.; Sunden Pikner, S.; Grondahl, K. Changes of Marginal Bone Level in Patients with "Progressive Bone Loss" at Branemark System(R) Implants: A Radiographic Follow-Up Study over an Average of 9 Years. *Clin. Implant Dent. Relat. Res.* **2015**, *17*, 619–628. [CrossRef]
10. Albrektsson, T.; Becker, W.; Coli, P.; Jemt, T.; Molne, J.; Sennerby, L. Bone loss around oral and orthopedic implants: An immunologically based condition. *Clin. Implant Dent. Relat. Res.* **2019**. [CrossRef]
11. Harris, W. *Vanishing Bone—Conquering a Stealth Disease Caused by Total Hip Replacements*; Oxford Press: Oxford, UK, 2018.
12. Landgraeber, S.; Jäger, M.; Jacobs, J.J.; Hallab, N.J. The pathology of orthopedic implant failure is mediated by innate immune system cytokines. *Mediators Inflamm.* **2014**, *2014*, 185150. [CrossRef] [PubMed]
13. Jiang, Y.; Jia, T.; Wooley, P.H.; Yang, S.Y. Current research in the pathogenesis of aseptic implant loosening associated with particulate wear debris. *Acta. Orthop. Belg.* **2013**, *79*, 1–9. [PubMed]
14. Abrahamsson, I.; Berglundh, T.; Lindhe, J. Soft tissue response to plaque formation at different implant systems. A comparative study in the dog. *Clin. Oral Implants Res.* **1998**, *9*, 73–79. [CrossRef] [PubMed]
15. Lang, N.P.; Bragger, U.; Walther, D.; Beamer, B.; Kornman, K.S. Ligature-induced peri-implant infection in cynomolgus monkeys. I. Clinical and radiographic findings. *Clin. Oral Implants Res.* **1993**, *4*, 2–11. [CrossRef] [PubMed]
16. Watzak, G.; Zechner, W.; Tangl, S.; Vasak, C.; Donath, K.; Watzek, G. Soft tissue around three different implant types after 1.5 years of functional loading without oral hygiene: A preliminary study in baboons. *Clin. Oral Implants Res.* **2006**, *17*, 229–236. [CrossRef] [PubMed]

17. Reinedahl, D.; Chrcanovic, B.; Albrektsson, T.; Tengvall, P.; Wennerberg, A. Ligature-Induced Experimental Peri-Implantitis-A Systematic Review. *J. Clin. Med.* **2018**, *7*. [CrossRef] [PubMed]
18. Moest, T.; Wrede, J.; Schmitt, C.M.; Stamp, M.; Neukam, F.W.; Schlegel, K.A. The influence of different abutment materials on tissue regeneration after surgical treatment of peri-implantitis—A randomized controlled preclinical study. *J. Craniomaxillofac. Surg.* **2017**, *45*, 1190–1196. [CrossRef] [PubMed]
19. Carcuac, O.; Abrahamsson, I.; Albouy, J.P.; Linder, E.; Larsson, L.; Berglundh, T. Experimental periodontitis and peri-implantitis in dogs. *Clin. Oral Implants Res.* **2013**, *24*, 363–371. [CrossRef]
20. Rovin, S.; Costich, E.R.; Gordon, H.A. The influence of bacteria and irritation in the initiation of periodontal disease in germfree and conventional rats. *J. Periodontal Res.* **1966**, *1*, 193–204. [CrossRef]
21. Martins, O.; Ramos, J.C.; Baptista, I.P.; Dard, M.M. The dog as a model for peri-implantitis: A review. *J. Investig. Surg.* **2014**, *27*, 50–56. [CrossRef]
22. Baron, M.; Haas, R.; Dortbudak, O.; Watzek, G. Experimentally induced peri-implantitis: A review of different treatment methods described in the literature. *Int. J. Oral Maxillofac. Implants* **2000**, *15*, 533–544.
23. Nguyen Vo, T.N.; Hao, J.; Chou, J.; Oshima, M.; Aoki, K.; Kuroda, S.; Kaboosaya, B.; Kasugai, S. Ligature induced peri-implantitis: Tissue destruction and inflammatory progression in a murine model. *Clin. Oral Implants Res.* **2017**, *28*, 129–136. [CrossRef]
24. Donath, K.; Breuner, G. A method for the study of undecalcified bones and teeth with attached soft tissues. The Sage-Schliff (sawing and grinding) technique. *J. Oral Pathol.* **1982**, *11*, 318–326. [CrossRef]
25. Johansson, C.B.; Morberg, P. Importance of ground section thickness for reliable histomorphometrical results. *Biomaterials* **1995**, *16*, 91–95. [CrossRef]
26. Johansson, C.B.; Morberg, P. Cutting directions of bone with biomaterials in situ does influence the outcome of histomorphometrical quantifications. *Biomaterials* **1995**, *16*, 1037–1039. [CrossRef]
27. Wilson, T.G.; Valderrama, P.; Burbano, M.; Blansett, J.; Levine, R.; Kessler, H.; Rodrigues, D.C. Foreign bodies associated with peri-implantitis human biopsies. *J. Periodontol.* **2015**, *86*, 9–15. [CrossRef]
28. Wang, X.; Li, Y.; Feng, Y.; Cheng, H.; Li, D. Macrophage polarization in aseptic bone resorption around dental implants induced by Ti particles in a murine model. *J. Periodontal Res.* **2019**. [CrossRef]
29. Donath, K.; Laass, M.; Günzl, H.J. The histopathology of different foreign-body reactions in oral soft tissue and bone tissue. *Virchows. Arch. A* **1992**, *420*, 131–137. [CrossRef]
30. Mbalaviele, G.; Novack, D.V.; Schett, G.; Teitelbaum, S.L. Inflammatory osteolysis: A conspiracy against bone. *J. Clin. Invest.* **2017**, *127*, 2030–2039. [CrossRef]
31. Paiva, K.B.S.; Granjeiro, J.M. Matrix Metalloproteinases in Bone Resorption, Remodeling, and Repair. *Prog Mol. Biol. Transl. Sci.* **2017**, *148*, 203–303. [CrossRef]
32. Setzen, G.; Williams, E.F., 3rd. Tissue response to suture materials implanted subcutaneously in a rabbit model. *Plast. Reconstr. Surg.* **1997**, *100*, 1788–1795. [CrossRef]
33. Nair, P.N. Pathogenesis of apical periodontitis and the causes of endodontic failures. *Crit. Rev. Oral Biol. Med.* **2004**, *15*, 348–381. [CrossRef]
34. You, T.M.; Choi, B.H.; Zhu, S.J.; Jung, J.H.; Lee, S.H.; Huh, J.Y.; Lee, H.J.; Li, J. Treatment of experimental peri-implantitis using autogenous bone grafts and platelet-enriched fibrin glue in dogs. *Oral Surg. Oral Med. Oral Pathol. Oral Radiol. Endod.* **2007**, *103*, 34–37. [CrossRef]
35. Schou, S.; Holmstrup, P.; Jorgensen, T.; Stoltze, K.; Hjorting-Hansen, E.; Wenzel, A. Autogenous bone graft and ePTFE membrane in the treatment of peri-implantitis. I. Clinical and radiographic observations in cynomolgus monkeys. *Clin. Oral Implants Res.* **2003**, *14*, 391–403. [CrossRef]
36. Yu, X.; Hu, Y.; Freire, M.; Yu, P.; Kawai, T.; Han, X. Role of toll-like receptor 2 in inflammation and alveolar bone loss in experimental peri-implantitis versus periodontitis. *J. Periodontal Res.* **2018**, *53*, 98–106. [CrossRef]
37. Albouy, J.P.; Abrahamsson, I.; Berglundh, T. Spontaneous progression of experimental peri-implantitis at implants with different surface characteristics: An experimental study in dogs. *J.Clin. Periodontol.* **2012**, *39*, 182–187. [CrossRef]
38. Jovanovic, S.A.; Kenney, E.B.; Carranza, F.A., Jr.; Donath, K. The regenerative potential of plaque-induced peri-implant bone defects treated by a submerged membrane technique: An experimental study. *Int. J. Oral Maxillofac. Implants* **1993**, *8*, 13–18.
39. Hayek, R.R.; Araujo, N.S.; Gioso, M.A.; Ferreira, J.; Baptista-Sobrinho, C.A.; Yamada, A.M.; Ribeiro, M.S. Comparative study between the effects of photodynamic therapy and conventional therapy on microbial reduction in ligature-induced peri-implantitis in dogs. *J. Periodontol.* **2005**, *76*, 1275–1281. [CrossRef]

40. Machtei, E.E.; Kim, D.M.; Karimbux, N.; Zigdon-Giladi, H. The use of endothelial progenitor cells combined with barrier membrane for the reconstruction of peri-implant osseous defects: An animal experimental study. *J. Clin. Periodontol.* **2016**, *43*, 289–297. [CrossRef]
41. Abdul-Karim, F.W.; Benevenia, J.; Pathria, M.N.; Makley, J.T. Case report 736: Retained surgical sponge (gossypiboma) with a foreign body reaction and remote and organizing hematoma. *Skeletal Radiol.* **1992**, *21*, 466–469.
42. Puvanesarajah, V.; Fayad, L.M.; Rao, S.S.; McCarthy, E.F.; Morris, C.D. Extremity gossypiboma mimicking sarcoma: Case report and review. *Skeletal Radiol.* **2019**, *48*, 629–635. [CrossRef]
43. Sari, A.; Basterzi, Y.; Karabacak, T.; Tasdelen, B.; Demirkan, F. The potential of microscopic sterile sponge particles to induce foreign body reaction. *Int. Wound J.* **2006**, *3*, 363–368. [CrossRef]
44. Altman, G.H.; Diaz, F.; Jakuba, C.; Calabro, T.; Horan, R.L.; Chen, J.; Lu, H.; Richmond, J.; Kaplan, D.L. Silk-based biomaterials. *Biomaterials* **2003**, *24*, 401–416. [CrossRef]
45. Nooh, N.; Abdullah, W.A.; Grawish Mel, A.; Ramalingam, S.; Javed, F.; Al-Hezaimi, K. The effects of surgicel and bone wax hemostatic agents on bone healing: An experimental study. *Indian J. Orthop.* **2014**, *48*, 319–325. [CrossRef]
46. Spelzini, F.; Konstantinovic, M.L.; Guelinckx, I.; Verbist, G.; Verbeken, E.; De Ridder, D.; Deprest, J. Tensile strength and host response towards silk and type i polypropylene implants used for augmentation of fascial repair in a rat model. *Gynecol. Obstet. Invest.* **2007**, *63*, 155–162. [CrossRef]
47. Trindade, R.; Albrektsson, T.; Galli, S.; Prgomet, Z.; Tengvall, P.; Wennerberg, A. Osseointegration and foreign body reaction: Titanium implants activate the immune system and suppress bone resorption during the first 4 weeks after implantation. *Clin. Implant. Dent. Relat. Res.* **2018**, *20*, 82–91. [CrossRef]
48. Brodbeck, W.G.; Macewan, M.; Colton, E.; Meyerson, H.; Anderson, J.M. Lymphocytes and the foreign body response: Lymphocyte enhancement of macrophage adhesion and fusion. *J. Biomed. Mater. Res. A* **2005**, *74*, 222–229. [CrossRef]
49. Rodriguez, A.; Macewan, S.R.; Meyerson, H.; Kirk, J.T.; Anderson, J.M. The foreign body reaction in T-cell-deficient mice. *J. Biomed. Mater. Res. A* **2009**, *90*, 106–113. [CrossRef]
50. Selders, G.S.; Fetz, A.E.; Radic, M.Z.; Bowlin, G.L. An overview of the role of neutrophils in innate immunity, inflammation and host-biomaterial integration. *Regen. Biomater.* **2017**, *4*, 55–68. [CrossRef]
51. Jhunjhunwala, S.; Aresta-DaSilva, S.; Tang, K.; Alvarez, D.; Webber, M.J.; Tang, B.C.; Lavin, D.M.; Veiseh, O.; Doloff, J.C.; Bose, S.; et al. Neutrophil Responses to Sterile Implant Materials. *PLoS ONE* **2015**, *10*, e0137550. [CrossRef]
52. Laffey, J.G.; Boylan, J.F.; Cheng, D.C. The systemic inflammatory response to cardiac surgery: Implications for the anesthesiologist. *Anesthesiology* **2002**, *97*, 215–252. [CrossRef]
53. Chrcanovic, B.R.; Albrektsson, T.; Wennerberg, A. Diabetes and oral implant failure: A systematic review. *J. Dent. Res.* **2014**, *93*, 859–867. [CrossRef]
54. Chrcanovic, B.R.; Albrektsson, T.; Wennerberg, A. Reasons for failures of oral implants. *J. Oral Rehabil.* **2014**, *41*, 443–476. [CrossRef]

11

On the Cleanliness of Different Oral Implant Systems

Dirk U. Duddeck [1,2,*], Tomas Albrektsson [3], Ann Wennerberg [4], Christel Larsson [5] and Florian Beuer [5]

1 Department of Prosthodontics, Geriatric Dentistry and Craniomandibular Disorders, University Charité Berlin, 14197 Berlin, Germany
2 CleanImplant Foundation, Research Department, 10117 Berlin, Germany
3 Department of Biomaterials, Institute for Clinical Sciences, Sahlgrenska Academy, University of Gothenburg, 40530 Gothenburg, Sweden
4 Department of Prosthodontics, Institute of Odontology, The Sahlgrenska Academy, University of Gothenburg, 40530 Gothenburg, Sweden
5 Department of Prosthodontics, Faculty of Odontology, Malmö University, 20506 Malmö, Sweden
* Correspondence: dirk.duddeck@gmx.de

Abstract: (1) Background: This paper aimed to compare the cleanliness of clinically well-documented implant systems with implants providing very similar designs. The hypothesis was that three well-established implant systems from Dentsply Implants, Straumann, and Nobel Biocare were not only produced with a higher level of surface cleanliness but also provided significantly more comprehensive published clinical documentation than their correspondent look-alike implants from Cumdente, Bioconcept, and Biodenta, which show similar geometry and surface structure. (2) Methods: Implants were analyzed using SEM imaging and energy-dispersive X-ray spectroscopy to determine the elemental composition of potential impurities. A search for clinical trials was carried out in the PubMed database and by reaching out to the corresponding manufacturer. (3) Results: In comparison to their corresponding look-alikes, all implants of the original manufacturers showed within the scope of this analysis—a surface free of foreign materials and reliable clinical documentation, while the SEM analysis revealed significant impurities on all look-alike implants such as organic residues and unintended metal particles of iron or aluminum. Other than case reports, the look-alike implant manufacturers provided no reports of clinical documentation. (4) Conclusions: In contrast to the original implants of market-leading manufacturers, the analyzed look-alike implants showed significant impurities, underlining the need for periodic reviews of sterile packaged medical devices and their clinical documentation.

Keywords: dental implants; surface properties; titanium; materials testing; implant contamination; implant surface; scanning electron microscopy; energy-dispersive X-ray spectrometry

1. Introduction

The advent of osseointegration has led to a clinical breakthrough in oral implants. Minimally rough, turned implants were the first osseointegrated oral implants used, with the first patient treated in 1965 [1]. These turned screws remain the most clinically documented implants of all with 75% of all studies in long-term reports [2]. Over time, other clinically documented oral implant systems have increasingly begun to be used. Those systems may have preferred slightly different surfaces; moderately rough implants have been the treatment of choice since the turn of the millennium, since they have demonstrated improved clinical results [3]. The surface of moderately rough implant systems may be manufactured in different ways, by subtractive methods such as the combination of blasting and acid etching or anodization and by additive techniques, such as hydroxyapatite coating. Products from what are regarded as the three largest oral implant companies in the world including Osseo Speed implants from Dentsply–Sirona, SLA-implants from Straumann and TiUnite implants from Nobel Biocare, have been clinically documented in numerous papers spanning a period of over 5 to over 10 years of follow up with very high levels of survival and success [4–6].

Since some osseointegrated oral implant systems have been duly documented with a very good clinical outcome, numerous new implant manufacturers have tried to mimic the surfaces and geometries presented by the leading companies. These are so called copy-cat or at least "look-alike" implant systems which usually lack clinical documentation of their own but claim to be as good as the original implants they are trying to mimic. However, in clinical reality these implants lack the scientific evidence of similar performance.

One surface characteristic of sterile packaged oral implants is their cleanliness. Oral implants may display different surface of an inorganic or organic nature. These impurities may derive from the manufacturing handling and packaging processes and may remain on the commercially available implant. We are presently lacking in knowledge of the precise clinical risks of implant impurities. However, contaminations are technically avoidable and, generally speaking, the authors assume all of us would prefer clean implants to avoid potential problems from surface impurities.

The aim of the present paper was to compare the cleanliness of proper clinically documented implant systems with implants that are very similar in design and surface; OsseoSpeed from Dentsply Implants was compared to a German look-alike implant called Cumdente; Standard Plus Implant SLA from Straumann was compared to a Chinese look-alike implant called Bioconcept (claiming to be 100% compatible with Straumann); and a TiUnite-surfaced implant NobelActive from Nobel Biocare was compared to a Swiss/Taiwanese implant system called Biodenta. Our hypothesis was that the three major and well-established implant systems have significantly comprehensive clinical documentation and have their implants produced in a significantly cleaner manner than would the respective look-alike systems.

Every single dental implant has to be clean, as this is a medical device that could harm patients—even if we found one single implant with impurities, this implant was intentionally sold for the therapy of one real patient. This paper was not intended to show a statistically relevant number of average contaminations for specific implant types. All implants in this study were randomly purchased and labeled for clinical use. Each sample of these medical devices was produced using a certain regime of quality management. If the quality management of a manufacturer cannot ensure a certain level of cleanliness, a single implant with significant impurities, which are technically avoidable, is proof of a lack of quality.

2. Experimental Section

Implant types used for this analysis were the following: Astra Tech–Dentsply Implants (OsseoSpeed EV, Mölndal, Sweden), Straumann (Standard Plus SLA Implant, Zürich, Switzerland), Nobel Biocare (NobelActive Internal RP, Zürich, Switzerland), Cumdente (AS Implant, Tübingen, Germany), Bioconcept (Tissue Level Implant, Jiangsu, China), Biodenta (Dental Implant, Bernek, Switzerland). The three implants from market-leading manufacturers and the correspondent three look-alike implants were purchased in the period between March 2018 and May 2019, either by ghost-shopping, where the ordering practice was reimbursed from the research fund or by direct order. In all six cases, the manufacturers or the respective distributors were not informed about the purpose of the implant order. None of the samples were provided free of charge. Prices varied from 191 euro to 322 euro for the samples of market-leading brands and from 78 euro to 276 euro for the look-alike products.

All of the six samples collected were carefully unpacked, mounted on the sample holder on carbon tabs without touching the implant surface, and analyzed with a scanning electron microscope (SEM) in a particle-free clean room environment (according Class 100 US Federal Standard 209E, Class 5 DIN EN ISO 14644-1) to avoid artifacts from the ambient air (Figure 1).

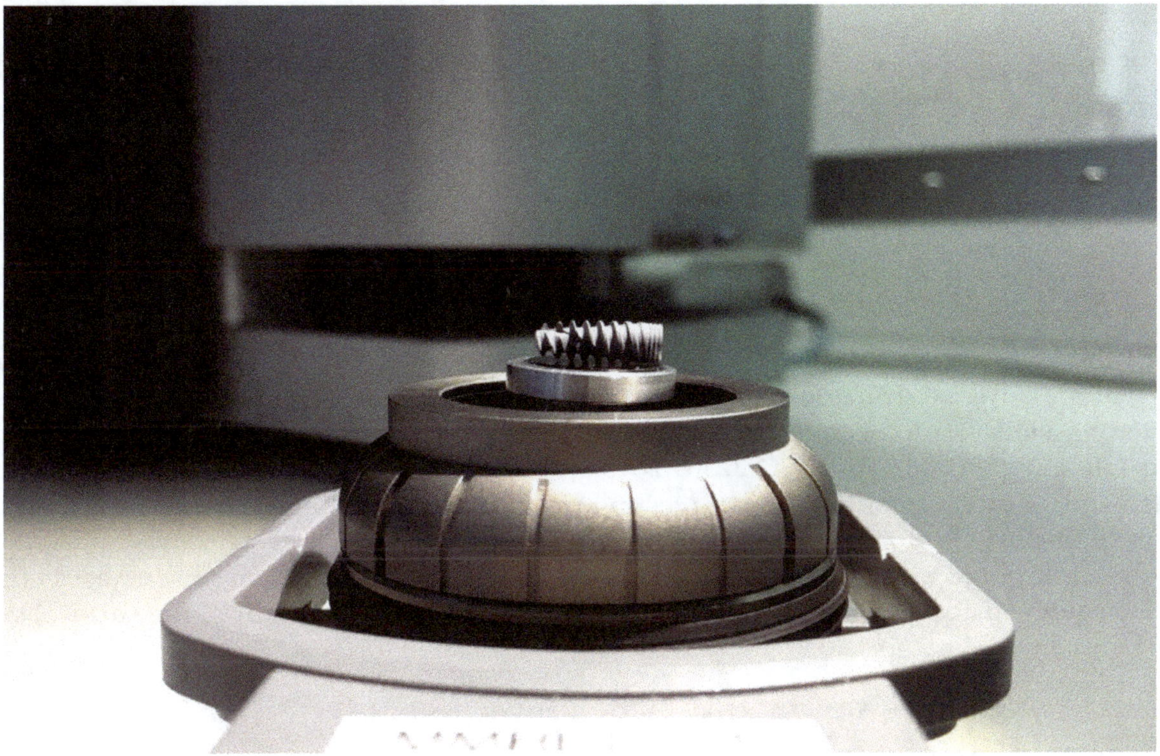

Figure 1. Implant sample with a length of 10 mm mounted on the SEM sample holder.

The scientific workstation used was a Phenom proX Scanning Electron Microscope (Eindhoven, Netherlands), equipped with a high-sensitivity backscattered electron (BSE) detector. The detector for the energy-dispersive X-ray spectroscopy (EDS) and elemental analysis was a thermoelectrically cooled silicon drift detector (SDD) type, with an active detector area of 25 mm^2.

The high-sensitivity BSE detector allows a magnification of up to 100,000× with a resolution down to 15 nm. This study used material-contrast images from 500× to a magnification of 5000×. Material-contrast imaging gave additional information about the chemical nature and allocation of different remnants or contaminations on the sample material.

In order to achieve a complete overview of the horizontally mounted implant sample and comprehensive surface quality information in high resolution, implants were scanned at a magnification of 500× in the "Image-Mapping" mode prior to the detailed analysis of potential impurities. This technique produces up to 600 single high-resolution SEM images of the implant surface that were digitally composed into one large image, with an extremely high resolution. The composed SEM image, showing the full size of the implant from shoulder to apex, made it possible to count particles in the visible field (viewing angle of approximately 120°) and to identify areas of interest for a subsequent EDS spot analysis. After the mapping process, SEM images of impurities and other regions of interest were produced with 500×, 1000× 2500×, and 5000× magnification. In the next step, the elemental composition of particles was determined and, where possible, the differential spectra of particles were achieved to subtract signals from the core material and such focus on signals from the superficial contamination (Figure 2).

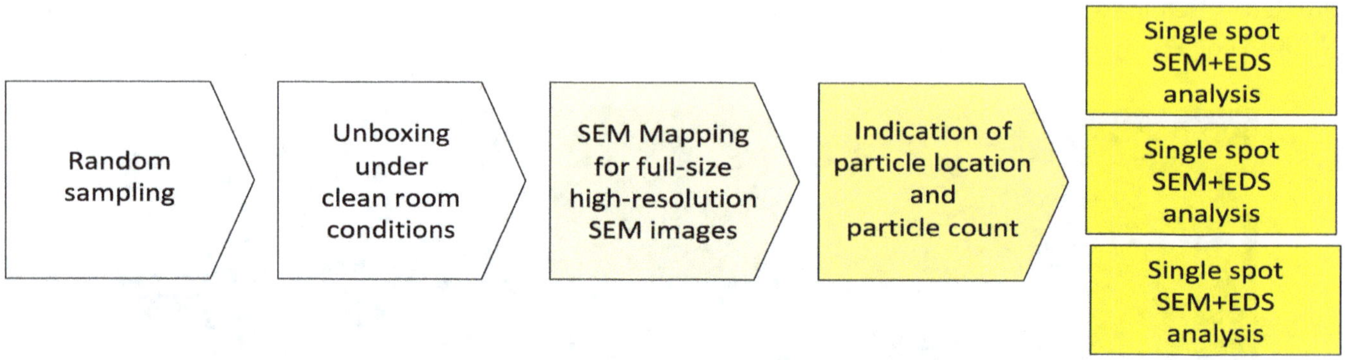

Figure 2. Workflow of the SEM/EDS analysis.

All of the analyses, as well as the complete setup, as described above were performed at the Medical Materials Research Institute, Berlin, Germany, which is an officially accredited (Deutsche Akkreditierungsstelle–DAkkS) and externally audited testing laboratory according to the international standards DIN EN ISO 9001:2015, ISO 22309:2015 and DIN EN ISO/IEC 17025. These standards were chosen as a precondition in order to assure testing procedures at the highest level of accuracy.

In addition to the SEM/EDS analysis, all of the implants in this study were provisionally evaluated from a surface topographical point of view by interferometry. All implants seemed to be in the moderately rough surface range, i.e., with Sa (Sa = arithmetical mean height of the surface) values of between 1 and 2 micrometers.

2.1. Clinical Documentation of Analyzed "Look-Alike" Implant Systems

A search for available clinical trial regarding the dental implant systems was carried out. Initially the website of each dental implant manufacturer was searched (www.biodenta.com, www.bioconcept.cn, www.cumdente.com). In addition, the manufacturers were contacted via their respective contact e-mail address on their websites, requesting any scientific documentation regarding clinical performance such as published papers or summaries of ongoing projects. If no response was received within one week, a reminder was sent.

Furthermore, a search for clinical trials was performed in the PubMed database (PubMed.gov, US National Library of Medicine, National Institutes of Health). The search terms "dental implants" (MeSH) and "dental implants" (free text) were used in combination with the product name "Biodenta", "Bioconcept", and "Cumdente". No limits were set. (("dental implants" [MeSH Terms] OR ("dental" [All Fields] AND "implants" [All Fields]) OR "dental implants" [All Fields]) AND biodenta [All Fields]), (("dental implants" [MeSH Terms] OR ("dental" [All Fields] AND "implants" [All Fields]) OR "dental implants" [All Fields]) AND bioconcept [All Fields], (("dental implants" [MeSH Terms] OR ("dental" [All Fields] AND "implants" [All Fields]) OR "dental implants" [All Fields]) AND cumdente [All Fields])).

2.2. Clinical Documentation of OsseoSpeed, SLA, and TiUnite Implant Systems

With respect to the implant systems OsseoSpeed from Dentsply-Sirona, SLA from Straumann, and TiUnite from Nobel Biocare, these belong to the most clinically documented oral implant systems in the world [2]. To remain brief, we decided to only quote five papers for each system as the total number of clinical reports on these devices amounts to several hundred scientific papers.

3. Results

3.1. SEM Imaging and Elemental Analysis

Implants were analyzed in three groups. In the first group, the implant from Astra Tech–Dentsply Implants (OsseoSpeed) and the implant from Cumdente (AS Implant) were compared. The full-size

SEM image of the Astra Tech implant—digitally composed of 455 single SEM images (tiles)—showed a homogenous surface with no foreign material (Figure 3).

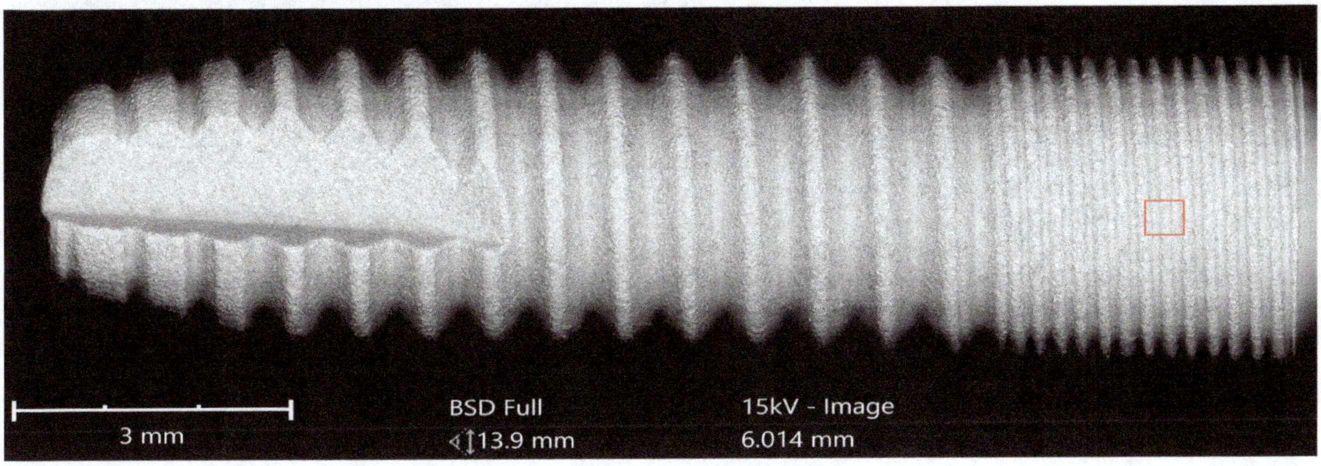

Figure 3. SEM mapping of OsseoSpeed implant (Astra Tech–Dentsply Implants). Magnification of the red marked area is shown in Figure 4.

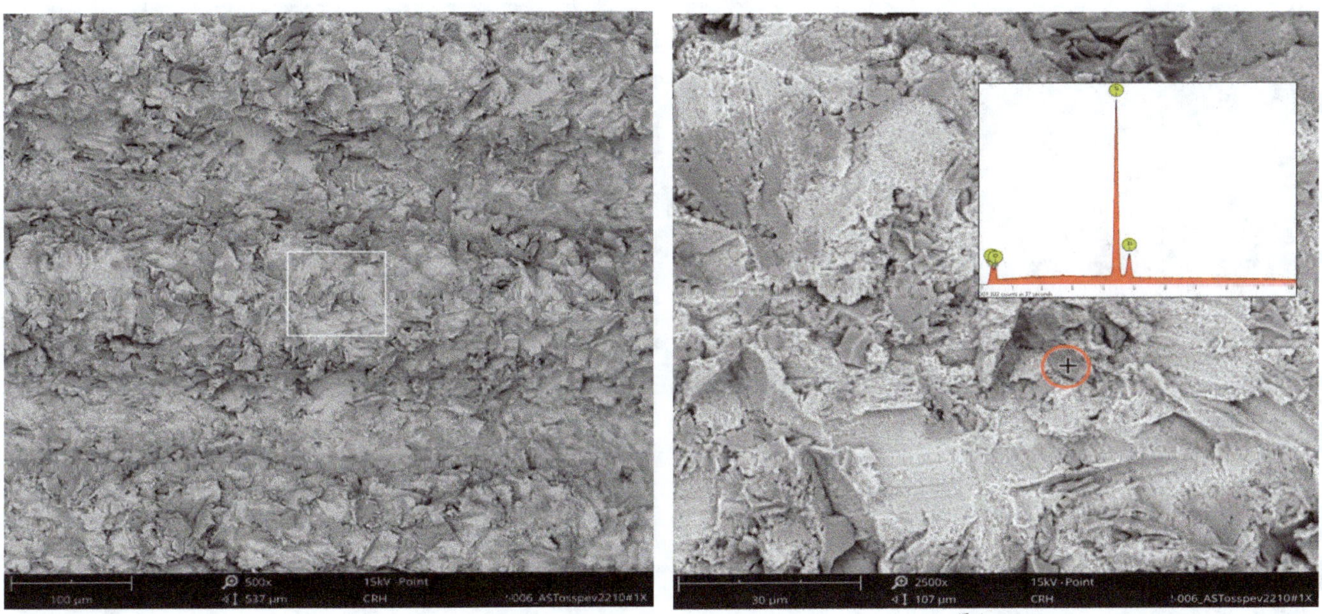

(a) (b)

Figure 4. OsseoSpeed surface: (**a**) the red marked area in Figure 3 magnified 500×; (**b**) higher magnification (2500×) of the white marked area in the left image with EDS spot analysis of an embedded TiO_2-particle (spot is marked with "+" in the red circle) showing only signals of the blasting material.

Higher magnification could identify the TiO_2 particles from the blasting process seen as sharp-edged particles of 5–10 mm embedded in the titanium surface. Elemental analysis of these particles only displayed signals of titanium and oxygen (Figure 4).

The Cumdente implant showed several anomalies in the correspondent full-size image, composed of 422 tiles (Figure 5).

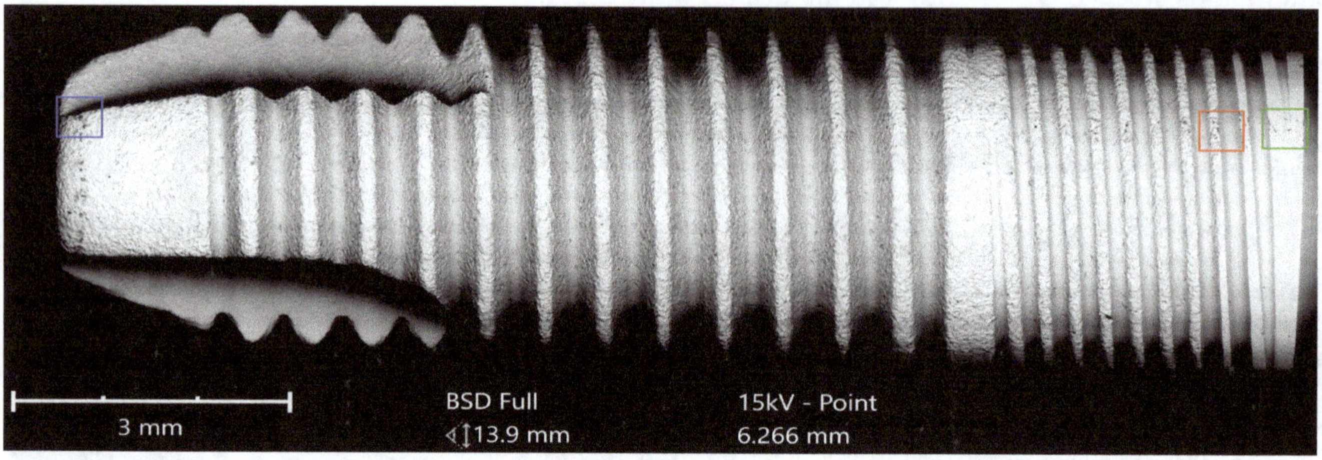

Figure 5. SEM mapping of the AS Implant (Cumdente); Red marked area—see magnification in Figure 6, blue marked area—see magnification in Figure 7, green marked area—see magnification in Figure 8.

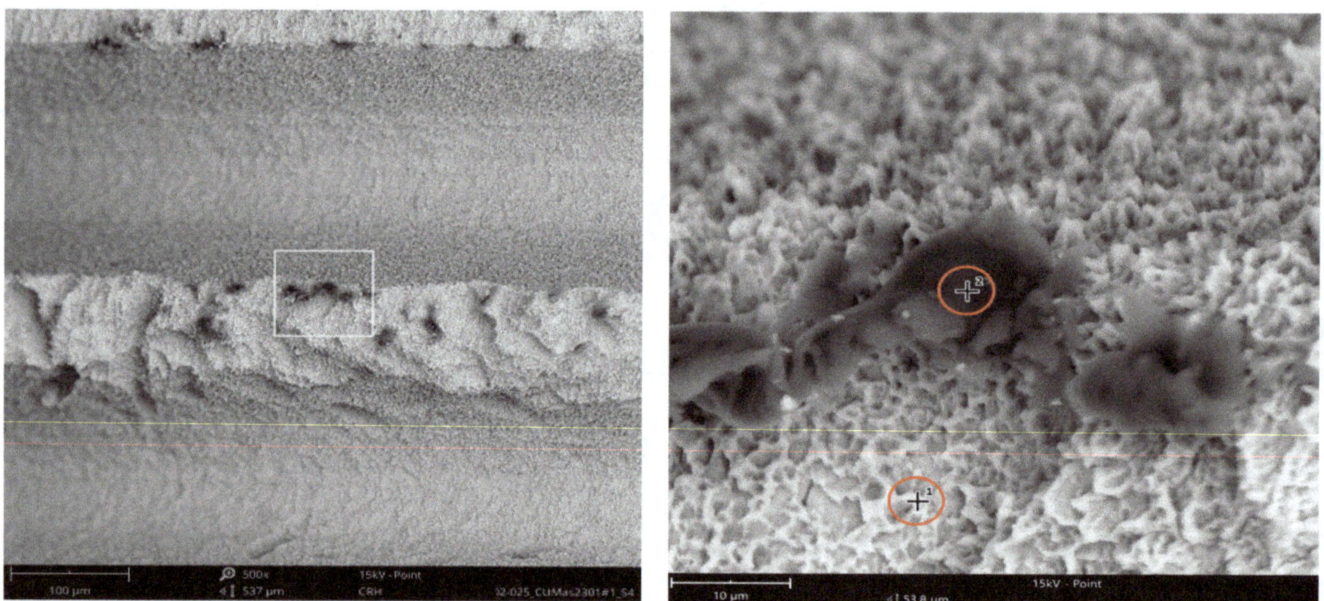

(a) (b)

Figure 6. AS Implant (Cumdente) with organic particles (10–50 μm) at the implant shoulder: (**a**) systematic contamination of exposed threads, red marked area of Figure 5 in 500×; (**b**) magnification (5000×) of white marked area in the left image. The EDS differential measurement of the marked spots was identical to the particles in Figure 7.

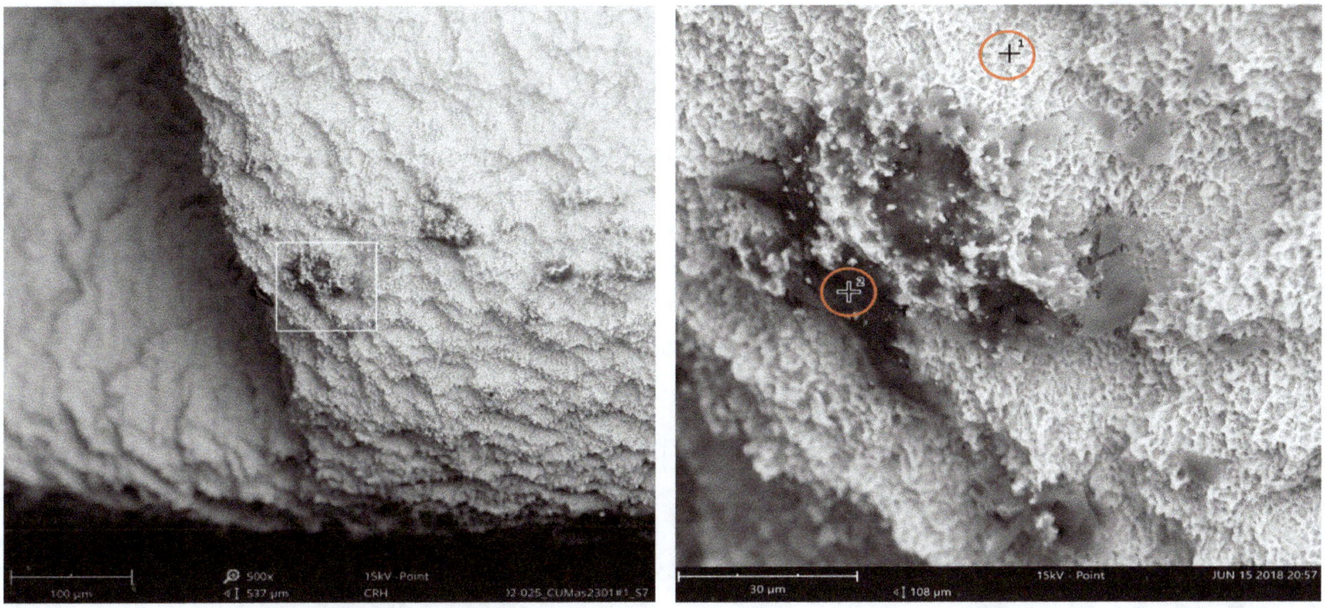

(a) (b)

Figure 7. AS Implant (Cumdente) with organic particles (5–70 µm) at the implant's apex: (**a**) blue marked area of Figure 5 in 500×; (**b**) magnification (5000×) of white marked area in Figure 7a; EDS differential measurement of marked spots is shown in Figure 8.

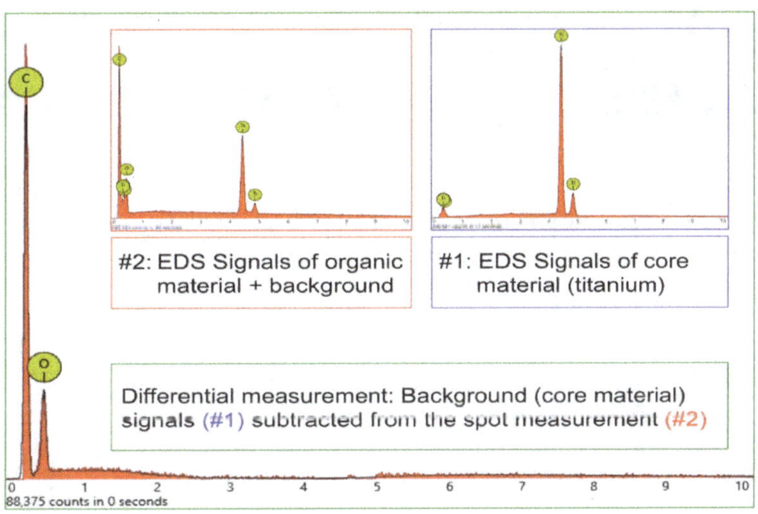

Figure 8. EDS differential measurement of the organic particle in Figure 7. Graph #1 shows titanium as the core material of this implant, with characteristic peaks at 0.452 KeV (La), 4.508 KeV (Lb), and 4.932 KeV (Kb). Graph #2 shows the spectrum of the particle with additional signals of the titanium background. The subtraction of X-ray quanta from the background material reveals the elemental composition of the impurity, which is carbon (characteristic Ka peak at 0.277 KeV) and oxygen (Ka peak at 0.523 KeV).

The SEM images with higher magnification revealed systematic contamination with multiple (>100) organic particles (5–60 µm) on exposed parts of the implant, as seen on the micro-threads next to the implant shoulder (Figure 6) and near the implant's apex (Figure 7).

In order to receive information about the particles' elemental composition, EDS measurement was performed with a spot focused on the foreign material, where background material was always detected as well, and another spot focused in direct proximity, where only the implant's core material was detected (spot #1 and #2 in Figures 6b and 7b, respectively). Using a software application, it was possible to subtract the signals of the core material so that the differential measurement revealed more precise information about the elemental composition of the foreign material. Figure 8 shows the differential EDS measurement of the particle in Figure 7, with a clear signal of carbon as the major element in this impurity.

One larger area at the implant shoulder showed numerous particles (5–40 μm) (Figure 9) with significant signals, not only of carbon but also of fluorine, as seen in the differential EDS analysis (Figure 10). The texture and elemental composition of the foreign material suggest that these particles are most likely remnants of polytetrafluoroethylene (PTFE), used at different implant production stages.

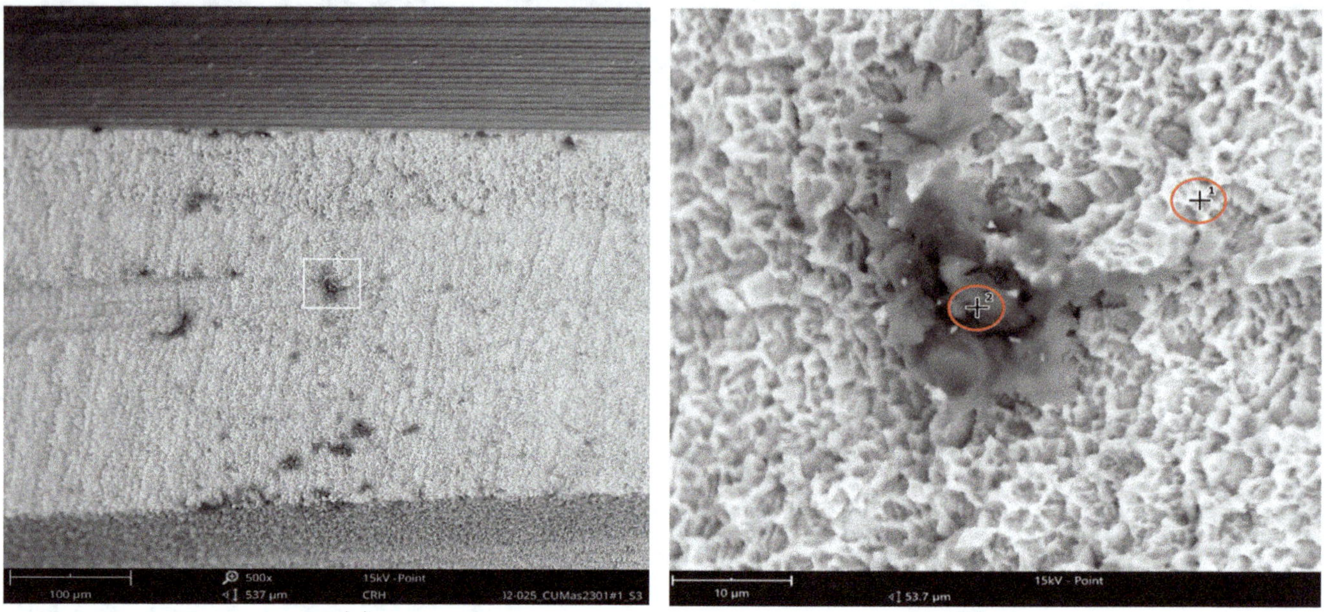

(a) (b)

Figure 9. Possible remnants of polytetrafluoroethylene (PTFE), AS Implant (Cumdente); (**a**) green marked area of Figure 5 in 500× shows a larger area of impurities; (**b**) magnification (5000×) of white marked area in the left image; EDS differential measurement of the marked spots is shown in Figure 10.

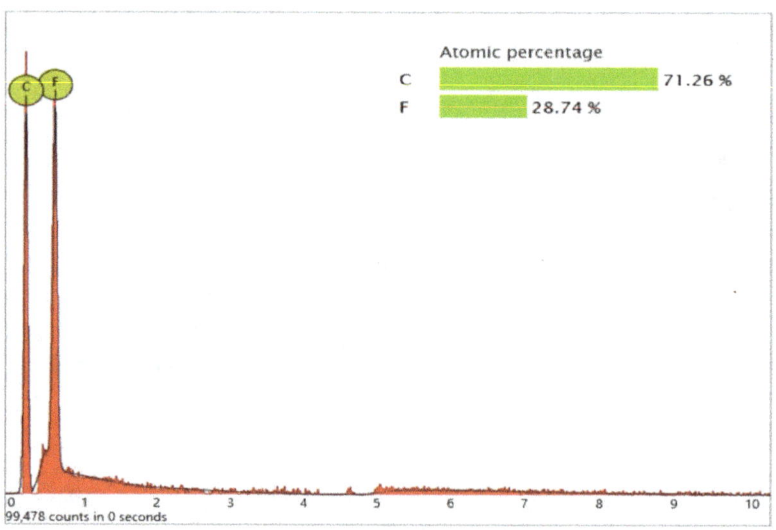

Figure 10. EDS differential measurement of the particles in Figure 9 with significant X-ray quanta of carbon and fluorine. Note that the quantitative information provided by the EDS analysis does not always reflect the precise stoichiometric relationship of the particle's chemical elements.

The second group compared the Straumann Standard Plus SLA Tissue Level Implant with an implant of the same geometry from Bioconcept, both made of commercially pure grade 4 titanium, which is a composition of 99% titanium, 0.50% iron (maximum), oxygen 0.40% (maximum), carbon 0.085 (maximum), hydrogen 0.015% (maximum), and nitrogen 0.05% (maximum), according to the ASTM F67 specification. The SEM imaging of the Straumann implant could not detect any organic or inorganic contaminants (Figures 11 and 12).

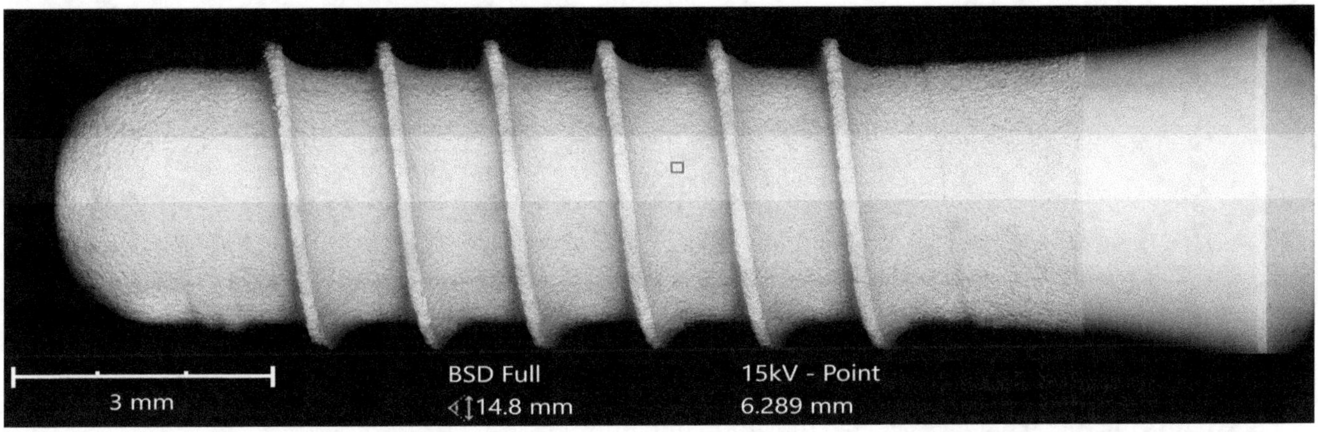

Figure 11. SEM mapping, Standard Plus SLA implant (Straumann); Magnification of red marked area is shown in Figure 12.

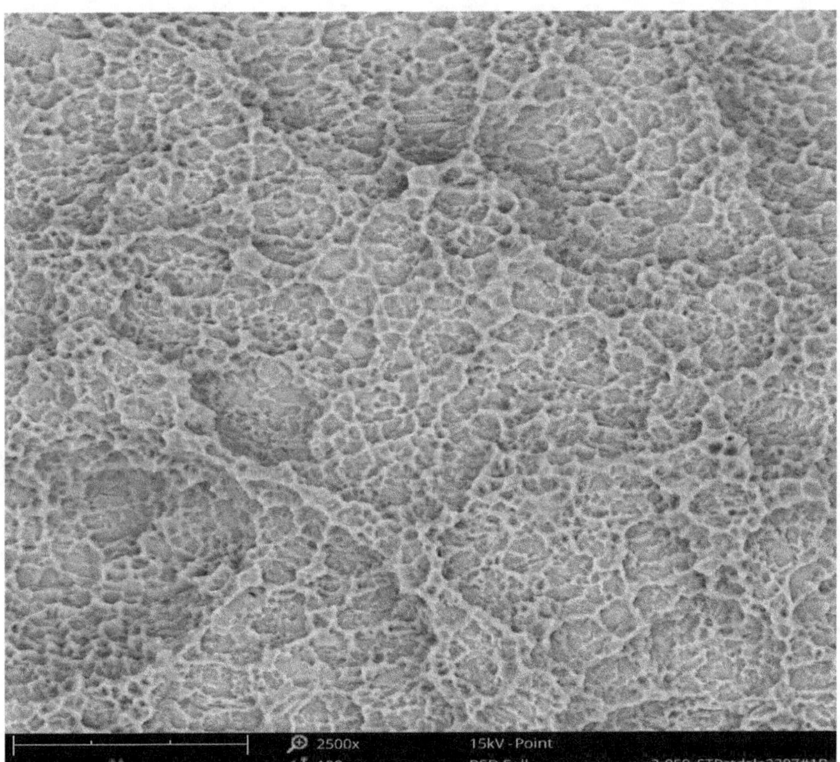

Figure 12. Surface of Standard Plus SLA implant (SEM 2500×); red marked area in Figure 11 with the typical texture of a sandblasted and acid-etched titanium surface, free of foreign materials.

While the Straumann implant can be rated as clean at the micron level, the analysis of the Bioconcept implant revealed several impurities, although the full-size image showed no systematic larger contamination (Figure 13). With higher magnification, approximately 20 small organic particles (10–20 µm) were found on the implant's surface, one particle showing additional signals of sulfur (Figure 15).

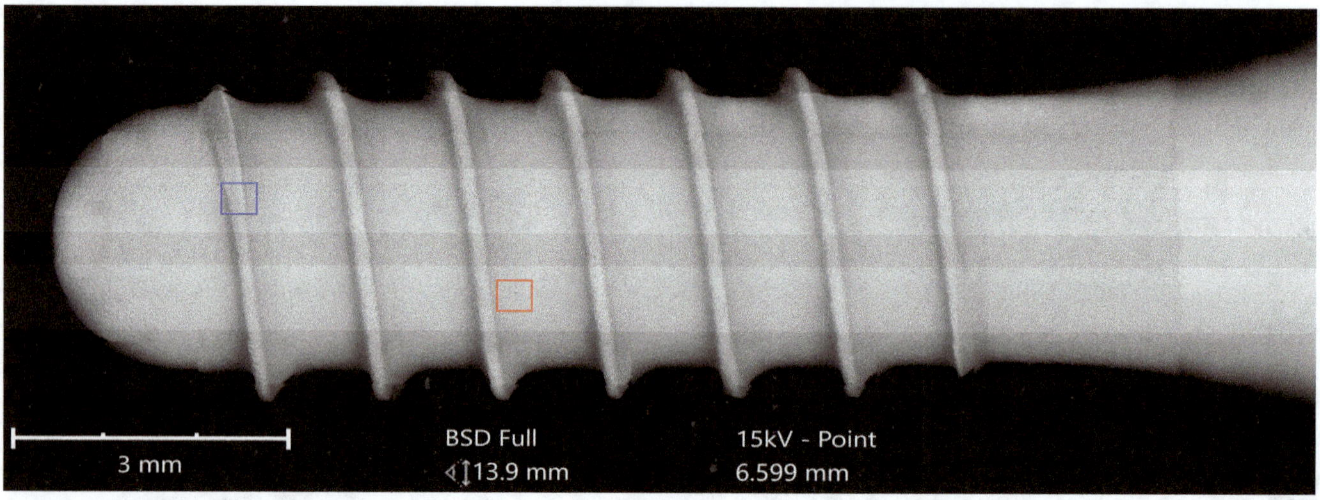

Figure 13. SEM mapping, Tissue Level Implant (Bioconcept); red marked area—see magnification in Figure 15, blue marked area—see magnification in Figure 14.

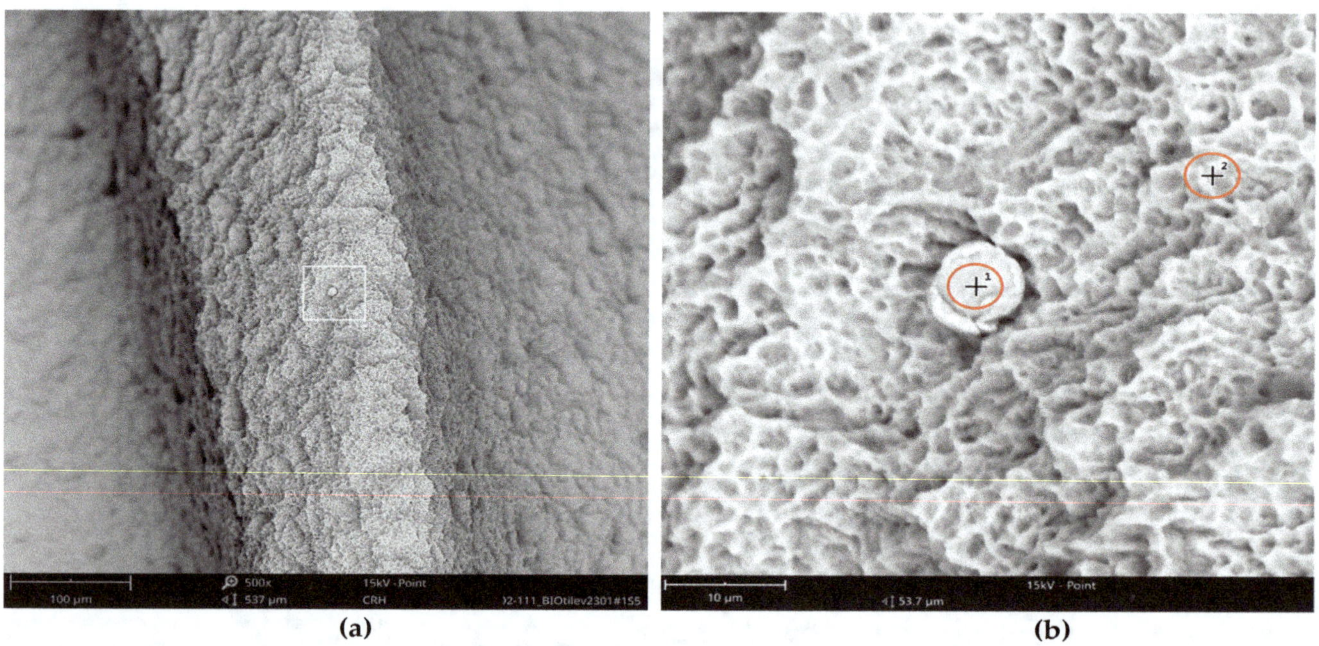

Figure 14. Metal particle on the surface of the Bioconcept implant; (**a**) blue marked area in Figure 13, SEM 500×; (**b**) magnification (5000×) of white marked area in the left image (**a**) showing bright metal impurity (8 µm) and 2 points of EDS spot measurement (#1 = metal particle, #2 = core material).

Surprisingly, one metal particle of 8 µm was found on the Bioconcept implant, seemingly entirely composed of iron, as the qualitative and quantitative elemental analysis and differential measurement of this particle revealed (Figures 14 and 16).

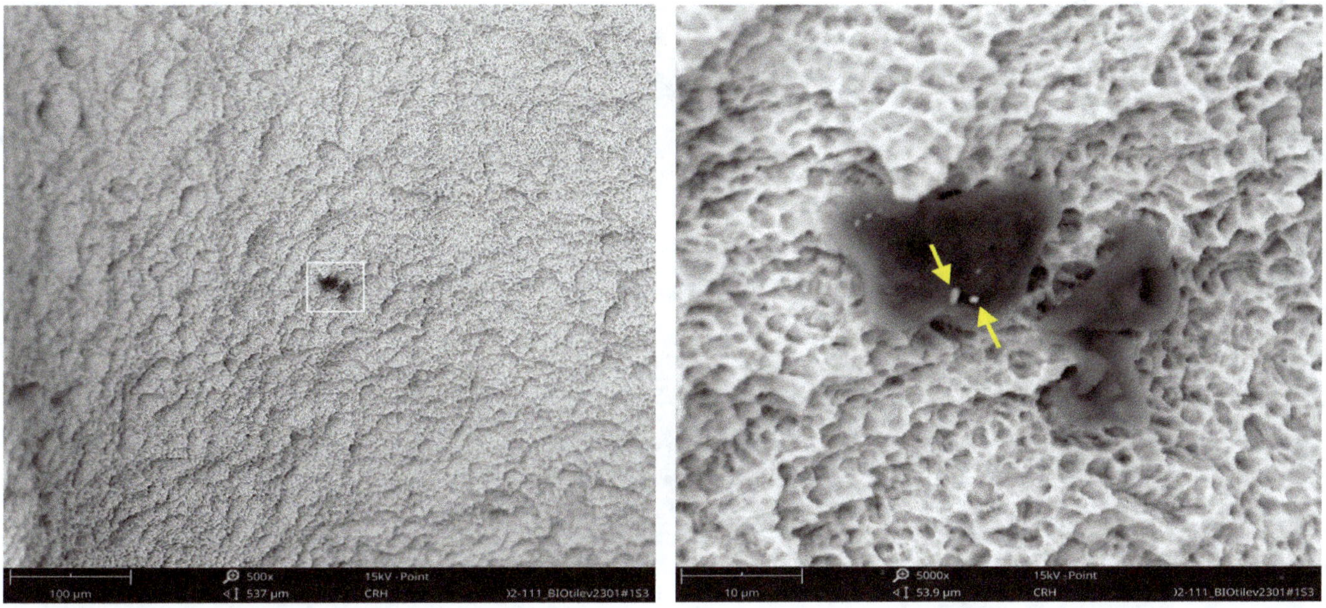

(a) (b)

Figure 15. Bioconcept implant with organic particles (10–15 μm); (**a**) red marked area in Figure 13, SEM 500×; (**b**) magnification (5000×) of white marked area in the left image (**a**); arrows indicate two embedded metal particles (0.5–1 μm) showing significant iron signals in the subsequent EDS differential measurement.

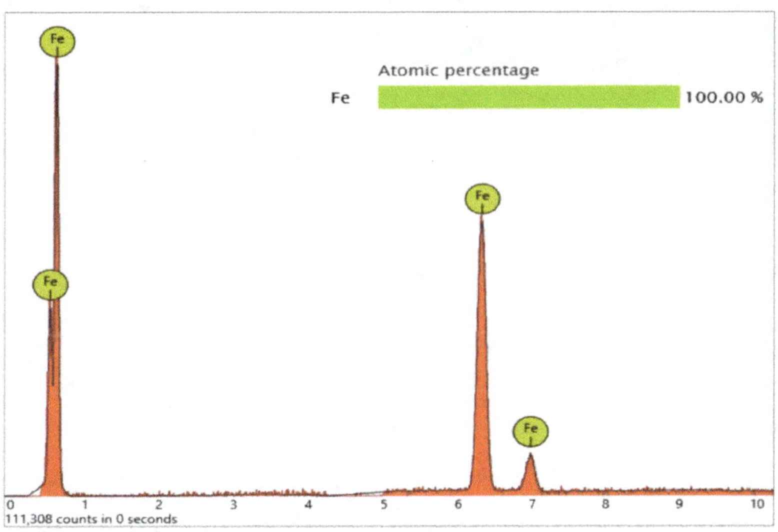

Figure 16. EDS differential measurement of the metal particle in Figure 14, revealing iron as the major element of the impurity.

The third group compared the NobelActive implant from Nobel Biocare with the Dental Implant from Biodenta. Both implants have an anodized surface with a characteristic titanium oxide layer. The area analysis of the NobelActive implant showed calcium and phosphorous signals in addition to titanium and oxygen. Within the scope of this analysis, neither inorganic nor organic particles were detected on the Nobel Biocare implant (Figures 17 and 18).

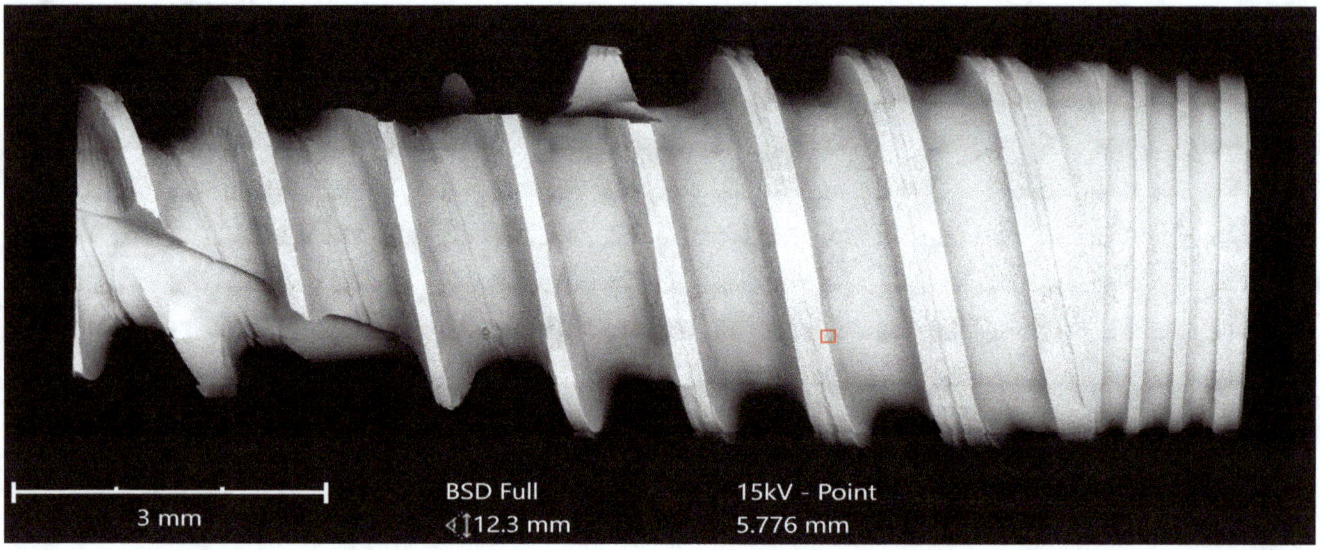

Figure 17. SEM mapping: NobelActive Internal RP implant (Nobel Biocare); red marked area—see magnification in Figure 18.

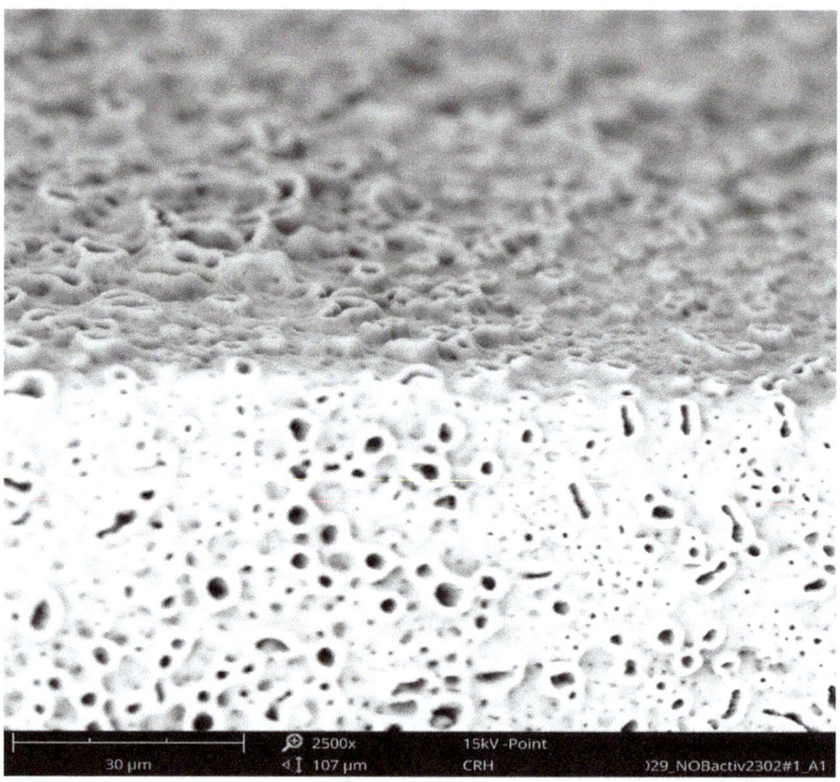

Figure 18. Surface of the NobelActive Internal RP implant (2500×); magnification of red marked area in Figure 17 with the typical texture of an anodized titanium surface, free of foreign materials.

While the full-size SEM image of the Biodenta implant exposed no significant organic contamination (Figure 19), the area analysis of the core material showed, in addition to calcium, phosphorous, titanium, and oxygen, high levels of magnesium in the EDS (Figure 20) that were not seen on the Nobel Biocare implant.

Significant traces of aluminum were detected in three areas of exposed threads and can be seen as bright particles (5–10 μm) in Figure 21. The graph in Figure 22 shows the correspondent EDS differential measurement of metal particles in Figure 20a.

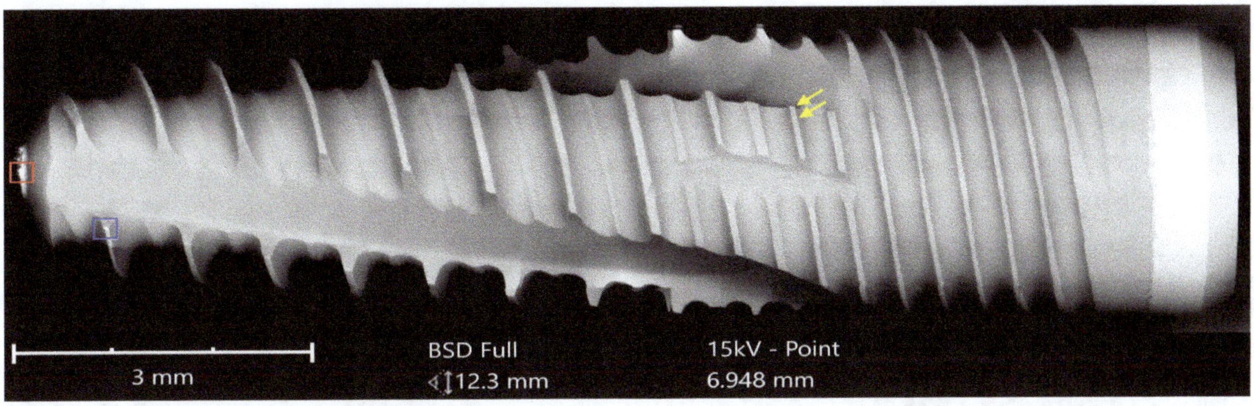

Figure 19. SEM mapping: Dental Implant (Biodenta); yellow arrows indicate spots with aluminum as shown in Figure 21. Magnifications of the blue and red marked areas are shown in Figure 23.

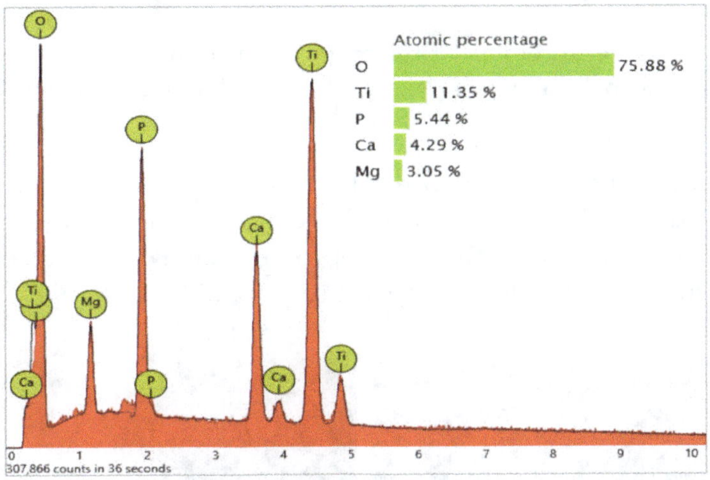

Figure 20. EDS area analysis of the implant's core material (Biodenta).

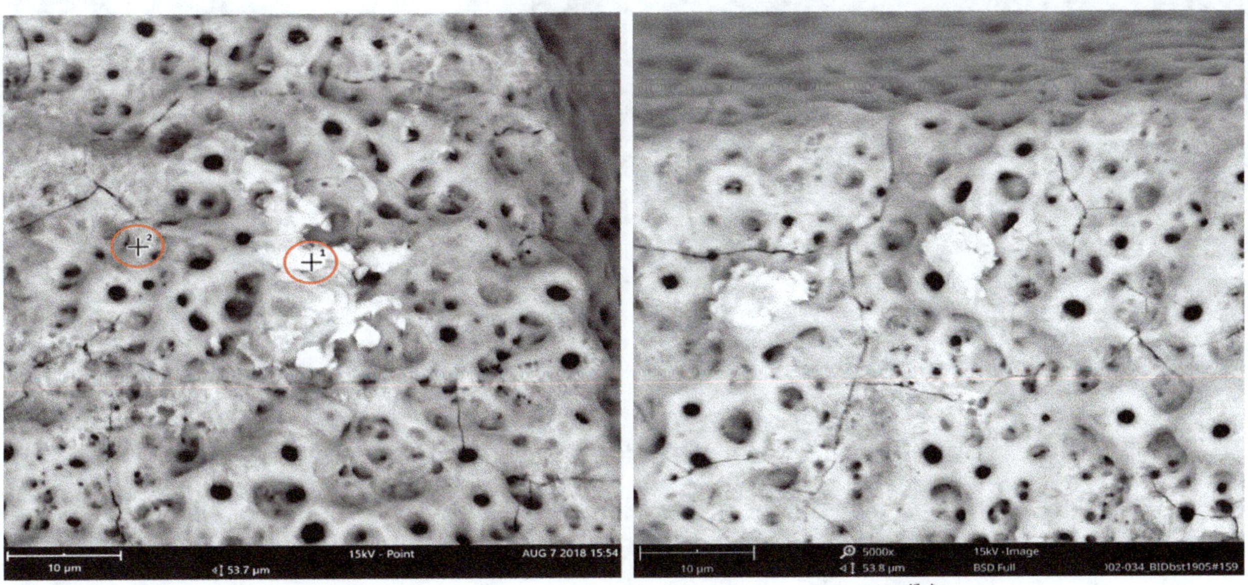

(a) **(b)**

Figure 21. Aluminum-containing particles (5–10 μm) on the surface of the Biodenta implant; location shown using yellow arrows in Figure 19; (**a**) SEM 5000× with 2 points of EDS spot measurement shown in Figure 22; (**b**) impurities with similar size in close proximity to particles shown in the left image (**a**).

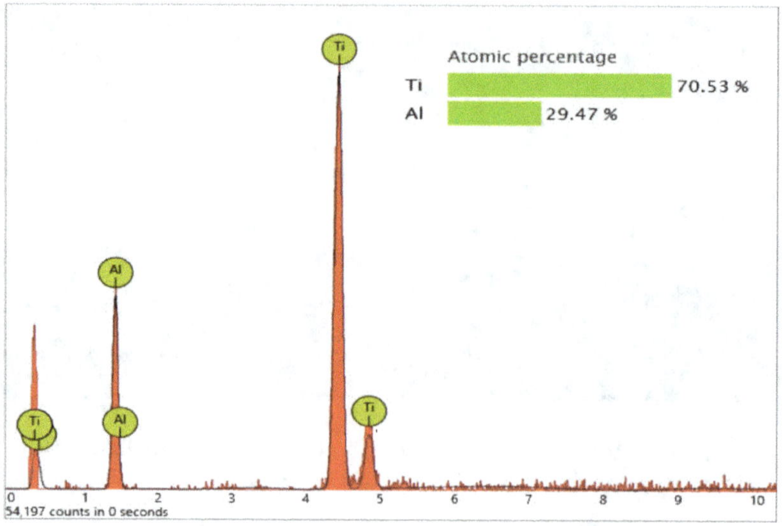

Figure 22. EDS differential measurement of the metal particle in Figure 20 (**a**), showing significant X-ray quanta of aluminum. The lack of oxygen signals indicates that these particles were not made of aluminum oxide.

These aluminum-containing particles must be rated as inorganic impurities as they are not comparable with sharp-edged aluminum oxide particles, used for blasting procedures of other implants. Apart from this, it is noticeable that the approximately 3 µm thick oxide layer was damaged at several exposed locations of the Biodenta implant (Figure 23).

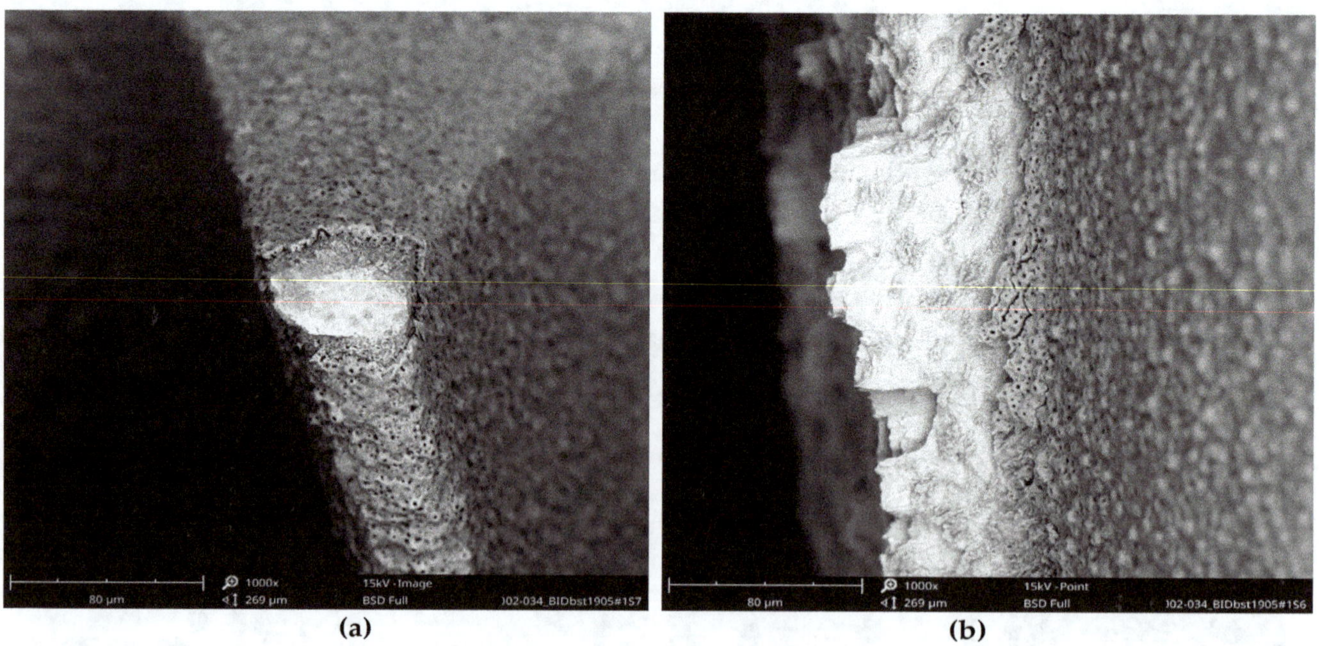

Figure 23. Damaged oxide layer of the Biodenta implant, SEM 1000×: (**a**) magnification of the blue marked area in Figure 19 showing the damage at the exposed implant thread; (**b**) magnification of the red marked area in Figure 19 demonstrates the large-area irregularity of the oxide layer at the implant apex.

3.2. Documentation of Clinical Results

None of the copy-cat manufacturers' websites contained any information regarding published clinical trials of the implant systems. No manufacturers responded to the email requesting scientific documentation regarding clinical performance. No manufacturers presented such documentation. The PubMed database search identified no papers regarding the Bioconcept or Cumdente system, but two papers for the Biodenta system. The two Biodenta papers were, however, in vitro trials that evaluated the company's CAD/CAM (computer-aided design/computer-aided manufacturing) system, not the clinical outcome of the implants [7,8]. Broadening the search by deleting "dental implants" and only using the respective company name did not identify any publications for the Cumdente system but one additional paper for the Biodenta system [9]. However, this paper did not report on the clinical outcome of implants. No clinical documentation of implant outcome was noticed for the Bioconcept system.

The OsseoSpeed implant has a very solid clinical documentation verifying excellent clinical results for up to 7 years in clinical function [10–14]. Similar excellent clinical results apply to the SLA implants from Straumann [4,15–18] and the TiUnite implants from Nobel Biocare [5,19–22], where these two implant systems have been documented for more than 10 years in numerous studies.

4. Discussion

In general, the implants OsseoSpeed (Astra Tech–Dentsply Implants), Standard Plus SLA Implant (Straumann), and NobelActive (Nobel Biocare) showed—within the scope of this analysis—a surface free of foreign materials in the SEM. The Cumdente AS Implant with a similar geometry compared to the Astra Tech OsseoSpeed implant demonstrated a surface with substantial organic contaminants and most likely remnants of Teflon. The Straumann look-alike implant from Bioconcept exposed numerous organic particles and two small particles containing significant amounts of iron. The Nobel Biocare look-alike implant from Biodenta showed high levels of magnesium and small particles with aluminum on the surface. These particles, with a diameter of 5 to 10 μm, and organic contaminants with a similar size, are small enough for phagocytosis by macrophages that would be theoretically possible for particles without a chemical bonding to the implant surface.

It may, therefore, be said that the original implants were cleaner than the correspondent look-alike devices. The price range for the look-alike implants indicated that the definition of a copy-cat product or look-alike implant is not necessarily based on a low price.

To the knowledge of the present authors, no defined thresholds have been published in peer reviewed journals until now, with respect to what may represent "acceptable" levels of impurities and what must be regarded as "unacceptable impurities". However, the non-profit CleanImplant Foundation (www.cleanimplant.org) has presented a consensus statement on surface impurities signed by Luigi Canullo (Rome, Italy), Jaafar Mouhyi (Marrakesh, Morroco), Michael Norton (London, UK), and four of the authors of this paper Tomas Albrektsson, Florian Beuer, Dirk Duddeck, and Ann Wennerberg [23]. In this consensus statement, surface anomalies and remnants of blasting materials were not considered clinically relevant, in contrast to the metal particles of tungsten, nickel, iron, chromium, copper, tin or antimony found on the surfaces of some implants. Single organic particles smaller than 50 μm in diameter were considered less vicious than numerous particles, with a maximum of 30 particles along the circumference of the implant. Major plaque-like organic contaminants exceeding the size of 50 μm and PTFE particles, presumably originating from Teflon baskets used during implant production, were considered unacceptable.

Other foreign bodies routinely seen adjacent to implants such as titanium particles [24–26] or the accidental presence of cement in the bone-to-implant interface that, according to some investigators, may be found in 59% of cemented implants [27], may combine to cause peri-implantitis [28].

Impurities on sterile packaged implants—caused by metal particles and contaminations with organic substances such as thermoplastic materials, synthetic polymers, or polysiloxanes—are technically avoidable, as this paper demonstrated. The academic discussion as to what extent implant pollution is acceptable normally ends quickly when dental professionals know about such contamination of an implant system and the next patient for an implant therapy is their partner or child. We should avoid using sterile packaged implants with verifiable impurities and therewith follow the well-established "precautionary principle" as an evolution of the ancient medical principle of "primum non nocere".

From a clinical point of view, it is obvious that Astra Tech–Dentsply Implants, Straumann, and Nobel Biocare have solidly documented clinical results reported in hundreds of scientific papers. On the other hand, a long history of clinical documentation representing high-quality efforts in the past is no guarantee for a high level of production quality and a clean surface at present, accentuating the need for periodic reviews by independent institutions. With respect to the look-alike systems, none of them had any properly documented clinical reports available. The absence of clinical documentation of look-alike systems may indicate either that they see themselves as identical to the implants they have copied or that they see implants as commodity products where all implant systems will work well clinically. The possibility first mentioned was critically analyzed in this paper comparing the cleanliness of different implant systems. The second possibility that implants are commodity products may be criticized against the knowledge of numerous implant systems that have been withdrawn from the market due to the unforeseen clinical problems over longer times of follow-up [29].

In essence, our hypothesis was verified in that the major implant systems displayed cleaner surfaces than those of their respective look-alike implants. However, whether the relative lack of cleanliness of look-alike implants indicates that they have an impaired clinical function in comparison to the major systems remains uncertain. Having said this, oral implants are placed in human beings and, therefore, it seems strongly advisable to present clinical results in peer-reviewed journals for every oral implant system to be used clinically. In this regard, the look-alike implants are clearly inferior to the major documented oral implant systems and none of the look-alike systems investigated had any clinical documentation of their own, which must be regarded as a major shortcoming. Since differences obviously exist between the major systems and the respective look-alike implants, clinicians using the latter devices must inform their patients of this fact and that the implants placed are totally un-documented with respect to clinical outcome.

5. Conclusions

In contrast to the original implants of market-leading manufacturers, the analyzed look-alike implants showed significantly more impurities, underlining the need for periodic reviews of the production quality by independent institutions. Multiple organic particles and remnants of PTFE (Cumdente), organic particles containing sulfur, particles containing iron (Bioconcept) or impurities with aluminum (Biodenta)—all particles small enough for possible phagocytosis—expose patients to unknown risks. In addition to the results of SEM/EDS analysis, the lack of clinical documentation of the analyzed look-alike implants raises concerns.

Author Contributions: Conceptualization, D.U.D., A.W., and T.A.; Investigation, D.U.D., C.L., and A.W.; Resources, D.U.D.; Writing—Original Draft Preparation, D.U.D., T.A., A.W., and C.L., Writing—Review and Editing, A.W., C.L., and F.B.; Supervision, D.U.D.; Project Administration, D.U.D.

Acknowledgments: SEM images and elemental analyses for this paper were performed with technical support from the Medical Materials Research Institute–mmri.berlin, Max-Planck-Str. 3, Zentrum für Mikrosysteme und Materialien (ZMM), 12489 Berlin–Adlershof, Germany.

References

1. Branemark, P.I.; Hansson, B.O.; Adell, R.; Breine, U.; Lindström, J.; Hallén, O.; Ohman, A. Osseointegrated implants in the treatment of the edentulous jaw. Experience from a 10-year period. *Scand. J. Plast. Reconstr. Surg. Suppl.* **1977**, *16*, 1–132. [PubMed]
2. Jimbo, R.; Albrektsson, T. Long-term clinical success of minimally and moderately rough oral implants: A review of 71 studies with 5 years or more of follow-up. *Implant Dent.* **2015**, *24*, 62–69. [CrossRef] [PubMed]
3. Wennerberg, A.; Albrektsson, T.; Chrcanovic, B. Long-term clinical outcome of implants with different surface modifications. *Eur. J. Oral Implantol.* **2018**, *11* (Suppl. 1), S123–S136. [PubMed]

4. Buser, D.; Janner, S.F.; Wittneben, J.G.; Bragger, U.; Ramseier, C.A.; Salvi, G.E. 10-year survival and success rates of 511 titanium implants with a sandblasted and acid-etched surface: A retrospective study in 303 partially edentulous patients. *Clin. Implant Dent. Relat. Res.* **2012**, *14*, 839–851. [CrossRef] [PubMed]
5. Glauser, R. Implants with an Oxidized Surface Placed Predominately in Soft Bone Quality and Subjected to Immediate Occlusal Loading: Results from an 11-Year Clinical Follow-Up. *Clin. Implant Dent. Relat. Res.* **2016**, *18*, 429–438. [CrossRef] [PubMed]
6. Toljanic, J.A.; Ekstrand, K.; Baer, R.A.; Thor, A. Immediate Loading of Implants in the Edentulous Maxilla with a Fixed Provisional Restoration without Bone Augmentation: A Report on 5-Year Outcomes Data Obtained from a Prospective Clinical Trial. *Int. J. Oral Maxillofac. Implant.* **2016**, *31*, 1164–1170. [CrossRef] [PubMed]
7. Katsoulis, J.; Muller, P.; Mericske-Stern, R.; Blatz, M.B. CAD/CAM fabrication accuracy of long- vs. short-span implant-supported FDPs. *Clin. Oral Implant. Res.* **2015**, *26*, 245–249. [CrossRef]
8. Rismanchian, M.; Shafiei, S.; Nourbakhshian, F.; Davoudi, A. Flexural strengths of implant-supported zirconia based bridges in posterior regions. *J. Adv. Prosthodont.* **2014**, *6*, 346–350. [CrossRef]
9. Rismanchian, M.; Shafiei, S.; Askari, N.; Khodaeian, N. Comparison of shear bond strength of two veneering ceramics to zirconia. *Dent. Res. J.* **2012**, *9*, 628–633. [CrossRef]
10. Boven, G.C.; Slot, J.W.A.; Raghoebar, G.M.; Vissink, A.; Meijer, H.J.A. Maxillary implant-supported overdentures opposed by (partial) natural dentitions: A 5-year prospective case series study. *J. Oral Rehabil.* **2017**, *44*, 988–995. [CrossRef]
11. Cooper, L.F.; Reside, G.; Raes, F.; Garriga, J.; Tarrida, L.; Wiltfang, J.; Kern, M.; Bruyn, H. Immediate provisionalization of dental implants in grafted alveolar ridges in the esthetic zone: A 5-year evaluation. *Int. J. Periodontics Restor. Dent.* **2014**, *34*, 477–486. [CrossRef]
12. Mertens, C.; Steveling, H.G. Early and immediate loading of titanium implants with fluoride-modified surfaces: Results of 5-year prospective study. *Clin. Oral Implant. Res.* **2011**, *22*, 1354–1360. [CrossRef]
13. Noelken, R.; Moergel, M.; Kunkel, M.; Wagner, W. Immediate and flapless implant insertion and provisionalization using autogenous bone grafts in the esthetic zone: 5-year results. *Clin. Oral Implant. Res.* **2018**, *29*, 320–327. [CrossRef]
14. Raes, S.; Raes, F.; Cooper, L.; Giner Tarrida, L.; Vervaeke, S.; Cosyn, J.; De Bruyn, H. Oral health-related quality of life changes after placement of immediately loaded single implants in healed alveolar ridges or extraction sockets: A 5-year prospective follow-up study. *Clin. Oral Implant. Res.* **2017**, *28*, 662–667. [CrossRef]
15. Fischer, K.; Stenberg, T. Prospective 10-year cohort study based on a randomized controlled trial (RCT) on implant-supported full-arch maxillary prostheses. Part 1: Sandblasted and acid-etched implants and mucosal tissue. *Clin. Implant Dent. Relat. Res.* **2012**, *14*, 808–815. [CrossRef]
16. French, D.; Larjava, H.; Ofec, R. Retrospective cohort study of 4591 Straumann implants in private practice setting, with up to 10-year follow-up. Part 1: Multivariate survival analysis. *Clin. Oral Implant. Res.* **2015**, *26*, 1345–1354. [CrossRef]
17. Roccuzzo, M.; Grasso, G.; Dalmasso, P. Keratinized mucosa around implants in partially edentulous posterior mandible: 10-year results of a prospective comparative study. *Clin. Oral Implant. Res.* **2016**, *27*, 491–496. [CrossRef]
18. Zhang, X.X.; Shi, J.Y.; Gu, Y.X.; Lai, H. Long-Term Outcomes of Early Loading of Straumann Implant-Supported Fixed Segmented Bridgeworks in Edentulous Maxillae: A 10-Year Prospective Study. *Clin. Implant Dent. Relat. Res.* **2016**, *18*, 1227–1237. [CrossRef]
19. Degidi, M.; Nardi, D.; Piattelli, A. 10-year follow-up of immediately loaded implants with TiUnite porous anodized surface. *Clin. Implant Dent. Relat. Res.* **2012**, *14*, 828–838. [CrossRef]
20. Imburgia, M.; Del Fabbro, M. Long-Term Retrospective Clinical and Radiographic Follow-up of 205 Branemark System Mk III TiUnite Implants Submitted to Either Immediate or Delayed Loading. *Implant Dent.* **2015**, *24*, 533–540. [CrossRef]
21. Karl, M.; Albrektsson, T. Clinical Performance of Dental Implants with a Moderately Rough (TiUnite) Surface: A Meta-Analysis of Prospective Clinical Studies. *Int. J. Oral. Maxillofac. Implant.* **2017**, *32*, 717–734. [CrossRef]

22. Ostman, P.O.; Hellman, M.; Sennerby, L. Ten years later. Results from a prospective single-centre clinical study on 121 oxidized (TiUnite) Branemark implants in 46 patients. *Clin. Implant Dent. Relat. Res.* **2012**, *14*, 852–860. [CrossRef]
23. Duddeck, D.; Albrektsson, T.; Wennerberg, A.; Mouhyi, J.; Norton, M.; Canullo, L.; Beuer, F. CleanImplant Trusted Quality Mark 2017–2018—Guideline and Consensus Paper. Available online: www.cleanimplant.org (accessed on 26 June 2019).
24. Albrektsson, T.; Becker, W.; Coli, P.; Jemt, T.; Mölne, J.; Sennerby, L. Bone loss around oral and orthopedic implants: An immunologically based condition. *Clin. Implant Dent. Relat. Res.* **2019**, *21*, 786–795. [CrossRef]
25. Tawse-Smith, A.; Ma, S.; Siddiqi, A.; Duncan, W.J.; Girvan, L.; Hussaini, H.M. Titanium Particles in the Peri-Implant Tissues: Surface Analysis and Histological Response. *Clin. Adv. Periodontics* **2012**, *2*, 232–238. [CrossRef]
26. Wennerberg, A.; Ide-Ektessabi, A.; Hatkamata, S.; Sawase, T.; Johansson, C.; Albrektsson, T.; Martinelli, A.; Södervall, U.; Odelius, H. Titanium release from implants prepared with different surface roughness. *Clin. Oral Implant. Res.* **2004**, *15*, 505–512. [CrossRef]
27. Korsch, M.; Obst, U.; Walther, W. Cement-associated peri-implantitis: A retrospective clinical observational study of fixed implant-supported restorations using a methacrylate cement. *Clin. Oral Implant. Res.* **2014**, *25*, 797–802. [CrossRef]
28. Wilson, T.G., Jr.; Valderrama, P.; Burbano, M.; Blansett, J.; Levine, R.; Kessler, H.; Rodrigues, D.C. Foreign bodies associated with peri-implantitis human biopsies. *J. Periodontol.* **2015**, *86*, 9–15. [CrossRef]
29. Qian, J.; Wennerberg, A.; Albrektsson, T. Reasons for marginal bone loss around oral implants. *Clin. Implant Dent. Relat. Res.* **2012**, *14*, 792–807. [CrossRef]

12

Ligature-Induced Experimental Peri-Implantitis

David Reinedahl [1,*], Bruno Chrcanovic [2], Tomas Albrektsson [2,3], Pentti Tengvall [3] and Ann Wennerberg [1]

1 Department of Prosthodontics, Institute of Odontology, Sahlgrenska Academy, Gothenburg University, Gothenburg 405 30, Sweden; ann.wennerberg@odontologi.gu.se
2 Department of Prosthodontics, Faculty of Odontology, Malmö University, Malmö 205 06, Sweden; brunochrcanovic@hotmail.com (B.C.); tomas.albrektsson@biomaterials.gu.se (T.A.)
3 Department of Biomaterials, Institute of Clinical Sciences, Sahlgrenska Academy, Gothenburg University, Gothenburg 405 30, Sweden; pentti.tengvall@gu.se
* Corresponsence: d.reinedahl@gmail.com

Abstract: This systematic review sought to analyze different experimental peri-implantitis models, their potential to induce marginal bone resorption (MBR) and the necessity of bacteria for bone loss to occur in these models. An electronic search in PubMed/Medline, Web of Science, and ScienceDirect was undertaken. A total of 133 studies were analyzed. Most studies induced peri-implantitis with ligatures that had formed a biofilm, sometimes in combination with inoculation of specific bacteria but never in a sterile environment. Most vertical MBR resulted from new ligatures periodically packed above old ones, followed by periodically exchanged ligatures and ligatures that were not exchanged. Cotton ligatures produced the most MBR, followed by steel, "dental floss" (not further specified in the studies) and silk. The amount of MBR varied significantly between different animal types and implant surfaces. None of the analyzed ligature studies aimed to validate that bacteria are necessary for the inducement of MBR. It cannot be excluded that bone loss can be achieved by other factors of the model, such as an immunological reaction to the ligature itself or trauma from repeated ligature insertions. Because all the included trials allowed plaque accumulation on the ligatures, bone resorbing capacity due to other factors could not be excluded or evaluated here.

Keywords: osseointegration; dental implant; peri-implantitis; ligature-induced peri-implantitis; aseptic loosening; systematic review

---

1. Introduction

Experiments that aimed to mimic peri-implantitis were first introduced in the early 1990s in response to reports on progressive peri-implant bone loss around dental implants [1,2]. These experiments have mainly been based on the infectious model of explanation where bacteria are the presumed cause of the phenomenon [2,3]. The view of peri-implantitis as a strictly infectious condition, as suggested in the studies these models were based on, is currently a matter of debate. Albrektsson and co-workers recently proposed that tissue responses to dental implants should be viewed similarly to other biomaterials; primarily as an immune mediated inflammatory and foreign body reaction (FBR), indicating that immunological reactions may be important also for MBR [4]. The initial, and most frequently used experimental peri-implantitis model was adopted from the ligature-induced periodontitis model. In short, ligatures made of silk, cotton, stainless-steel wire, or other materials, are placed around the neck of dental implants, usually in a sub-marginal position. The ligatures are then allowed to accumulate plaque for a few months, after which a certain amount of marginal bone resorption (MBR) can be expected. Previous authors have claimed that plaque accumulation is necessary for bone resorption to occur in response to ligation [2,5], but Baron et al. pointed out a lack of validation for this claim in their review from year 2000 and concluded that other factors, such as a foreign body reaction to the ligature may also trigger a peri-implant inflammatory response [6]. The aims of the present review were to categorize (1) the models that induce experimental peri-implantitis described in literature and (2) to verify whether the amount of vertical MBR varies between different ligature techniques (exchanged or non-exchanged ligature), material and size of ligatures, animals or implant surfaces used in these studies. With this information in mind, we then (3) critically analyzed the attempts to validate the presence of bacteria containing biofilms as a cause of MBR in ligature-induced peri-implantitis models.

2. Materials and Methods

The present study followed the PRISMA Statement for Transparent Reporting of Systematic Reviews and Meta-analyses [7].

2.1. Search Strategies

An electronic search without time restrictions for publications in English was undertaken in January 2018 in the following databases: PubMed/Medline, Web of Science, and ScienceDirect. The following terms were used in the search strategies:

(((dental implant) OR oral implant)) AND (experimentally induced periimplantitis) OR experimentally induced peri-implantitis) OR experimental periimplantitis) OR experimental peri-implantitis) OR ligature induced periimplantitis) OR ligature induced peri-implantitis) OR ligature) OR plaque induced periimplantitis) OR plaque induced peri-implantitis) OR plaque accumulation) OR mechanical overload) OR bacterial inoculation)

An additional manual search of related journals was conducted. The reference list of the identified studies and the relevant reviews on the subject were scanned for possible additional studies.

2.2. Inclusion and Exclusion Criteria

The inclusion criteria comprised in vivo studies performing experimentally induced peri-implantitis. All animal species used for the experiments and all methods to induce peri-implantitis were considered. Studies inducing periodontitis (around teeth) were not included, unless they were also investigating peri-implantitis around implants. Studies evaluating only mucositis around implants were excluded.

2.3. Study Selection

The titles and abstracts of all reports identified through the electronic searches were read independently by the authors. For studies appearing to meet the inclusion criteria, or for which there were insufficient data in the title and abstract to make a clear decision, the full report was obtained. Disagreements were resolved by discussion between the authors and the authors rapidly reached a consensus.

2.4. Data Extraction

Two review authors independently searched for trials aiming to validate the necessity of biofilm in order to induce MBR by means of ligatures. They then independently extracted data using specially designed data extraction forms. The data extraction forms were piloted on several papers, which were modified as required before use.

From the studies included in the final analysis, the following data was extracted (when available): Year of publication, animal species used in the experiments, number of animals, jaw receiving the implants, number of extracted teeth (to make room for the implants), implants' healing period, study design (split design, inter-quadrant, other), implant characteristics (shape, dimensions, material, surface, bone/tissue level), number of implants per animal, number of surgery stages, time between abutment connection and peri-implantitis induction, use or not of randomization, use or not of loading, pre- and post-operative care (antibiotic, and plaque control method, timing, and duration), method of induction of peri-implantitis (ligature, overload, bacterial inoculation, other), ligature (material, size, exchange regimen, duration, control side protocol), diagnostic markers (clinical measurements, mobility, microbiological sampling, radiographies, histometric measurements, histological evaluation, other), peri-implant bone defect (time of registration, vertical MBR, horizontal MBR, measurement method, development after ligature removal, number of lost implants). Contact with authors for possible missing data was performed.

2.5. Analyses

Descriptive statistics were utilized to report the data. In order to standardize and clarify ambiguous data, vertical MBR was reported for each publication. Vertical MBR was the continuous outcome evaluated, and the statistical unit was the implant (the implants used in the animals). The untransformed proportion (random-effects DerSimonian–Laird (1986) method) for vertical bone loss was calculated [8] with consideration for the different implant surfaces, the different animal species, the different methods to induce peri-implantitis and, when ligature was the method used, the different regimen applied, i.e., application of only one ligature, exchange of ligatures over time, and application of a new ligature on the top of an old one. Meta-regression was performed for the outcome of vertical MBR, using the time period of peri-implantitis induction as covariate. Statistical significance was set at $p < 0.05$. The data were analyzed using the software OpenMeta (Analyst) (MetaMorph Inc., Nashville, TN, USA) [9].

3. Results

3.1. Literature Search

The study selection process is summarized in Figure 1. The search strategy in the databases returned 3525 papers. A number of 745 articles were cited in more than one database (duplicates). The reviewers independently screened the abstracts for those articles related to the aim of the review. Of the resulting 2780 studies, 2642 were excluded for not being related to the topic or for not being induced peri-implantitis animal studies. Additional hand-searching of journals and of the reference lists of selected studies yielded 10 additional papers. The full-text reports of the remaining 148 articles led to the exclusion of 15 because they did not meet the inclusion criteria. Thus, a total of 133 publications were included in the review (see References S1).

3.2. Description of the Studies and Analyses

Regarding ligature-induced peri-implantitis; none of the included publications attempted to validate the presence of a bacterial biofilm in order to achieve MBR.

Detailed data of the 133 included studies are listed in Tables S1 and S2. Dogs were the most commonly used animal for the experiments (being the case of 94 studies) followed by monkeys (26 studies), mice (8 studies), micro-/mini-pigs (3 studies), and rats (2 studies).

Concerning the method of peri-implantitis induction, most of the studies (n = 91) induced peri-implantitis with the use of ligatures alone. Ligatures of cotton were used in 50 studies, silk in 31 studies, 3 metallic ligatures, one the resorbable suture Vicryl, one "dental floss", and 5 studies used a combination of ligatures of different materials. Thirteen studies applied a period of ligature and then a period of plaque accumulation (or vice-versa), 8 studies compared two or more groups concerning the method of peri-implantitis induction (ligature and/or overload and/or plaque accumulation), 5 studies used cotton ligatures followed by inoculation of *Porphyromonas gingivalis*. Seven studies provided a time of plaque accumulation alone, 4 studies exposed the implants to overload, 2 studies applied ligatures plus cyanoacrylate, 2 studies used bacterial inoculation alone, and 1 study immunized the animals followed by an injection of lipopolysaccharides.

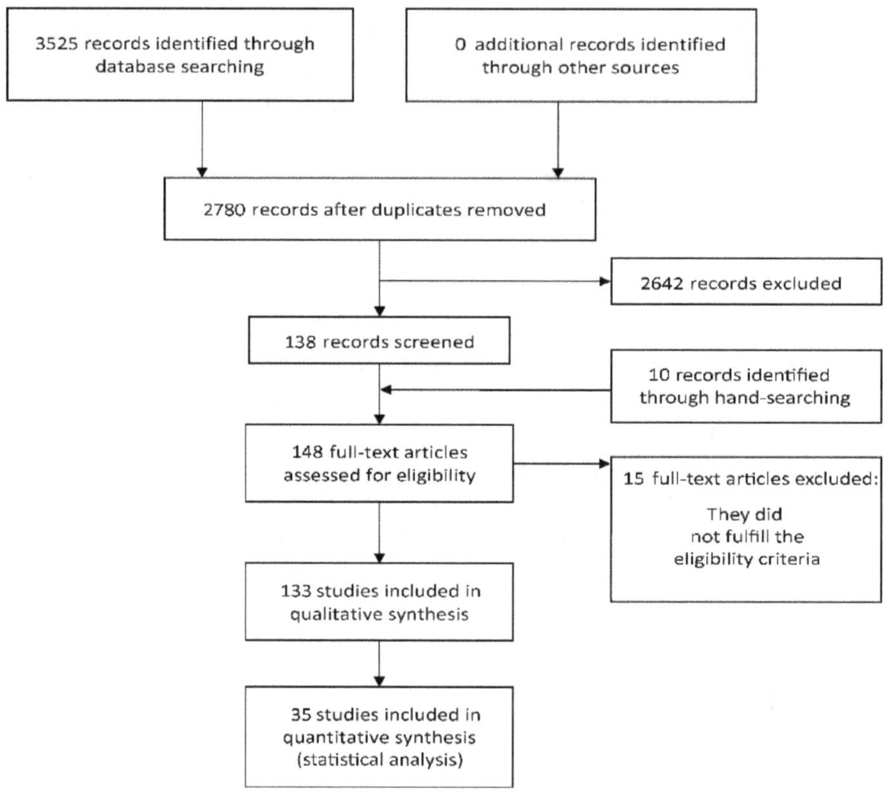

Figure 1. Study selection.

The implant healing period before the induction of experimental peri-implantitis was at average 96.0 ± 57.1 days (min–max, 0–365). Seventy-nine studies used bone-level implants, 46 tissue-level implants, 5 studies used both types of implants, 2 studies installed the implants at the sub-crestal level, and proper information was not provided in one study.

The ligature methods were of three different regimens: One ligature not replaced (n = 53), exchange of ligatures (n = 43), and periodical replacement of ligatures on top of old ones (n = 11). Information was not available in 4 studies. Only 30 studies provided information on ligature size, varying from suture size 7–0 to 2–0 United States Pharmacopeia (USP). Other examples included 0.010 inch, 0.254 mm, and 1.58 mm. The duration of ligature placement time varied between 7 and 660 days, and some studies intercalated the use of ligatures between periods of plaque accumulation or of plaque control.

Plaque control maintenance was performed in 111 studies, where the period varied between "only once" to 2 years. Information about plaque control was not available in 8 studies. The plaque control methods used varied considerably among studies and included one or a combination of two or more of the following activities: Daily brushing with toothpaste, interdental brushing, electric pencil brush, application of chlorhexidine, scrubbing with chlorhexidine, implant scaling with plastic scaler, gentle mechanical cleaning of pockets, manual irrigation with syringe, dental water jet, flossing, and curettage. The plaque control maintenance also varied considerably among studies concerning the duration period, the number of maintenance periods, and timing (for example; after teeth extraction, after implant installation, at abutment connection, and after ligature removal).

The studies usually made use of several diagnostic markers listed in Table S2, but the present review focused on the analysis of the vertical MBR. Table 1 shows the estimated vertical bone loss in relation to implant surface type, species, method of peri-implantitis induction, and ligature regimen, according to the untransformed proportion using the DerSimonian–Laird method (1986) analysis [6].

Only studies providing the number of implants used, mean value and standard deviation for bone loss were included here (n = 35 of the 133 reviewed studies) because these values are necessary for the analyses. Detailed data for these 35 studies are listed in Tables S3 and S4 and a reference list is available in References S2.

Table 1. Estimated vertical bone resorption in relation to implant surface type, species, method of peri-implantitis induction and ligature regimen.

Factor	MBR (in mm) (95% CI), p-Value, SE	Heterogeneity	Number of Measurements * Included for the Meta Regression (Number of Studies)
Surface			
Turned	2.265 (1.786, 2.745), $p < 0.001$, 0.245	$I^2 = 99.5\%$, $p < 0.001$	29 (21)
Acid-etched	2.864 (2.491, 3.237), $p < 0.001$, 0.190	$I^2 = 94.72\%$, $p < 0.001$	12 (6)
SB	2.509 (1.555, 3.463), $p < 0.001$, 0.487	$I^2 = 98.03\%$, $p < 0.001$	6 (5)
SB+F	1.697 (-0.640, 4.034), $p = 0.155$, 1.193	$I^2 = 98.94\%$, $p < 0.001$	3 (2)
SBAE	2.175 (1.658, 2.693), $p < 0.001$, 0.264	$I^2 = 98.44\%$, $p < 0.001$	21 (10)
SBAE/HA-coated	2.700 (2.174, 3.226), NA, 0.268	NA	1 (1)
HA-coated	2.349 (1.254, 3.444), $p < 0.001$, 0.559	$I^2 = 98.58\%$, $p < 0.001$	12 (7)
HA-plasma	1.650 (1.410, 1.890), $p < 0.001$, 0.122	$I^2 = 0\%$, $p = 0.683$	2 (1)
CaP-plasma sprayed	0.469 (-0.010, 0.949), $p = 0.055$, 0.245	$I^2 = 75.67\%$, $p < 0.043$	2 (1)
TPS	2.184 (1.523, 2.844), $p < 0.001$, 0.337	$I^2 = 98.16\%$, $p < 0.001$	13 (9)
Cancellous	1.932 (1.432, 2.431), $p < 0.001$, 0.255	$I^2 = 0\%$, $p = 0.990$	4 (1)
Anodized	3.462 (3.273, 3.651), $p < 0.001$, 0.097	$I^2 = 16.1\%$, $p = 0.311$	4 (2)
Overall	**2.295 (2.042, 2.548), $p < 0.001$, 0.129**	**$I^2 = 99.18\%$, $p < 0.001$**	**109 (35 **)**
Species			
Dog	2.389 (2.152, 2.626), $p < 0.001$, 0.121	$I^2 = 98.3\%$, $p < 0.001$	98 (30)
Monkey	1.649 (1.254, 2.044), $p < 0.001$, 0.202	$I^2 = 96.75\%$, $p < 0.001$	9 (4)
Rat	0.800 (0.393, 1.207), NA, 0.208	NA	1 (1)
Mouse	0.579 (0.549, 0.609), NA, 0.015	NA	1 (1)
Overall	**2.295 (2.042, 2.548), $p < 0.001$, 0.129**	**$I^2 = 99.18\%$, $p < 0.001$**	**109 (35 **)**
Method			
Plaque	0.689 (0.507, 0.871), $p < 0.001$, 0.093	$I^2 = 66.17\%$, $p = 0.007$	7 (2)
Inoculation	0.800 (0.393, 1.207), NA, 0.208	NA	1 (1)
Ligature			
Cotton	2.730 (2.478, 2.982), $p < 0.001$, 0.129	$I^2 = 97.88\%$, $p < 0.001$	66 (22)
Silk	1.683 (1.296, 2.070), $p < 0.001$, 0.197	$I^2 = 98.98\%$, $p < 0.001$	28 (8)
"Dental floss"	2.361 (1.675, 3.046), $p < 0.001$, 0.350	$I^2 = 86.05\%$, $p = 0.007$	2 (1)
Steel	2.607 (1.359, 3.856), $p < 0.001$, 0.637	$I^2 = 98.08\%$, $p < 0.001$	5 (2)
Overall	**2.295 (2.042, 2.548), $p < 0.001$, 0.129**	**$I^2 = 99.18\%$, $p < 0.001$**	**109 (35 **)**
Ligature regimen			
Only one	2.000 (1.647, 2.352), $p < 0.001$, 0.180	$I^2 = 98.91\%$, $p < 0.001$	37 (13)
Exchange	2.303 (2.030, 2.576), $p < 0.001$, 0.139	$I^2 = 97.89\%$, $p < 0.001$	48 (14)
New on top	3.123 (2.409, 3.838), $p < 0.001$, 0.365	$I^2 = 98.66\%$, $p < 0.001$	20 (6)
Overall	**2.395 (2.098, 2.620), $p < 0.001$, 0.133**	**$I^2 = 99.2\%$, $p < 0.001$**	**105 (33) *****

CI—confidence interval, SE—standard error, MBL—marginal bone loss, SB—sandblasted, SB+F—sandblasted + fluoride modified, SBAE—Sandblasted/acid-etched, HA—hydroxyapatite, NA—not applicable (there is only one study for this category), TPS—Titanium plasma-sprayed. * Some studies performed measurements of MBL in different implant surfaces, and/or different time points, and/or different methods. ** The total number of studies is always 35 for the factors "surface", "species", and "method", even though the sum of the studies for all categories under the same factor is higher than 35. The reason for this is that some studies performed measurements of MBL in different conditions, as explained in the footnote "*" above. An exception is made for "ligature regimen" (see footnote "***" below). *** The ligature regimen was not clearly informed in four measurements performed in two studies.

4. Discussion

This systematic review presents a broad inclusion of experimental peri-implantitis studies that were all based on the infectious model except for a few studies that exposed the implants to overload. The infectious model of explanation for peri-implantitis stems from the traditional view that osseointegration results from ordinary bone healing adjacent to an inert implant and where all subsequent marginal bone loss is due to bacterial challenge [3,10]. Currently, it is becoming more and more clear that osseointegration is an FBR of demarcation type that is dependent on local and systemic factors [11–13]. Even though the demarcation type reaction serves a functional purpose by enabling dental implants to carry chewing forces, its immunological purpose is to shield off the material and limit its tissue damage. It has been well established that an FBR is initiated at the time of implantation of all biomaterials and that its expression may vary between encapsulation, dissolution, resorption or rejection, depending on the properties of the material or the trauma associated with its insertion. Its expression type may also vary over time in response to changing local or systemic factors [14,15].

Sub-marginal ligation remains the most commonly used means to induce experimental peri-implantitis and provides a relatively rapid and effective MBR. Plaque accumulation alone on the other hand, provides minimal or absent MBR as evident from the dog (n = 5) and monkey (n = 2) studies which used that technique in the present review [16–22]. Prior to its introduction in dental implant research in the early 1990s, the model had been used extensively in experimental periodontitis studies [23]. While it has been realized that ligature-induced peri-implantitis may not completely mimic the onset and progression of disease in humans [24], it is still generally regarded as a solely infectious model as evident from repeated claims that bone resorption results from exposition to biofilm, not the ligature per se [2,4,25]. The earliest studies on experimental peri-implantitis revealed that the infectious model of explanation was adopted from studies on native tissues (experimental periodontitis), rather than implanted material. For example, Lindhe et al. referred to a 1966 study on germ-free vs. conventional rats to support the theory [2]. In the provided reference, Rovin et al. described an increased inflammatory response in the gingival tissues of conventional rats compared to germ free rats after ligation with USP 3-0 braided silk sutures. However, none of the rats lost any bone and neither did the distance between the epithelial attachment and cemento-enamel junction vary between these groups at any time interval until the termination of the experiment after 6 months of ligation. Rovin et al. concluded that their specific rat type appeared unsusceptible to periodontitis [26]. We failed to identify any experimental peri-implantitis studies that attempted to validate that ligatures cannot induce MBR without the presence of a biofilm. As concluded in a previous review by Baron et al., it still "remains uncertain whether the peri-implant inflammatory response is really only the result of increased plaque accumulation or if the thread itself, as a foreign body, also acts as a stimulus" [5].

In the present review dogs displayed more bone loss in response to ligation than monkeys, which points to differences in their susceptibility to ligature-induced peri-implantitis. The time required to achieve a certain amount of bone loss also varied greatly within the groups of dogs or monkeys in single studies [27,28]. The difference in MBR between rodents and large animals in the present review may be due to the small implants and ligatures used in rodents compared to dogs and monkeys. One must also consider the small number of rodent studies (n = 2) included in the analysis. Recently, different mouse strains and knock out models have been used to better understand why the marginal bone resorption in response to ligation differs between animals [29,30].

The significant differences in the MBR that resulted from different ligature materials in the present meta-analysis, may be due to differences between the FBRs provoked by these materials. They could also be related to varying plaque carriage potentials for these materials, but this can hardly explain why smooth stainless-steel ligatures induced more bone loss than twined silk. Consider also the significant differences in MBR between different ligature regimens, with more bone loss generated from regularly exchanged ligatures and new ligatures packed on top of old ones, as compared to only one ligature. Studies that utilized the exchanged ligature technique in the present review typically carried out the exchange every 3 weeks by first removing the old ligature and then pushing a new one into the bottom of the existing peri-implant pocket. Assuming that an anaerobic flora exists in the apical part of a lesion prior to ligature exchange, it is likely that the removal procedure will disrupt the biofilm and also introduce air into the lesion (aeration is generally considered an important part of the surgical treatment of an anaerobic infection). It would also take some time for a new anaerobic biofilm to develop on the new, presumably clean ligature. This may indicate that a close proximity between ligature and bone, is more critical for continuous bone loss to occur than the type and composition of its bacterial flora. The general disregard of the ligature itself as a potential inducer of bone loss may perhaps explain why details about ligature size, material, structure, and sometimes composition, were left out in many studies. In fact, none of the included studies compared the effect of different ligature types or regimens.

The addition of ligature around a dental implant introduces a new foreign body on another foreign body. It is plausible to assume that the new foreign body will alter the biological response of adjacent tissues to a type more specific for the introduced ligature material. Because bacteria were always present on the ligatures of the included studies, their isolated effect could not be evaluated in the present review. However, the FBRs to some of the most common ligature materials have been described elsewhere in the literature. Silk, for example, is commonly used in in vivo applications and produced the least amount of marginal bone loss in the present review. Setzen et al. reported that twined silk sutures, identical with those commonly used in the trials of the present review, produced a relatively extensive foreign body reaction and the thickest fibrous capsule of 11 sterile suture materials that were placed subcutaneously in a rabbit model [31]. Cotton on the other hand, has been shown to induce intense FBRs and also produced the most vertical MBL in the present review. Even though cotton is generally avoided in vivo, it has sometimes been used as a negative control in studies that compared the FBR to different biomaterials [32]. From reports on iatrogenic injuries following surgery, it is known that retained sterile cotton sponges can cause large lesions of foreign body type in both hard and soft tissues, sometimes referred to as "cottonballomas". For example, Kalbermatten et al. reported a massive osteolytic process surrounded by a thin rim of bone next to a sterile cotton sponge that had been left 25 years earlier during the stabilization of a femoral fracture [33]. The case exemplifies the slow progression often seen in foreign body type lesions, as well as their potential to induce both bone resorption and bone remodelling. Even microscopic remnants of sterile lint retained from cotton sponges during routine surgery have been shown to cause considerable foreign body granulomas with ingested lint particles visible within macrophages and foreign body giant cells after 4 weeks in rats [34]. It is plausible that similar particles can disseminate from the cotton ligatures used to induce experimental peri-implantitis, but their presence or eventual role does not appear to have been investigated in experimental peri-implantitis models. Within the orthopedic field, macrophage activation after phagocytosis or cell-surface contact with wear particles is considered the key causal reason for aseptic implant loosening, which is the main cause for revision surgery over the mid- and long-term [35,36].

The addition of bacteria on ligatures, as was the case in all reviewed studies, will obviously alter the inflammatory reaction to the ligature and likely plays an important role in the initiation and progression of MBR, i.e. it is an offer to bacteria to invade new space. Bacteria may however not be the only cause, as indicated by the results of this meta-analysis and other cited literature. It therefore remains uncertain whether a ligature-induced lesion represents clinical peri-implantitis better than a man-made defect would, perhaps created at implant insertion and then allowed to accumulate biofilm for a short time. A man-made defect would probably decrease animal suffering significantly, considering that ligatures have sometimes been left in place for as long as 1 year to induce a few millimeters of bone loss [37–39]. A few experiments with man-made defects have been reported. For example, Takasaki et al. combined manually created bone defects with a shorter ligature period of 5 weeks [40].

It also remains uncertain as to what extent a ligature-induced lesion can represent clinical peri-implantitis and until further validation has been provided, clinical conclusions from ligature-induced peri-implantitis studies should be drawn with great care and the experimental and clinical conditions should be treated as separate entities at all times.

Author Contributions: Conceptualization, D.R., B.C., T.A., P.T., A.W.; Methodology, D.R., B.C., T.A., P.T., A.W.; Formal Analysis, B.C., D.R.; Investigation D.R., B.C.; Writing—Original Draft Preparation, D.R., B.C.; Writing—Review & Editing, all authors; Supervision, A.W., T.A., P.T.; Funding Acquisition, A.W.

References

1. Hickey, J.S.; O'Neal, R.B.; Scheidt, M.J.; Strong, S.L.; Turgeon, D.; Van Dyke, T.E. Microbiologic characterization of ligature-induced peri-implantitis in the microswine model. *J. Periodontol.* **1991**, *62*, 548–553. [CrossRef] [PubMed]
2. Lindhe, J.; Berglundh, T.; Ericsson, I.; Liljenberg, B.; Marinello, C. Experimental breakdown of peri-implant and periodontal tissues. A study in the beagle dog. *Clin. Oral Implants Res.* **1992**, *3*, 9–16. [CrossRef] [PubMed]

3. Lindhe, J.; Meyle, J.; D.o.E.W.o.P. Group. Peri-implant diseases: Consensus Report of the Sixth European Workshop on Periodontology. *J. Clin. Periodontol.* **2008**, *35*, 282–285. [CrossRef] [PubMed]
4. Albrektsson, T.; Dahlin, C.; Jemt, T.; Sennerby, L.; Turri, A.; Wennerberg, A. Is marginal bone loss around oral implants the result of a provoked foreign body reaction? *Clin. Implant Dent. Relat. Res.* **2014**, *16*, 155–165. [CrossRef] [PubMed]
5. Carcuac, O.; Abrahamsson, I.; Albouy, J.P.; Linder, E.; Larsson, L.; Berglundh, T. Experimental periodontitis and peri-implantitis in dogs. *Clin. Oral Implants Res.* **2013**, *24*, 363–371. [CrossRef] [PubMed]
6. Baron, M.; Haas, R.; Dortbudak, O.; Watzek, G. Experimentally induced peri-implantitis: a review of different treatment methods described in the literature. *Int. J. Oral Maxillofac. Implants* **2000**, *15*, 533–544. [PubMed]
7. Moher, D.; Liberati, A.; Tetzlaff, J.; Altman, D.G.; Group, P. Preferred reporting items for systematic reviews and meta-analyses: the PRISMA statement. *Ann. Intern. Med.* **2009**, *151*, 264–269. [CrossRef] [PubMed]
8. DerSimonian, R.; Laird, N. Meta-analysis in clinical trials. *Control Clin. Trials.* **1986**, *7*, 177–188. [CrossRef]
9. Wallace, B.C.; Trikalinos, T.A.; Lau, J.; Trow, P.; Schmid, C.H. Closing the Gap between Methodologists and End-Users: R as a Computational Back-End. *J. Stat. Softw.* **2012**, *49*, 1–15. [CrossRef]
10. Zitzmann, N.U.; Berglundh, T. Definition and prevalence of peri-implant diseases. *J. Clin. Periodontol.* **2008**, *35*, 286–291. [CrossRef] [PubMed]
11. Albrektsson, T.; Chrcanovic, B.; Ostman, P.O.; Sennerby, L. Initial and long-term crestal bone responses to modern dental implants. *Periodontol 2000.* **2017**, *73*, 41–50. [CrossRef] [PubMed]
12. Trindade, R.; Albrektsson, T.; Tengvall, P.; Wennerberg, A. Foreign Body Reaction to Biomaterials: On Mechanisms for Buildup and Breakdown of Osseointegration. *Clin. Implant Dent. Relat. Res.* **2014**, *18*, 192–203. [CrossRef] [PubMed]
13. Trindade, R.; Albrektsson, T.; Galli, S.; Prgomet, Z.; Tengvall, P.; Wennerberg, A. Osseointegration and foreign body reaction: Titanium implants activate the immune system and suppress bone resorption during the first 4 weeks after implantation. *Clin. Implant Dent. Relat. Res.* **2018**, *20*, 82–91. [CrossRef] [PubMed]
14. Donath, K.; Laass, M.; Günzl, H.J. The histopathology of different foreign-body reactions in oral soft tissue and bone tissue. *Virchows Arch. A Pathol. Anat. Histopathol.* **1992**, *420*, 131–137. [CrossRef] [PubMed]
15. Anderson, J.M.; Rodriguez, A.; Chang, D.T. Foreign body reaction to biomaterials. *Semin. Immunol.* **2008**, *20*, 86–100. [CrossRef] [PubMed]
16. Abrahamsson, I.; Berglundh, T.; Lindhe, J. Soft tissue response to plaque formation at different implant systems. A comparative study in the dog. *Clin. Oral Implants Res.* **1998**, *9*, 73–79. [CrossRef] [PubMed]
17. Ericsson, I.; Berglundh, T.; Marinello, C.; Liljenberg, B.; Lindhe, J. Long-standing plaque and gingivitis at implants and teeth in the dog. *Clin. Oral Implants Res.* **1992**, *3*, 99–103. [CrossRef] [PubMed]
18. Ericsson, I.; Persson, L.G.; Berglundh, T.; Marinello, C.P.; Lindhe, J.; Klinge, B. Different types of inflammatory reactions in peri-implant soft tissues. *J. Clin. Periodontol.* **1995**, *22*, 255–261. [CrossRef] [PubMed]
19. Lang, N.P.; Brägger, U.; Walther, D.; Beamer, B.; Kornman, K.S. Ligature-induced peri-implant infection in cynomolgus monkeys. I. Clinical and radiographic findings. *Clin. Oral Implants Res.* **1993**, *4*, 2–11. [CrossRef] [PubMed]
20. Lang, N.P.; Wetzel, A.C.; Stich, H.; Caffesse, R.G. Histologic probe penetration in healthy and inflamed peri-implant tissues. *Clin. Oral Implants Res.* **1994**, *5*, 191–201. [CrossRef] [PubMed]
21. Watzak, G.; Zechner, W.; Tangl, S.; Vasak, C.; Donath, K.; Watzek, G. Soft tissue around three different implant types after 1.5 years of functional loading without oral hygiene: a preliminary study in baboons. *Clin. Oral Implants Res.* **2006**, *17*, 229–236. [CrossRef] [PubMed]
22. Saito, A.; Hosaka, Y.; Sekiguchi, K.; Kigure, T.; Isobe, S.; Shibukawa, Y.; Sumii, H.; Ito, T.; Nakagawa, T.; Yamada, S. Responses of peri-implant tissues to undisturbed plaque formation in dogs: clinical, radiographic, and microbiological findings. *Bull. Tokyo Dent. Coll.* **1997**, *38*, 13–20. [PubMed]
23. Oz, H.S.; Puleo, D.A. Animal models for periodontal disease. *J. Biomed. Biotechnol* **2011**, *2011*, 754857. [CrossRef] [PubMed]
24. Berglundh, T.; Stavropoulos, A. Preclinical in vivo research in implant dentistry. Consensus of the eighth European workshop on periodontology. *J. Clin. Periodontol.* **2012**, *39*, 1–5. [CrossRef] [PubMed]
25. Moest, T.; Wrede, J.; Schmitt, C.M.; Stamp, M.; Neukam, F.W.; Schlegel, K.A. The influence of different abutment materials on tissue regeneration after surgical treatment of peri-implantitis—A randomized controlled preclinical study. *J. Craniomaxillofac. Surg.* **2017**, *45*, 1190–1196. [CrossRef] [PubMed]

26. Rovin, S.; Costich, E.R.; Gordon, H.A. The influence of bacteria and irritation in the initiation of periodontal disease in germfree and conventional rats. *J. Period. Res.* **1966**, *1*, 193–204. [CrossRef] [PubMed]
27. You, T.M.; Choi, B.H.; Zhu, S.J.; Jung, J.H.; Lee, S.H.; Huh, J.Y.; Lee, H.J.; Li, J. Treatment of experimental peri-implantitis using autogenous bone grafts and platelet-enriched fibrin glue in dogs. *Oral Surg. Oral Med. Oral Pathol. Oral Radiol. Endod.* **2007**, *103*, 34–37. [CrossRef] [PubMed]
28. Schou, S.; Holmstrup, P.; Jørgensen, T.; Stoltze, K.; Hjørting-Hansen, E.; Wenzel, A. Autogenous bone graft and ePTFE membrane in the treatment of peri-implantitis. I. Clinical and radiographic observations in cynomolgus monkeys. *Clin. Oral Implants Res.* **2003**, *14*, 391–403. [CrossRef] [PubMed]
29. Hiyari, S.; Naghibi, A.; Wong, R.; Sadreshkevary, R.; Yi-Ling, L.; Tetradis, S.; Camargo, P.M.; Pirih, F.Q. Susceptibility of different mouse strains to peri-implantitis. *J. Period. Res.* **2018**, *53*, 107–116. [CrossRef] [PubMed]
30. Yu, X.; Hu, Y.; Freire, M.; Yu, P.; Kawai, T.; Han, X. Role of toll-like receptor 2 in inflammation and alveolar bone loss in experimental peri-implantitis versus periodontitis. *J. Period. Res.* **2018**, *53*, 98–106. [CrossRef] [PubMed]
31. Setzen, G.; Williams, E.F., 3rd. Tissue response to suture materials implanted subcutaneously in a rabbit model. *Plast. Reconstruct. Surg.* **1997**, *100*, 1788–1795. [CrossRef]
32. Ibrahim, M.; Bond, J.; Medina, M.A.; Chen, L.; Quiles, C.; Kokosis, G.; Bashirov, L.; Klitzman, B.; Levinson, H. Characterization of the Foreign Body Response to Common Surgical Biomaterials in a Murine Model. *Eur. J. Plast. Surg.* **2017**, *40*, 383–392. [CrossRef] [PubMed]
33. Kalbermatten, D.F.; Kalbermatten, N.T.; Hertel, R. Cotton-induced pseudotumor of the femur. *Skeletal Radiol.* **2001**, *30*, 415–417. [CrossRef] [PubMed]
34. Sari, A.; Basterzi, Y.; Karabacak, T.; Tasdelen, B.; Demirkan, F. The potential of microscopic sterile sponge particles to induce foreign body reaction. *Int. Wound J.* **2006**, *3*, 363–368. [CrossRef] [PubMed]
35. Landgraeber, S.; Jäger, M.; Jacobs, J.J.; Hallab, N.J. The pathology of orthopedic implant failure is mediated by innate immune system cytokines. *Mediat. Inflamm.* **2014**, *2014*, 185150. [CrossRef] [PubMed]
36. Jiang, Y.; Jia, T.; Wooley, P.H.; Yang, S.Y. Current research in the pathogenesis of aseptic implant loosening associated with particulate wear debris. *Acta Orthop. Belg.* **2013**, *79*, 1–9. [PubMed]
37. Akagawa, Y.; Matsumoto, T.; Hashimoto, M.; Tsuru, H. Clinical evaluation of the gingiva around single crystal sapphire endosseous implant after experimental ligature-induced plaque accumulation in monkeys. *J. Prosthet. Dent.* **1992**, *68*, 111–115. [CrossRef]
38. Akagawa, Y.; Matsumoto, T.; Kawamura, M.; Tsuru, H. Changes of subgingival microflora around single-crystal sapphire endosseous implants after experimental ligature-induced plaque accumulation in monkeys. *J. Prosthet. Dent.* **1993**, *69*, 594–598. [CrossRef]
39. Kozlovsky, A.; Tal, H.; Laufer, B.Z.; Leshem, R.; Rohrer, M.D.; Weinreb, M.; Artzi, Z. Impact of implant overloading on the peri-implant bone in inflamed and non inflamed peri-implant mucosa. *Clin. Oral Implants Res.* **2007**, *18*, 601–610. [CrossRef] [PubMed]
40. Takasaki, A.A.; Aoki, A.; Mizutani, K.; Kikuchi, S.; Oda, S.; Ishikawa, I. Er:YAG laser therapy for peri-implant infection: A histological study. *Lasers Med. Sci.* **2007**, *22*, 143–157. [CrossRef] [PubMed]

13

Intraosseous Temperature Change during Installation of Dental Implants with Two Different Surfaces and Different Drilling Protocols: An In Vivo Study in Sheep

Michele Stocchero [1], Yohei Jinno [1,*], Marco Toia [1], Marianne Ahmad [1], Evaggelia Papia [2], Satoshi Yamaguchi [3] and Jonas P. Becktor [1]

1 Department of Oral & Maxillofacial Surgery and Oral Medicine, Faculty of Odontology, Malmö University, 20506 Malmö, Sweden
2 Department of Materials Science and Technology, Faculty of Odontology, Malmö University, 20506 Malmö, Sweden
3 Department of Biomaterials Science, Osaka University Graduate School of Dentistry, Osaka 565-0871, Japan
* Correspondence: yohei.jinno@mau.se

Abstract: Background: The intraosseous temperature during implant installation has never been evaluated in an in vivo controlled setup. The aims were to investigate the influence of a drilling protocol and implant surface on the intraosseous temperature during implant installation, to evaluate the influence of temperature increase on osseointegration and to calculate the heat distribution in cortical bone. Methods: Forty Brånemark implants were installed into the metatarsal bone of Finnish Dorset crossbred sheep according to two different drilling protocols (undersized/non-undersized) and two surfaces (moderately rough/turned). The intraosseous temperature was recorded, and Finite Element Model (FEM) was generated to understand the thermal behavior. Non-decalcified histology was carried out after five weeks of healing. The following osseointegration parameters were calculated: Bone-to-implant contact (BIC), Bone Area Fraction Occupancy (BAFO), and Bone Area Fraction Occupancy up to 1.5 mm (BA1.5). A multiple regression model was used to identify the influencing variables on the histomorphometric parameters. Results: The temperature was affected by the drilling protocol, while no influence was demonstrated by the implant surface. BIC was positively influenced by the undersized drilling protocol and rough surface, BAFO was negatively influenced by the temperature rise, and BA1.5 was negatively influenced by the undersized drilling protocol. FEM showed that the temperature at the implant interface might exceed the limit for bone necrosis. Conclusion: The intraosseous temperature is greatly increased by an undersized drilling protocol but not from the implant surface. The temperature increase negatively affects the bone healing in the proximity of the implant. The undersized drilling protocol for Brånemark implant systems increases the amount of bone at the interface, but it negatively impacts the bone far from the implant.

Keywords: oral implants; osseointegration; implant installation; anchorage technique; histology; osteotomy; intraosseous temperature; in vivo study; finite element model

---

1. Introduction

Despite the high success rate of dental implants [1,2], early and late implant failures are still encountered [3,4]. It is known that the surgical approach is one key-factor for successful implant treatment [5]. It was advocated that an optimal surgical technique should provide initial mechanical implant stability necessary for the initiation of the osseointegration process [6,7]. Simultaneously, implants should be installed with a gentle and atraumatic surgical technique, avoiding excessive biomechanical and thermal stresses to the bone [8].

Undersized drilling is one of the most common surgical techniques for increasing primary implant stability. With this technique, an implant is installed in a substantially smaller osteotomy than its diameter [9]. The rationale of such a procedure is to maximize the initial implant contact with the bone locally and, thus, secure the implant stability [10]. This approach increases the implant rotational resistance, measured as the insertion torque value (ITV) [11]. This condition is often considered desirable [12], especially when immediate or early loading protocols are applied [13].

However, there are some concerns among researchers and clinicians regarding the host bone reaction to increased lateral compression, especially when the cortical bone layer is involved [14]. Excessive stresses and strains beyond bone physiological limits can have disadvantageous effects on the local microcirculation and bone cellular responses, leading to so-called bone compression necrosis [15]. In vivo studies and clinical research reported an extensive area of apoptotic osteocytes, tissue damage, and ultimately peri-implant bone loss [16–18]. Moreover, previous consensus reports indicated compression necrosis as a possible risk factor for peri-implant tissues disease [19,20].

Besides the over-compression of the pristine bone, a thermal injury may be an additional factor inducing bone necrosis. When the bone is heated above 53 °C, irreversible tissue damage was observed [21], while 47 °C for 1 min is considered as the border condition for the occurrence of an injury [22]. Although the risk of bone overheating during the drilling procedure was extensively investigated [23], the increase of temperature during implant installation, was seldom reported [24]. During the seating into an osteotomy site, energy is supplied to the bone and part of it is transferred as frictional heat [25]. According to thermodynamics, thermal energy is partially absorbed and conducted by the implant itself, and by the bone, in the form of temperature increase [26].

It is unknown whether the frictional heat generated during implant installation can cause an increase in bone temperature exceeding the threshold of initiating irreversible tissue damage. The temperature may be influenced by several factors, including implant-osteotomy size discrepancy and implant micro-design. One could postulate that the installation of an implant in an undersized osteotomy and the use of a moderately rough surface would generate a greater temperature increase in the bone than a larger osteotomy and a turned surface.

However, the in vivo intraosseous temperature during implant installation was never previously evaluated in a controlled experimental setting. Besides that, the effect of such temperature on histomorphometric parameters is unknown.

The primary aim of this in vivo study was to investigate the influence of the drilling protocol and implant surface on the intraosseous temperature change during dental implant installation. The secondary aims were to evaluate the influence of the temperature on osseointegration and peri-implant bone healing and to calculate the heat distribution in cortical bone.

2. Materials and Methods

2.1. Study Design and Samples

This study was approved by the ethical committee of the Ecole Nationale Vétérinaire d'Alfort, Paris, France, (reference number: 02343.03) and it is reported according to the ARRIVE (Animal Research Reporting of in Vivo Experiments) guidelines [27]. Ten female Finnish Dorset crossbred sheep (average; years old and 54 kg) were used and housed together for one week before surgery. A total of forty 3.75 mm × 7 mm dental implants (Brånemark system® MKIII RP implant, Nobel Biocare AB, Göteborg, Sweden) were installed, including 20 implants with moderately rough oxidized titanium surface (TiUnite® surface) and 20 implants with a turned surface. The present implant surfaces, investigated by a broad variety of preclinical and clinical research [28–30], presents the following surface characteristics according to Wennerberg and Albrektsson with the parameters Sa (the arithmetic average height deviation from mean plane) and Sdr (the developed surface ratio): 1.1 μm and 0.9 μm (Sa); 37% and 34% (Sdr) for TiUnite® and turned surface, respectively [31].

2.2. Surgical Procedures

All surgeries were done under general anesthesia with ketamine (Imalgene 1000®, Merial, Villeurbanne, France), and diazepam (Valium, Roche, Boulogne-Billancourt, France) for injection, and with 2.5% isoflurane (Forane®/Forene®, Drägerverk AG, Lubeck, Germany) for inhalation. The surgical room had a controlled temperature set at 19 °C.

In each sheep, the metatarsal bone of one leg was shaved and disinfected with 40% ethanol and 0.5% chlorhexidine. After skin incision, the bone was exposed with periosteal elevator, and 4 implants were installed in the ventral metatarsal bone plate, consisting of approximately 4 mm of cortical bone, along the longitudinal direction.

Based on the drilling protocol and implant surface topography, four experimental groups were designed as showed in Table 1.

Table 1. Description of the experimental groups.

	Drilling Protocol	Implant Surface
Group A (n = 10)	Undersized	Moderately rough
Group B (n = 10)	Non-undersized	Moderately rough
Group C (n = 10)	Undersized	Turned
Group D (n = 10)	Non-undersized	Turned

Each metatarsal bone received one implant per group. The sequence of the implantation for each metatarsal bone, according to the experimental group (A, B, C, D) was randomized by a computer-generated method, Microsoft® excel (Version 15.30). The sequential implant osteotomies were free-hand prepared at approximately 20 mm inter-implant distance.

The surgical instrumentation sequence was performed following two different drilling protocols. In all groups, a 2.0 mm drill, 2.8 mm step drill, and 3.0 mm drill were used. Hereafter, the osteotomy was finalized based on the group (Figure 1a):

- Group A and C (undersized drilling protocol): 3.2 drill and tap drill were subsequently used for the preparation of the coronal 1.5 mm, in order to favor the engagement of the first threads during the implant installment.
- Group B and D (non-undersized drilling protocol): 3.2 drill and tap drill were subsequently used for the entire thickness of the cortical bone.

All drilling procedures were performed at 1200 rpm under abundant saline irrigation using a total of two new drill sets. Implant installation was carried out at 25 rpm without saline irrigation. Both the drilling procedure and implant installation were performed using a SA-310 W&H Elcomed implant unit (W&H, Burmoos, Austria). The insertion torque value (ITV) was recorded using the specific function and saved to a USB memory. Implants where ITV exceeded 80 Ncm during installation were manually installed by a manual torque wrench. Based on the ITV, three classes were distinguished: ITV $\leq$ 45 Ncm; 45 < ITV < 80 Ncm; ITV $\geq$ 80 Ncm. The flap was closed using a resorbable suture (Vicryl™, Ethicon®, Sommerville, NJ, USA) for the inner layer and non-absorbable suture for the external layer (Ethicon™, Ethicon®, Sommerville, NJ, USA). Morphine (0.1 mg/kg) was given intravenously every second hour during the operation and subcutaneously for the three first postoperative days.

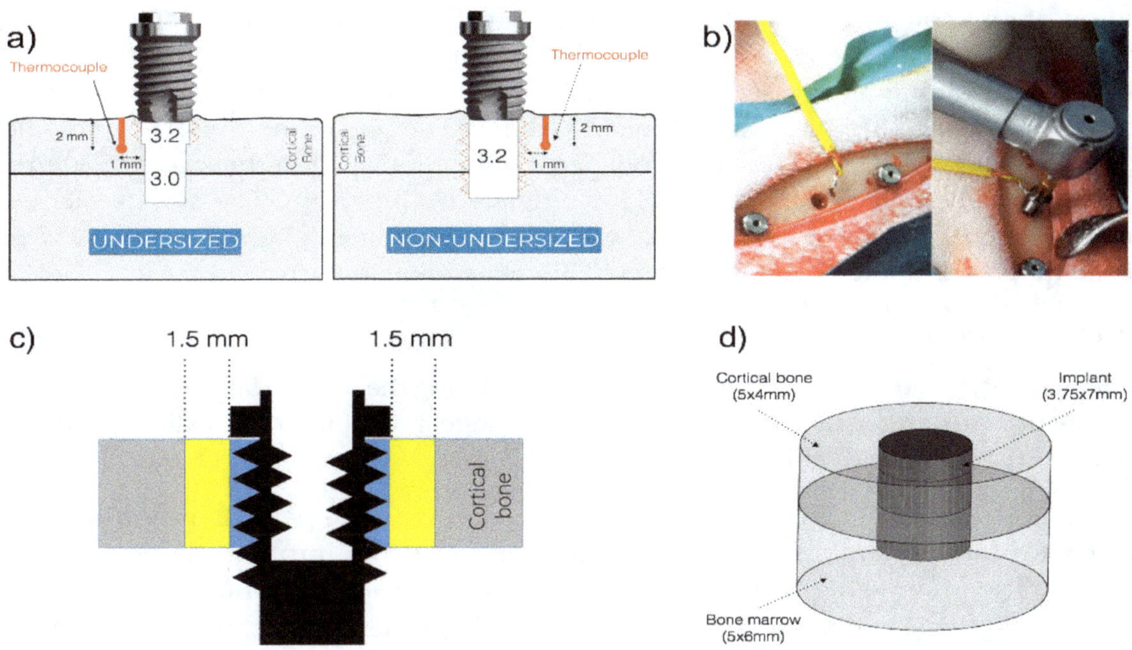

Figure 1. (**a**) Representation of the osteotomy preparation: the undersized drilling protocol on the left and non-undersized drilling protocol on the right. The osteotomy dimensions are depicted in the figures. The thermocouple site was prepared 2 mm deep into the cortical bone and 1 mm from the implant surface. (**b**) Overview of the surgical field with the thermocouple in position before implant installation (**left**) and during implant installation (**right**). (**c**) Representation of the regions of interest for histomorphometrical parameters. Bone-to-implant Contact (BIC) was calculated only for the cortical portion. Bone Area Fraction Occupancy (BAFO) was calculated in the blue part. Bone Area 1.5 (BA1.5) was calculated in the yellow part. (**d**) The Finite Element Model (FEM) was composed of three cylindrical elements: Cortical bone, bone marrow, and implant.

2.3. Temperature Measurement

Intraosseous temperature was measured using the type-K thermocouple (Omega Engineering Limited, Manchester, UK) with a 0.5 mm tip, coupled to a HH12C handheld thermometer (Omega Engineering Limited, Manchester, UK). This dual-channel meter device is able to record the lower and maximum temperature with 2.5 measurements per second and a resolution of 0.1 °C. The tip of the thermocouple was inserted in a prepared drilled hole in the proximity of the implant osteotomy. More in details, the thermocouple site was prepared in a predetermined position in a proximal or distal site at 1 mm from the implant surface (Figure 1a) with the aid of a metal surgical template. To prepare the site, which had a diameter of 0.5 mm and a depth of 2 mm, a lance drill (Precision Drill, Nobel Biocare AB, Göteborg, Sweden) was used. To ensure the reproducibility of the hole depth, the drill was inserted until the marked line met the upper border of the template. Once the osteotomy was prepared, the thermocouple was inserted and kept the position until the thermometer showed a stable value (basal temperature). The installation of the implants was carried out approximately 1 min after the finalization of the drilling procedure. During the implant installation, the temperature was measured, and the maximum value was recorded as the maximum value (Figure 1b). The difference between the maximum and basal temperature for each site was calculated as the temperature change.

2.4. Preparation of Samples

After a healing period of five weeks, all animals were euthanized with an intravenous injection of a combination of 4000 mg embutramide, 538.4 mg mebezonium, and 87.8 mg tetracaine (T61, Intervet International, Unterschleißheim, Germany) and metatarsal bone blocks containing the implants were retrieved. Blocks were fixed in 4% formalin for seven days before dehydration by ascending concentration of ethanol, and embedded in light-curing methylmethacrylate (Technovit 7200 VLC, Heraeus Kulzer, Wehrheim, Germany) for undecalcified ground section procedures. The embedded bone samples with implant were sectioned parallel to the long axis at the center position of the implant using a diamond saw cutting machine (EXAKT 300, EXAKT Advanced Technologies GmbH, Norderstedt, Germany), and grinded and polished until a final section thickness of 30 μm (EXAKT 400CS, EXAKT Advanced Technologies GmbH, Norderstedt, Germany). The non-decalcified sections were stained in toluidine blue and pyronin G, and photographed using light microscopy with a digital imaging system (NanoZoomer S210, HAMAMATSU, Shizuoka, Japan).

2.5. Histomorphometric Analysis

Quantitative histomorphometry was performed considering the cortical layer only. All measurements were carried out with an image analysis software (Image J v.1.43u, National Institute of Health). The following variables were calculated:

- Bone-to-implant contact (BIC): On each side of the implant, the percentage of the bone in direct contact with the implant surface in the entire length of the implant placed in the bone was calculated. The mean value of the two sides was used for each implant.
- Bone Area Fraction Occupancy (BAFO): On each side of the implant, the percentage of the area within the implant threads occupied by visibly distinguishable bone was calculated. The mean value of the two sides was used for each implant.
- Bone Area Fraction Occupancy up to 1.5 mm (BA1.5): On each side of the implant a region of interest up to 1.5 mm from the implant outer diameter line was considered (Figure 1c). The percentage of the area occupied by visibly distinguishable bone was calculated. The mean value of the two sides was used for each implant.

2.6. Finite Element Model

In order to have a deeper understanding of the thermal behavior at the peri-implant bone, a Finite Element Model (FEM) was generated (Figure 1d). The model was composed of three cylindrical elements: Cortical bone (dimensions: 5 mm × 4 mm), bone marrow (dimensions: 5 mm × 6 mm), and implant (dimensions: 3.75 mm × 7 mm) designed by the CAD software (Solidworks Simulation 2011, Dassault Systèmes Solidworks, Waltham, MA, USA). Two different calorific values were set to the upper and bottom surface of the fixture related to the drilling hole with different diameters.

Steady conduction analysis was conducted by voxel-based Finite Element Analysis (FEA) software (VOXELCON2015, Quint, Fuchu, Japan). The thermal conductivity of cortical bone, bone marrow, and implant were set to 0.6 W/mK, 0.3 W/mK, and 20 W/mK, respectively [32,33]. The air temperature around those models was set to 19 °C.

The temperature change in the location of the thermocouple (2 mm depth from cortical bone surface and 1 mm away from the fixture surface) was approximated to 8 °C and 4 °C for the undersized drilling protocol groups and non-undersized drilling protocol groups, respectively. Until converging the calorific value, the steady conduction analysis was repeatedly conducted.

2.7. Statistical Methods

Categorical variables were reported as relative frequency, while continuous variables were reported as mean ± standard deviation after checking the normality of the distribution. Wilcoxon rank-sum test was used to test the influence of the drilling protocol and implant surface on temperature change.

Multiple regression models were used to evaluate the effect of the drilling protocol, implant surface, temperature change on the histomorphometric parameters (BIC, BAFO, BA1.5). p-values < 0.05 were considered statistically significant. The R statistical software package was used for the statistical evaluation and modelling (available at www.r-project.org/).

3. Results

3.1. *ITV, General Healing and Temperature*

All animals survived during surgical procedures and the experimental period. No implant was lost during the healing period. Signs of minor periosteal reaction were noted in three metatarsal bone samples. Such a response did not undermine the peri-implant bone healing and was limited to the periosteal area, which was not considered in this study. All implants were included in the statistical analysis. The relative distribution of the ITV class among the groups is displayed in Figure 2a.

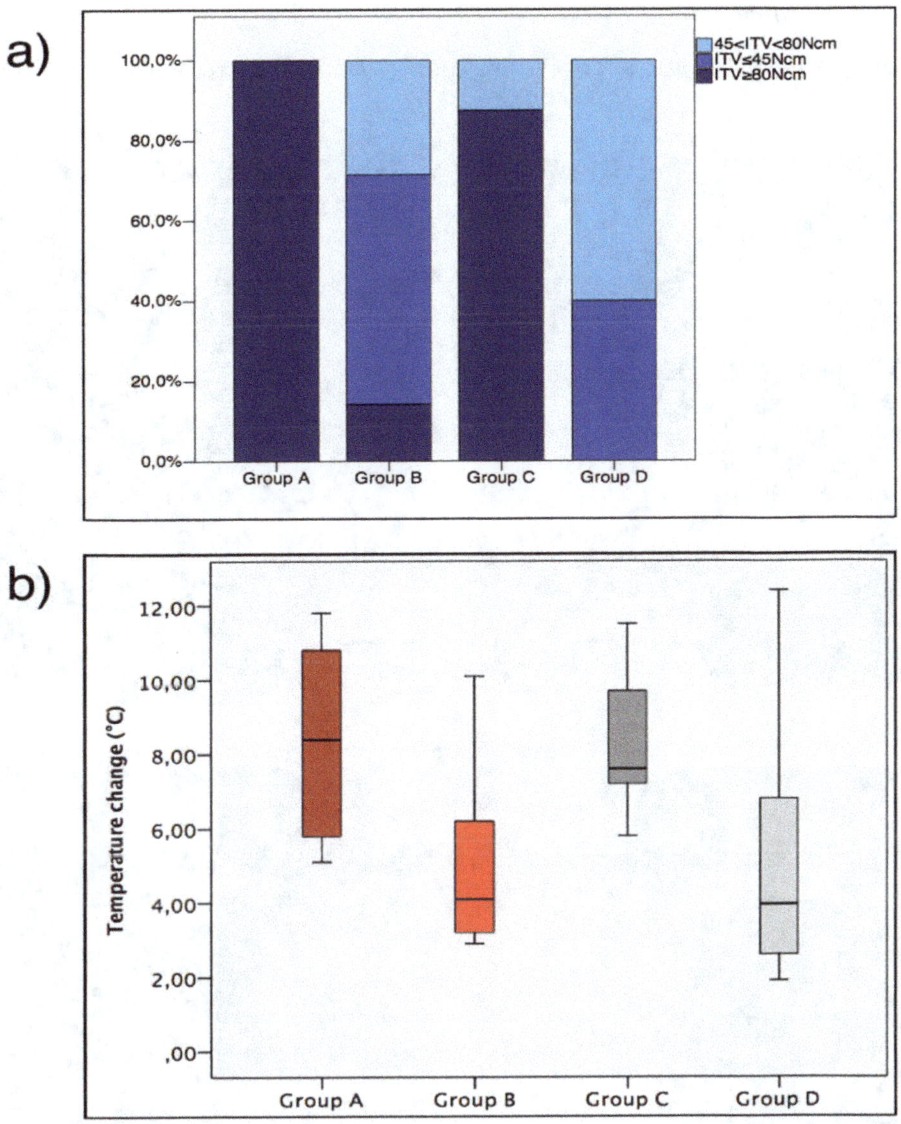

Figure 2. (**a**) Cumulative percentage of insertion torque value (ITV) classes divided per group. Note that all implants installed for group A had a ITV ≥ 80 Ncm. (**b**) Temperature change represented in box-plots.

The values for basal and maximum temperature are indicated in Table 2. Temperature change values are shown in Figure 2b. The temperature change was affected by the drilling protocol ($p < 0.001$), while it was not influenced by the surface topography ($p = 0.879$).

Table 2. Basal temperature and maximum temperature for the different groups are shown in °C. SD: Standard deviation; Max: maximum value; Min: minimum value.

	Basal Temperature				Maximum Temperature			
	Mean	**SD**	**Max**	**Min**	**Mean**	**SD**	**Max**	**Min**
Group A	31.3	2.3	34.5	28.4	39.6	3.3	45.3	34.7
Group B	31.0	3.4	34.7	23.7	36.0	3.4	41.5	28.6
Group C	31.0	3.3	34.0	23.6	39.1	3.7	44.0	33.4
Group D	31.3	2.3	34.2	27.5	36.4	1.8	39.9	33.6

3.2. Histomorphometric Parameters

Representation of the histologic sections are displayed in Figure 3.

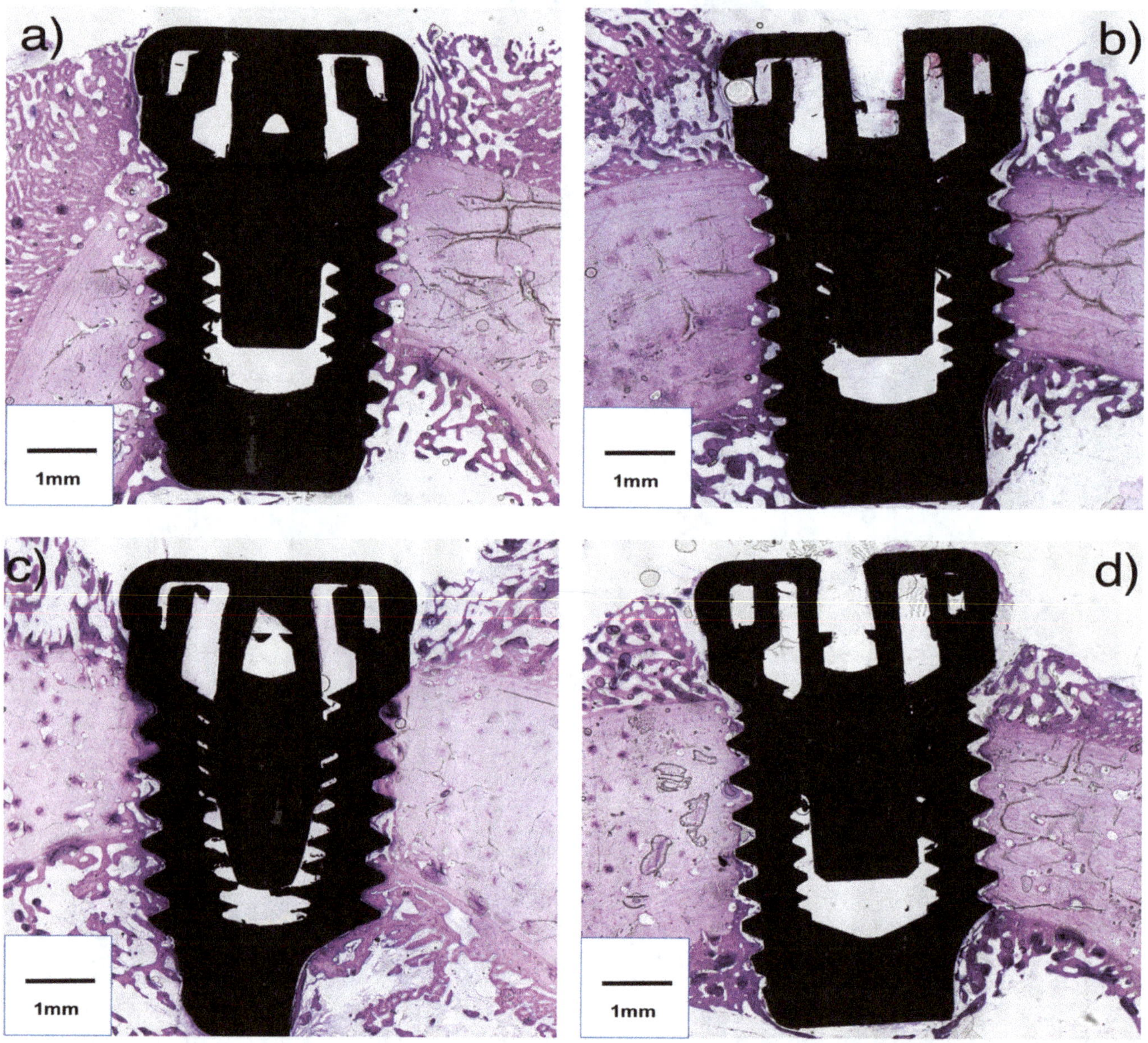

Figure 3. Histologic sections of the implant and peri-implant bone (original magnification 20×). Representations of group A, B, C, and D are depicted in (**a**), (**b**), (**c**), and (**d**), respectively.

Mean values and standard deviation for BIC, BAFO, and BA1.5 are presented in Figure 4.

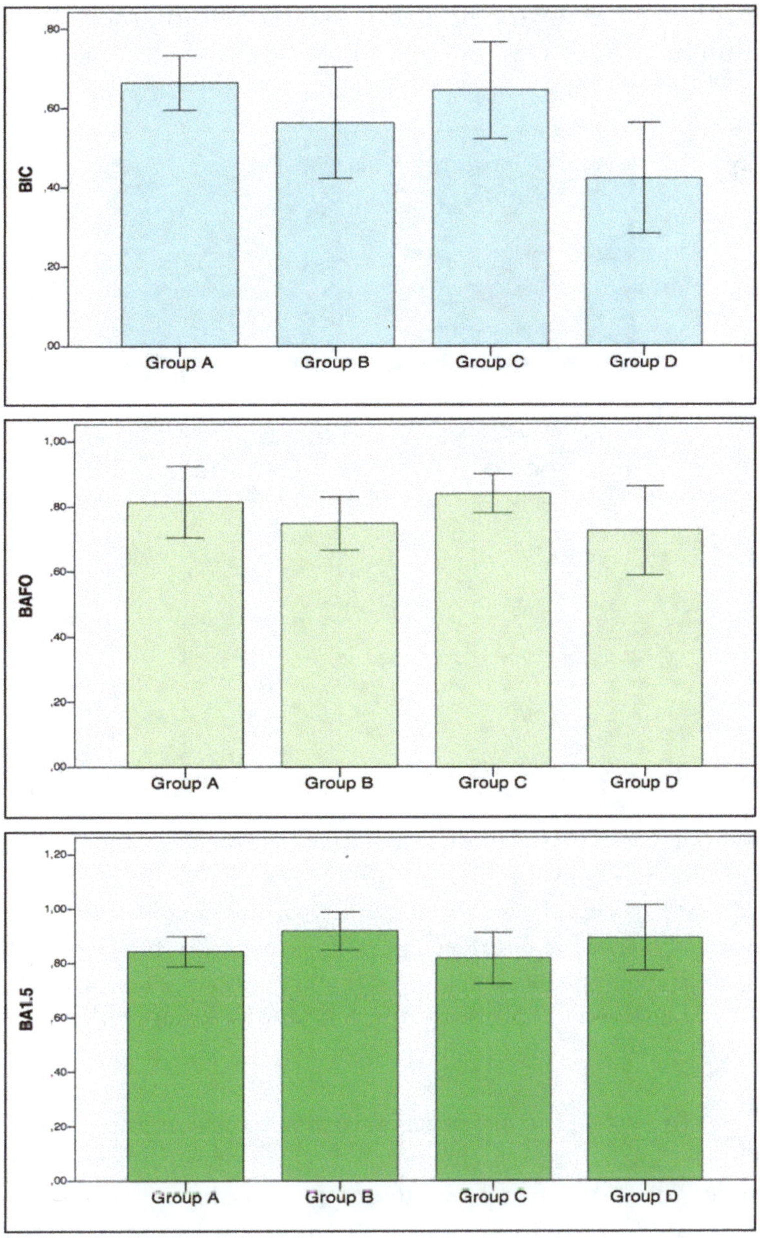

Figure 4. Bone to Implant Contact (**BIC**), Bone Area Fraction Occupancy (**BAFO**), and Bone Area Fraction Occupancy up to 1.5 mm (**BA1.5**) results represented as mean values. Error bars represent the standard deviation.

According to robust multiple regression analysis (Adjusted R^2: 0.37, p = 0.0001), BIC was statistically significantly influenced by the implant surface (p = 0.01) and the drilling protocol (p = 0.0001). More specifically, BIC was increased with a moderately rough surface and undersized drilling protocol. BAFO was negatively affected by temperature increase (p = 0.01). Moreover BAFO was positively affected by the undersized drilling protocol (p = 0.0006) (Adjusted R^2: 0.24, p = 0.005). BA1.5 was moderately affected by the undersized drilling protocol ($p < 0.001$) (Adjusted R^2: 0.11, p = 0.06 for the model). No significant influence on BA1.5 was noted for the temperature change.

3.3. Finite Element Model

Temperature distribution at the center section is shown in Figure 5. The calorific value of the normal model was 30.8 W/m^3. The calorific values of the upper fixture and bottom fixture were 30.8 W/m^3 and 60.4 W/m^3, respectively. The calorific value of fixture for the undersized drilling model showed 1.96 times greater than that for the non-undersized drilling model. The bone temperature at the interface with the implant surface was calculated for both models.

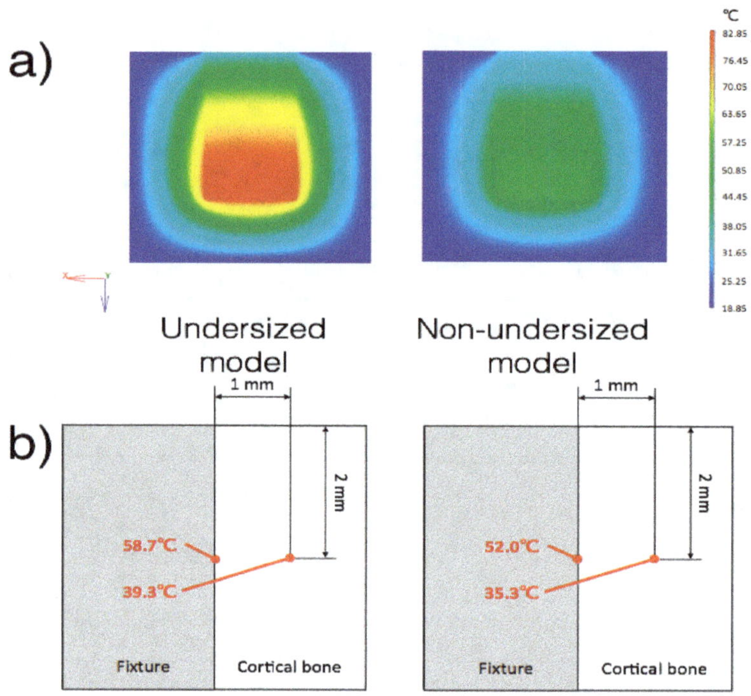

Figure 5. (**a**) The temperature distribution calculated on the Finite Element Model (FEM). The undersized drilling model and non-undersized model are displayed on the left and on the right, respectively. The temperature is displayed in °C. Note how the heat is poorly distributed around the implant surface. This means that the overheating risk is limited to the bone in the proximity to the implant. (**b**) Calculation of the bone temperature at the implant interface according to the FEM. This value was calculated by entering the value recorded with the thermocouple in the experimental part.

4. Discussion

In the present in vivo study, the intraosseous temperature was measured during dental implant installation into cortical bone, following two different drilling protocols and with two different implant surfaces. In addition, histomorphometric parameters of osseointegration were evaluated in relation to the bone temperature recorded during the implant installation and a computational model was created to examine the thermal distribution. To the knowledge of the authors, the current investigation represents the first in vivo experiment with this setup.

4.1. Bone Temperature

In the present study, it was discovered that the intraosseous temperature during implant installation was influenced by the drilling protocol. During implant installation, a certain amount of energy is also dissipated into heat [25]. As previous in vitro studies have observed, the rotational torque is positively related to bone heating during implant installation [24,34]. Accordingly, in this study, the installation of implants into undersized sites developed a great friction resistance, resulting in both in a higher ITV (Figure 3) and temperature increase, compared with non-undersized osteotomies. Specifically, the undersized drilling protocol groups resulted in a median increase of temperature of approximately 8 °C, while in the non-undersized drilling protocol groups, it was approximately 4 °C. The maximum recorded temperature of 45.3 °C exceeded the limit of cell damage, which is 45 °C according to Ludewig [35], but it was lower than the critical value for bone necrosis, which is 50 °C according to Lundskog [36]. In the early 1980s, Eriksson, whose doctoral thesis greatly contributed to the knowledge on bone tissue regeneration, stated that the threshold level for bone survival was 47 °C for 1 min [37]. However, the temperature recorded in the present study was detected at 1 mm from the implant surface. To have a better understanding of the temperature behavior in the proximity of the implant, a FEM was designed. It was estimated that the temperature at the bone-implant interface for the undersized groups and non-undersized groups reached 58.7 °C and 52.0 °C respectively (Figure 5). Thus, according to the FEM calculation, the installation of the implant caused a frictional heat over the critical temperature for bone injury at the bone-implant interface. One may expect that implants installed with an undersized drilling protocol would create a major extent of tissue damage. Still, such an overheating condition is restricted to the proximity of the implant, as shown by the model. Since the temperature change was affected by the drilling protocol ($p < 0.001$), but was not influenced by the surface topography ($p = 0.879$), the surface characteristics (parameters Sa and Sdr) were not included in the design of the FEM.

Such results are confirmed by histomorphometry. In effect, it was demonstrated that the temperature generated during implant installation has a tangible biologic impact, since the amount of bone between the threads, namely BAFO, is negatively affected by the temperature increase. This finding is in accordance with Eriksson's study, in which they observed a loss of 10% of bone tissue after 30 days when a rabbit tibia was heated to 47 °C for 1 min [22]. This study supports the conclusion that the portion of the bone in proximity with the implant surface might be the most sensitive to heating at the implant installation. Moreover, based on the FEM analysis and histomorphometric results, this heating might induce bone damage if the undersized drilling protocol is applied. The influence of the heat generated by the drilling procedures was likely to be excluded since one minute elapsed before the implant installation. Previous research indicated that the bone returned to baseline temperature after approximately 30 s [38].

Nevertheless, due to the low thermal conductivity properties of cortical bone, we could expect a low grade of heat distribution through the bone [39]. Thus, the risk of bone overheating is limited to the bone in the proximity to the bone-to-implant interface.

It has to be said that Eriksson observed how bone cells are susceptible to the exposure time, other than peak temperature [40]. In the present experiment, the maximum temperature endured for a few seconds, then it gradually descended. However, the actual temperature/time curve was not recorded, representing a limitation of the study.

4.2. Drilling Protocol

The present findings showed that an undersized drilling protocol per se might not be detrimental to osseointegration for the Brånemark implant. In a previous study by the authors, implants were inserted in sheep mandible according to two different drilling techniques [41]. The results showed that implants inserted into an undersized osteotomy caused tissue damage to the peri-implant bone. In particular, large remodeling cavities with resorption activity were noted, and a lower amount of bone was identified up to 1.5 mm distance from the implant, both from histomorphometric μ-CT analysis. In addition, the drilling protocol seemed not to influence the amount of total BIC. Such findings are partially confirmed by the present results, since the amount of bone up to 1.5 mm from implant surface (BA1.5), was negatively influenced by the undersized drilling protocol. An explanation could be that the bone compression during the implant installation in a tight osteotomy would trigger a remodeling process at a distance from the implant interface. On the other hand, the temperature change does not influence this parameter, since the thermal conductivity of the bone would prevent the heat from being transferred at such a distance from the implant.

Compared with the previous sheep study [41], a number of differences were noted. In the former study, an implant with a micro-threaded neck was used, while the Brånemark type implant was utilized in the present investigation. A previous FEA study on the press-fit phenomena at the implant insertion, [42] affirmed that the micro-thread portion, induced more relevant strains compared to the situation without microthreads. Thus, one could expect greater bone damage after undersized drilling in such a scenario. On the contrary, the undersized drilling protocol positively influenced the amount of bone in close proximity to the implant, i.e., BIC and BAFO, in the present study. It could be assumed that a large portion of the bone in contact with the implant might be the original bone that was forced to the implant surface during the implant installation and still not removed. This finding was observed in several previous studies, which used a similar implant design [5,43,44]. In normal conditions, such tissue will be gradually resorbed with time and eventually substituted with vital bone, according to the remodeling process [45].

4.3. Surface

An interesting finding of the present study was that the type of implant surface did not influence the bone temperature. It could be expected that a moderately rough surface could increase the friction and thereby the heat [46,47]. However, no differences were noticed in the temperature increase between moderately rough and turned surfaced implants. According to the results, a moderately rough surface had a positive effect on the amount of bone in contact with the implant. This finding confirms that such surface topography is able to promote the osteoconductive properties of the implant, compared to turned surfaced implants, as reported by animal and human histologic reports by Ivanoff et al. and Zechner et al. [28,48].

4.4. Clinical Applications and Limitations

The study represents one of the first attempts to study the implant insertion temperature in an in vivo setting. Results demonstrated that an undersized drilling protocol causes an increase of intraosseous temperature during implant seating. A temperature increase negatively affected the amount of peri-implant bone. Thus, it may be suggested to reduce the friction overheating during implant installation. This would include decreasing the rotational speed [49], the use of the self-tapping implant design [24], the use of irrigation during implant installation, and the selection of the proper drilling protocol based on the implant design and the bone quality.

Considering the limitations in the present study, the record of the temperature was limited to the peak value during each insertion. Further studies are needed to evaluate the exact duration of the heat. In addition, from the present study, we cannot confirm whether the increase of the temperature caused tissue necrosis, since no specific stain for cell metabolism and tissue turnover was used. Moreover, the relationship between the compression and the heat, following undersized drilling was not explored. Future studies should be designed in order to indicate whether there is a predominant factor in the generation of tissue damage in the proximity of the implant. Finally, it must be stated that the sheep model, which has been broadly used in dental implant research, presents similarities and differences compared to human bone [50]. The thickness and density of cortical bone may approximate clinical scenarios, such as encountered in the mandible. In addition, sheep bone turnover resembles bone processes in humans, even though it is slightly more rapid. The healing period of five weeks was selected according to our previous research [41], since the influence of the surgical protocol is more evident at this stage in the peri-implant bone. However, the metatarsal bone, while it represents an accessible and convenient substrate for orthopedic and dental implant research, presents quite large anatomical and physiological differences compared with the human jaw, and it may display slightly divergent thermal properties. Therefore the present findings must be taken with reasonable caution.

5. Conclusions

Within the limitations of the present study, it was shown that different drilling protocol for the Brånemark implant system affects both the intraosseous temperature during implant installation and the peri-implant bone healing. The undersized drilling protocol provokes a greater increase of bone temperature in the proximity of the implant compared with non-undersized drilling. The temperature at the bone-implant interface may exceed the critical value for thermal necrosis, and it may have negative effects on peri-implant bone healing. The present results indicate that undersized drilling increases the amount of bone in the proximity of the implant, but it has a negative impact on the bone area far from the implant surface. The moderately rough surface does not influence the bone temperature, while it increased the bone attached to the implant. Further studies are needed to confirm the present results and to deeply investigate the thermal behavior and the biologic effect of peri-implant bone overheating during implant installation and to provide guidelines on the clinical decisions for the proper drilling protocol, based on the bone quality and implant design.

Author Contributions: Conceptualization—M.S. and J.B.; Data curation—M.S., Y.J. and S.Y.; Formal analysis—M.S. and S.Y.; Funding acquisition—J.B.; Investigation—M.S., Y.J., M.T., M.A. and E.P.; Methodology—M.S., Y.J., M.A., E.P. and S.Y.; Project administration—E.P. and J.B.; Resources—Y.J., M.T. and M.A.; Software—S.Y.; Supervision—J.B.; Validation—Y.J., M.T., E.P. and J.B.; Visualization—M.T. and E.P.; Writing—Original draft—M.S., Y.J. and S.Y.; Writing—Review & Editing—M.T., M.A., E.P., S.Y. and J.B.

Acknowledgments: The authors are grateful to Benoit Lecuelle and Thomas Lilin from Ecole Nationale Vétérinaire d'Alfort, Paris, France and Simone Selvaggio, Italy for their valuable help during the surgical procedures.

References

1. Chrcanovic, B.R.; Kisch, J.; Albrektsson, T.; Wennerberg, A. A retrospective study on clinical and radiological outcomes of oral implants in patients followed up for a minimum of 20 years. *Clin. Implant. Dent. Relat. Res.* **2018**, *20*, 199–207. [CrossRef] [PubMed]
2. Donati, M.; Ekestubbe, A.; Lindhe, J.; Wennstrom, J.L. Marginal bone loss at implants with different surface characteristics A 20-year follow-up of a randomized controlled clinical trial. *Clin. Oral Implants Res.* **2018**, *29*, 480–487. [CrossRef] [PubMed]
3. Chrcanovic, B.R.; Kisch, J.; Albrektsson, T.; Wennerberg, A. Factors Influencing Early Dental Implant Failures. *J. Dent. Res.* **2016**, *95*, 995–1002. [CrossRef] [PubMed]
4. Derks, J.; Hakansson, J.; Wennstrom, J.L.; Tomasi, C.; Larsson, M.; Berglundh, T. Effectiveness of implant therapy analyzed in a Swedish population: Early and late implant loss. *J. Dent. Res.* **2015**, *94*, 44s–51s. [CrossRef] [PubMed]
5. Albrektsson, T.; Branemark, P.I.; Hansson, H.A.; Lindstrom, J. Osseointegrated titanium implants. Requirements for ensuring a long-lasting, direct bone-to-implant anchorage in man. *Acta Orthop. Scand.* **1981**, *52*, 155–170. [CrossRef] [PubMed]
6. Esposito, M.; Hirsch, J.M.; Lekholm, U.; Thomsen, P. Biological factors contributing to failures of osseointegrated oral implants. Success criteria and epidemiology. *Eur. J. Oral Sci.* **1998**, *106*, 527–551. [CrossRef] [PubMed]
7. Szmukler-Moncler, S.; Salama, H.; Reingewirtz, Y.; Dubruille, J.H. Timing of loading and effect of micromotion on bone-dental implant interface: Review of experimental literature. *J. Biomed. Mater. Res.* **1998**, *43*, 192–203. [CrossRef]
8. Albrektsson, T.; Zarb, G.; Worthington, P.; Eriksson, A.R. The long-term efficacy of currently used dental implants: A review and proposed criteria of success. *Int. J. Oral Maxillofac. Implants* **1986**, *1*, 11–25.
9. Friberg, B.; Sennerby, L.; Grondahl, K.; Bergstrom, C.; Back, T.; Lekholm, U. On cutting torque measurements during implant placement: A 3-year clinical prospective study. *Clin. Implant. Dent. Relat. Res.* **1999**, *1*, 75–83. [CrossRef]
10. Bilhan, H.; Geckili, O.; Mumcu, E.; Bozdag, E.; Sunbuloglu, E.; Kutay, O. Influence of surgical technique, implant shape and diameter on the primary stability in cancellous bone. *J. Oral Rehabil.* **2010**, *37*, 900–907. [CrossRef]
11. Stocchero, M.; Toia, M.; Cecchinato, D.; Becktor, J.P.; Coelho, P.G.; Jimbo, R. Biomechanical, Biologic, and Clinical Outcomes of Undersized Implant Surgical Preparation: A Systematic Review. *Int. J. Oral Maxillofac. Implants* **2016**, *31*, 1247–1263. [CrossRef] [PubMed]
12. O'Sullivan, D.; Sennerby, L.; Meredith, N. Measurements comparing the initial stability of five designs of dental implants: A human cadaver study. *Clin. Implant. Dent. Relat. Res.* **2000**, *2*, 85–92. [CrossRef] [PubMed]
13. Esposito, M.; Grusovin, M.G.; Willings, M.; Coulthard, P.; Worthington, H.V. The effectiveness of immediate, early, and conventional loading of dental implants: A Cochrane systematic review of randomized controlled clinical trials. *Int. J. Oral Maxillofac. Implants* **2007**, *22*, 893–904. [PubMed]

14. Stocchero, M. *On Influence of Undersized Implant Site On Implant Stability and Osseointegration*; Malmö University: Malmö, Sverige, 2018.
15. Bashutski, J.D.; D'Silva, N.J.; Wang, H.L. Implant compression necrosis: Current understanding and case report. *J. Periodontol.* **2009**, *80*, 700–704. [CrossRef] [PubMed]
16. Duyck, J.; Corpas, L.; Vermeiren, S.; Ogawa, T.; Quirynen, M.; Vandamme, K.; Jacobs, R.; Naert, I. Histological, histomorphometrical, and radiological evaluation of an experimental implant design with a high insertion torque. *Clin. Oral Implants Res.* **2010**, *21*, 877–884. [CrossRef] [PubMed]
17. Cha, J.Y.; Pereira, M.D.; Smith, A.A.; Houschyar, K.S.; Yin, X.; Mouraret, S.; Brunski, J.B.; Helms, J.A. Multiscale analyses of the bone-implant interface. *J. Dent. Res.* **2015**, *94*, 482–490. [CrossRef]
18. Toia, M.; Stocchero, M.; Cecchinato, F.; Corra, E.; Jimbo, R.; Cecchinato, D. Clinical Considerations of Adapted Drilling Protocol by Bone Quality Perception. *Int. J. Oral Maxillofac. Implants* **2017**, *32*, 1288–1295. [CrossRef]
19. Berglundh, T.; Armitage, G.; Araujo, M.G.; Avila-Ortiz, G.; Blanco, J.; Camargo, P.M.; Chen, S.; Cochran, D.; Derks, J.; Figuero, E.; et al. Peri-implant diseases and conditions: Consensus report of workgroup 4 of the 2017 World Workshop on the Classification of Periodontal and Peri-Implant Diseases and Conditions. *J. Clin. Periodontol.* **2018**, *45*, S286–S291. [CrossRef]
20. Schwarz, F.; John, G.; Schmucker, A.; Sahm, N.; Becker, J. Combined surgical therapy of advanced peri-implantitis evaluating two methods of surface decontamination: A 7-year follow-up observation. *J. Clin. Periodontol.* **2017**, *44*, 337–342. [CrossRef]
21. Eriksson, A.; Albrektsson, T.; Grane, B.; McQueen, D. Thermal injury to bone. A vital-microscopic description of heat effects. *Int. J. Oral Surg.* **1982**, *11*, 115–121. [CrossRef]
22. Eriksson, A.R.; Albrektsson, T. Temperature threshold levels for heat-induced bone tissue injury: A vital-microscopic study in the rabbit. *J. Prosthet. Dent.* **1983**, *50*, 101–107. [CrossRef]
23. Augustin, G.; Zigman, T.; Davila, S.; Udilljak, T.; Staroveski, T.; Brezak, D.; Babic, S. Cortical bone drilling and thermal osteonecrosis. *Clin. Biomech. (Bristol, Avon)* **2012**, *27*, 313–325. [CrossRef]
24. Markovic, A.; Misic, T.; Milicic, B.; Calvo-Guirado, J.L.; Aleksic, Z.; Ethinic, A. Heat generation during implant placement in low-density bone: Effect of surgical technique, insertion torque and implant macro design. *Clin. Oral Implants Res.* **2013**, *24*, 798–805. [CrossRef] [PubMed]
25. Matsuoka, M.; Motoyoshi, M.; Sakaguchi, M.; Shinohara, A.; Shigeede, T.; Saito, Y.; Matsuda, M.; Shimizu, N. Friction heat during self-drilling of an orthodontic miniscrew. *Int. J. Oral Maxillofac. Surg.* **2011**, *40*, 191–194. [CrossRef] [PubMed]
26. Wong, K.; Boyde, A.; Howell, P.G. A model of temperature transients in dental implants. *Biomaterials* **2001**, *22*, 2795–2797. [CrossRef]
27. Berglundh, T.; Stavropoulos, A. Preclinical in vivo research in implant dentistry. Consensus of the eighth European workshop on periodontology. *J. Clin. Periodontol.* **2012**, *39*, 1–5. [CrossRef]
28. Ivanoff, C.J.; Widmark, G.; Johansson, C.; Wennerberg, A. Histologic evaluation of bone response to oxidized and turned titanium micro-implants in human jawbone. *Int. J. Oral Maxillofac. Implants* **2003**, *18*, 341–348.
29. Karl, M.; Albrektsson, T. Clinical Performance of Dental Implants with a Moderately Rough (TiUnite) Surface: A Meta-Analysis of Prospective Clinical Studies. *Int. J. Oral Maxillofac. Implants* **2017**, *32*, 717–734. [CrossRef]
30. Wennerberg, A.; Albrektsson, T. Effects of titanium surface topography on bone integration: A systematic review. *Clin. Oral Implants Res.* **2009**, *20*, 172–184. [CrossRef]
31. Wennerberg, A.; Albrektsson, T. On implant surfaces: A review of current knowledge and opinions. *Int. J. Oral Maxillofac. Implants* **2010**, *25*, 63–74.
32. Davidson, S.R.; James, D.F. Measurement of thermal conductivity of bovine cortical bone. *Med. Eng. Phys.* **2000**, *22*, 741–747. [CrossRef]
33. Aghvami, M.; Brunski, J.B.; Serdar Tulu, U.; Chen, C.H.; Helms, J.A. A Thermal and Biological Analysis of Bone Drilling. *J. Biomech. Eng.* **2018**, *140*. [CrossRef]
34. Wikenheiser, M.A.; Markel, M.D.; Lewallen, D.G.; Chao, E.Y. Thermal response and torque resistance of five cortical half-pins under simulated insertion technique. *J. Orthop. Res.* **1995**, *13*, 615–619. [CrossRef]
35. Ludewig, R. *Temperaturmessungen Beim Knochensagen*; University of Gissen: Gissen, Germany, 1972.
36. Lundskog, J. Heat and bone tissue. An experimental investigation of the thermal properties of bone and threshold levels for thermal injury. *Scand. J. Plast. Reconstr. Surg.* **1972**, *9*, 72–74.

37. Eriksson, A.R. *Heat-Induced Bone Tissue Injury: An in Vivo Investigation of Heat Tolerance of Bone Tissue and Temperature Rise in the Drilling of Cortical Bone*; University of Göteborg: Gothenburg, Sweden, 1984.
38. Gurdan, Z.; Vajta, L.; Toth, A.; Lempel, E.; Joob-Fancsaly, A.; Szalma, J. Effect of pre-drilling on intraosseous temperature during self-drilling mini-implant placement in a porcine mandible model. *J. Oral Sci.* **2017**, *59*, 47–53. [CrossRef]
39. Flanagan, D. Heat generated during seating of dental implant fixtures. *J. Oral Implantol.* **2014**, *40*, 174–181. [CrossRef]
40. Eriksson, R.A.; Albrektsson, T. The effect of heat on bone regeneration: An experimental study in the rabbit using the bone growth chamber. *J. Oral Maxillofac. Surg.* **1984**, *42*, 705–711. [CrossRef]
41. Stocchero, M.; Toia, M.; Jinno, Y.; Cecchinato, F.; Becktor, J.P.; Naito, Y.; Halldin, A.; Jimbo, R. Influence of different drilling preparation on cortical bone: A biomechanical, histological, and micro-CT study on sheep. *Clin. Oral Implants Res.* **2018**. [CrossRef]
42. Natali, A.N.; Carniel, E.L.; Pavan, P.G. Dental implants press fit phenomena: Biomechanical analysis considering bone inelastic response. *Dent. Mater.* **2009**, *25*, 573–581. [CrossRef]
43. Roberts, W.E. Bone tissue interface. *J. Dent. Educ.* **1988**, *52*, 804–809.
44. Roberts, W.E.; Garetto, L.P.; DeCastro, R.A. Remodeling of devitalized bone threatens periosteal margin integrity of endosseous titanium implants with threaded or smooth surfaces: Indications for provisional loading and axially directed occlusion. *J. Indiana Dent. Assoc.* **1989**, *68*, 19–24.
45. Osborn, J.F. Dynamic aspects of the implant-bone-interface. In *Dental implants. Materials and systems*; Heimke, G., Ed.; Carl Hanser Verlag: Munchen, Germany, 1980; pp. 111–123.
46. Shalabi, M.M.; Wolke, J.G.; Jansen, J.A. The effects of implant surface roughness and surgical technique on implant fixation in an in vitro model. *Clin. Oral Implants Res.* **2006**, *17*, 172–178. [CrossRef]
47. Dos Santos, M.V.; Elias, C.N.; Lima, C.J.H. The effects of superficial roughness and design on the primary stability of dental implants. *Clin. Implant. Dent. Relat. Res.* **2011**, *13*, 215–223. [CrossRef]
48. Zechner, W.; Tangl, S.; Furst, G.; Tepper, G.; Thams, U.; Mailath, G.; Watzek, G. Osseous healing characteristics of three different implant types. *Clin. Oral Implants Res.* **2003**, *14*, 150–157. [CrossRef]
49. Sumer, M.; Keskiner, I.; Mercan, U.; Misir, F.; Cankaya, S. Assessment of heat generation during implant insertion. *J. Prosthet. Dent.* **2014**, *112*, 522–525. [CrossRef]
50. Pearce, A.I.; Richards, R.G.; Milz, S.; Schneider, E.; Pearce, S.G. Animal models for implant biomaterial research in bone: A review. *Eur. Cell Mater.* **2007**, *13*, 1–10. [CrossRef]

14

Is Complete Re-Osseointegration of an Infected Dental Implant Possible? Histologic Results of a Dog Study

Markus Schlee [1,2], Loubna Naili [3], Florian Rathe [1,4], Urs Brodbeck [5] and Holger Zipprich [6,*]

1 Private Practice, Forchheim, Germany; markus.schlee@32schoenezaehne.de (M.S.); florian.rathe@32schoenezaehne.de (F.R.)
2 Department of Maxillofacial Surgery, Goethe University, 60590 Frankfurt am Main, Germany
3 Private Practice, Kirchbachstraße 186, 28211 Bremen, Germany; lnaili@students.uni-mainz.de
4 Private Practice and Department of Prosthodontics, Danube University, 3500 Krems, Austria
5 Private Practice, 8051 Zürich, Switzerland; ursbrodbeck@bluewin.ch
6 Department of Prosthodontics, Goethe University, 60590 Frankfurt am Main, Germany
* Correspondence: zipprich@em.uni-frankfurt.de

Abstract: Complete reosseointegration after treatment of periimplantitis was never published yet. This short scientific communication reports about results of a randomized controlled preclinical study. An electrolytic approach was compared to a classical modality (ablative, cotton pellets soaked with sodium chloride solution and H_2O_2. For electrolytic cleaning a complete reosseointegration was achieved in several cases serving as a proof of concept.

Keywords: periimplantitis; electrolytic cleaning; augmentation; air flow; re-osseointegration; dog study

1. Introduction

Ligature-induced inflammation and bone loss in a dog model was introduced to imitate periimplantitis in humans and preclinically study different treatment approaches. Schwarz et al. [1] compared bone defects in 24 patients with advanced periimplantitis to ligature-induced bone defects at 30 implants in five beagle dogs. Defect morphology was similar in both entities. The authors concluded that the dog model would be an appropriate model for simulating periimplantitis in humans. Seong at al. reported the possibility of spontaneous healing after ligature removal in dogs [2]. The authors claimed that further clarification of differences between the forced acute bone loss induced by ligatures and the chronic process in clinical periimplantitis would be necessary. Nevertheless, the dog model provided valuable insights into the etiology and pathogenesis of periimplantitis [3] and may be a reasonable model for studying whether re-osseointegration of implant surfaces covered by bacterial biofilms is possible. Based on animal studies, re-osseointegration is feasible, although unpredictable, as it varies between studies and depends on implant surface characteristics and defect morphology [4,5].

In this preclinical randomized and controlled trial, electrolytic cleaning (EC) versus classical cleaning (CC, rubbing a gauze strip soaked in H_2O_2 (3%), followed by a strip soaked in saline (0.9%)) was employed to prove whether complete re-osseointegration is possible in a dog model. This approach was chosen on the basis of previous studies [5]. A custom-made pilot series device and the pilot electrolyte (sodium and potassium iodine) of the in vitro study of Ratka et al. [6] were used in this study. The aim of this short scientific communication is to share histologic results and to prove whether complete re-osseointegration is possible when EC has been used as a decontamination technique.

2. Experimental Section

The study was approved by the Internal Review Board of the University of São Paulo (2013.1.1193.58.3 by CEUA (Comissão de Ética no Uso de Animais)). No sample size calculation could be done because this was the first in vivo trial and no data were available. To have a high chance of achieving significance, we used a large number of dogs compared to existing literature (8 dogs). Two months after extraction (T1) of all premolars and the first molars in the left and right mandible, 4 implants per quadrant were placed (Figure 1). It was planned to place two different brands of implants: 48 BL implants (BL SLA® 3.3 × 8.0 mm, Straumann, Basel, Switzerland) and 16 Nobel Active implants (NA TiUnite® 3.5 × 8.5mm, Nobel Biocare, Kloten, Switzerland). In view of the expected bone defects, the inter-implant distance was at least 6 mm (Figure 1). In addition to the study implants, extra implants were placed, provided there was sufficient space and the study implants would not be impeded. Ligatures were pushed into the sulcus at T2 (4 months) and removed at T3 (7 months). A hygiene program was set up, and the implants were treated at T4 (8 months) by either CC or EC in a randomized manner with the use of sealed envelopes. The mode of action of EC has been described before [6,7]. In summary, the implants were negatively loaded with a current of around 5 V, and rinsed with an electrolyte which passed an anode inside a spray-head (Figure 4c). Sodium iodine (200 g/L), potassium iodine (200 g/L), and L (+)-lactic acid (20 g/L) were used as the electrolyte [6] and an early prototype of a spray-head (Figure 4c) as the source of current (5 min, 400 mA) in the present study. The current directs anions and cations to the electric field. While the anions at the anode form an iodine disinfecting solution, the cations penetrate the biofilm, take an electron from the implant surface, and the emerging hydrogen bubbles (H_2) lift off the bacterial biofilm. The CC implants were treated by rubbing a gauze strip soaked in H_2O_2 (3%), followed by a strip soaked in saline (0.9%, Braun Melsungen, Germany). All sites were augmented with autogenous bone harvested from the ramus area of the lateral mandible (Micross Safescraper, Zantomed, Duisburg, Germany), covered with a collagen membrane (Bio-Gide, Geistlich, Wohlhusen, Switzerland), and the flap was coronally advanced to cover the augmented area without tension. One implant per dog (2 Nobel, 4 Straumann) was randomly selected and not treated to serve as a negative control. The animals were sacrificed for histologic evaluation at T5 (11 months). Standardized x-rays were taken at T1, 2, 4, and 5. Bleeding on probing (BoP) as well as an assessment of pocket depth (PD) at T2, 4, and 5 (Figure 2) were performed. Preparation of samples followed the technique introduced by Donath [8], and staining was done with Stevenel's blue or Toluidine blue. Bone gain was assessed using a digital tool (NDP.view 2.5.19, (Hamamatsu Photonics KK, Shizuoka, Japan)) and analyzed histomorphometrically.

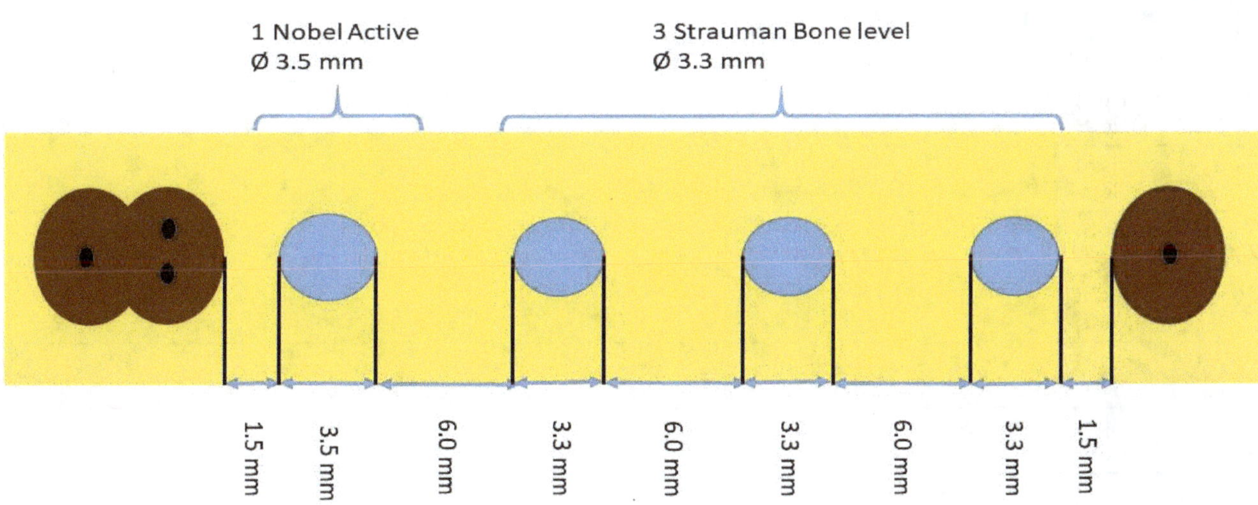

Figure 1. Allocation of implant positions.

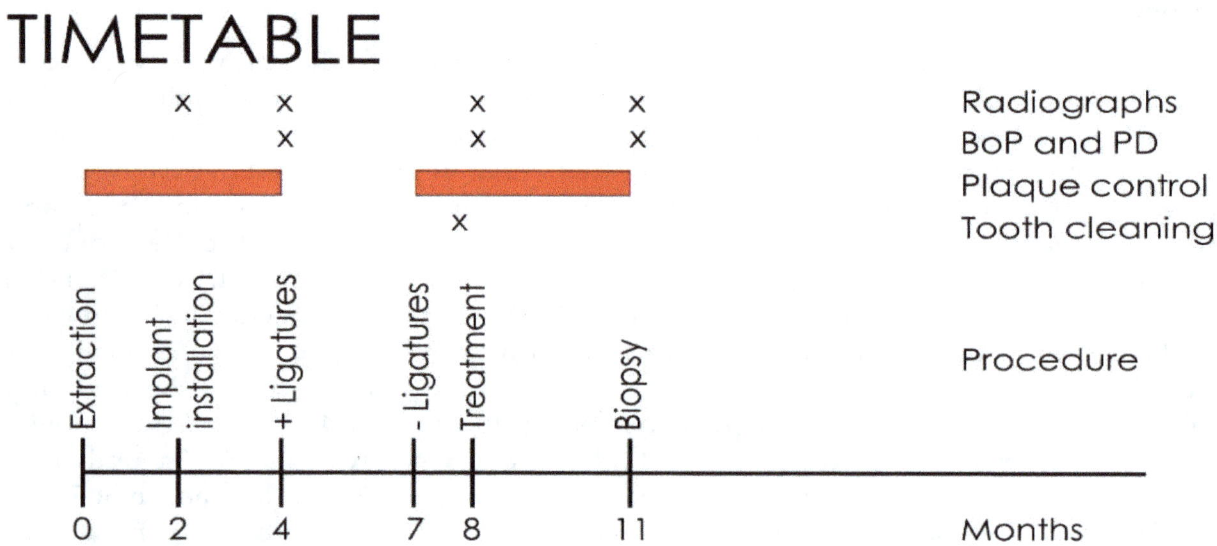

Figure 2. Timetable of the dog study.

3. Results

Sixty-five implants were finally placed (Table 1). Fourteen TiUnite® implants and 43 SLA® implants were treated (EC & CC) and eight implants (2 TiUnite® and 6 SLA®) were left untreated. Two implants could not be placed due to the required distances (Figure 1). All implants displayed massive horizontal bone loss before treatment, in most cases merging with neighboring defects (Figures 3 and 4), which left a site that was difficult to augment. Forty-eight implants were exposed during healing whereas nine EC (5 TiUnite® and 4 SLA®) and eight CC (3 TiUnite® and 5 SLA®) implants stayed covered until T5. Complete re-osseointegration could be demonstrated for implants treated by CC in one implant and for four TiUnite® and six SLA® implants treated by EC (Figures 5–8). The median bone gain for implants which healed submerged was 1.58 ± 0.76 in the case of EC and 1.19 ± 0.29 in the case of CC. The boxplot appears in Figure 9.

Table 1. Allocation of implant positions.

Dog	Quadrant	Straumann	Nobel	Straumann Not Treated	Nobel Not Treated	Total	Not Placed
1	right	2	1			3	1
	left	3	1	1		5	
2	right	3	1			4	
	left	3	1	1		5	
3	right	3	1			4	
	left	2	1	1		4	
4	right	3	0		1	4	
	left	3	1			4	
5	right	3	1			4	
	left	3	0		1	4	
6	right	3	1	1		5	
	left	3	1			4	
7	right	2	1			3	1
	left	2	1	1		4	
8	right	3	1			4	
	left	2	1	1		4	
total		43	14	6	2	65	2
Straumann						49	
Nobel						16	

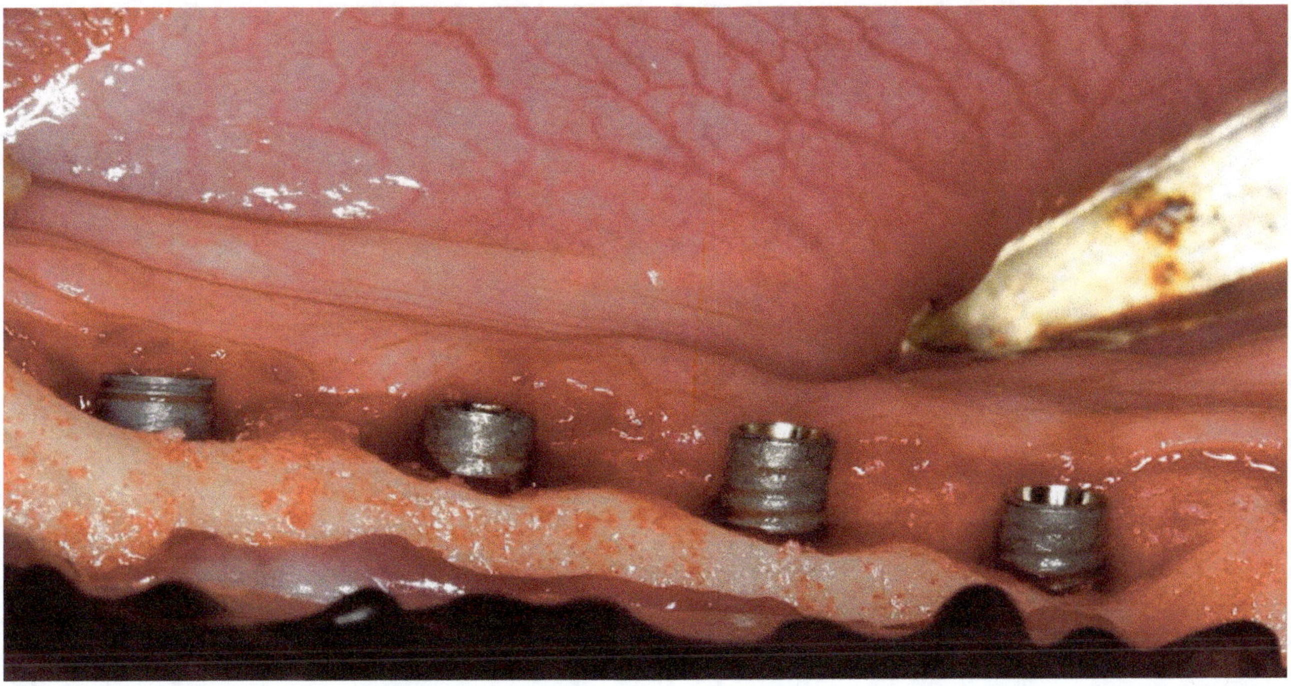

Figure 3. Massive horizontal bone loss results in merging bone defects and massive resorption of the whole ridge.

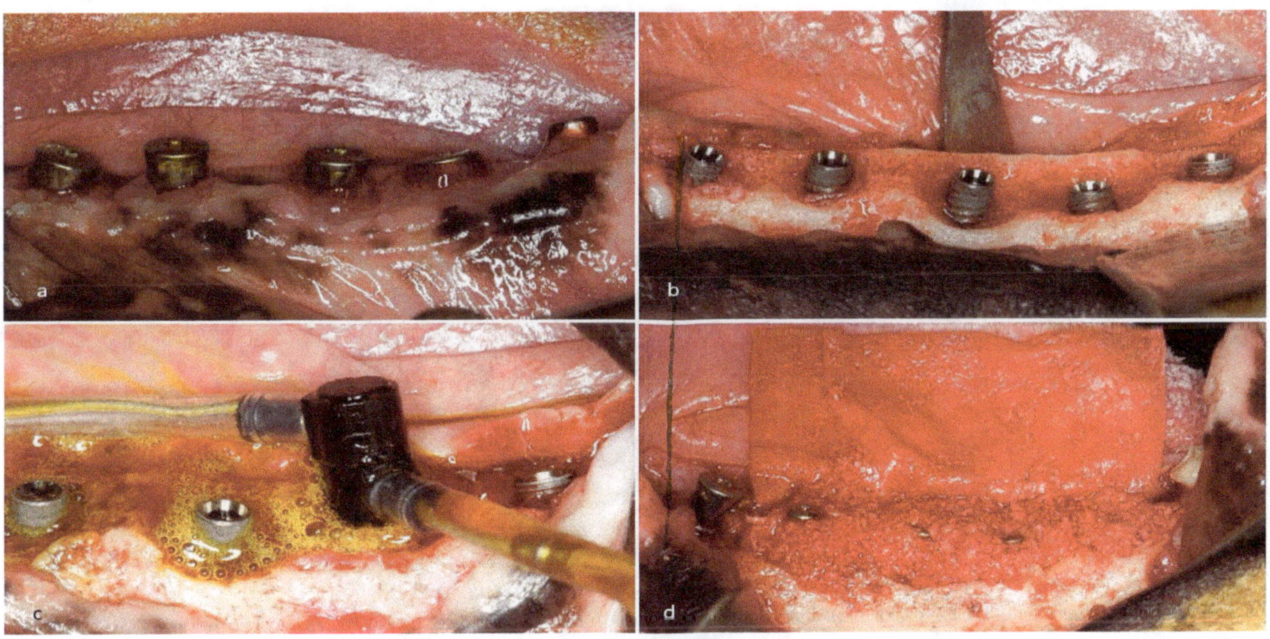

Figure 4. (**a**) Infected site prior to treatment, (**b**) reflected flap indicates a complex merged defect morphology, (**c**) electrolytic cleaning with a spray-head, (**d**) augmented site before collagen membrane was applied.

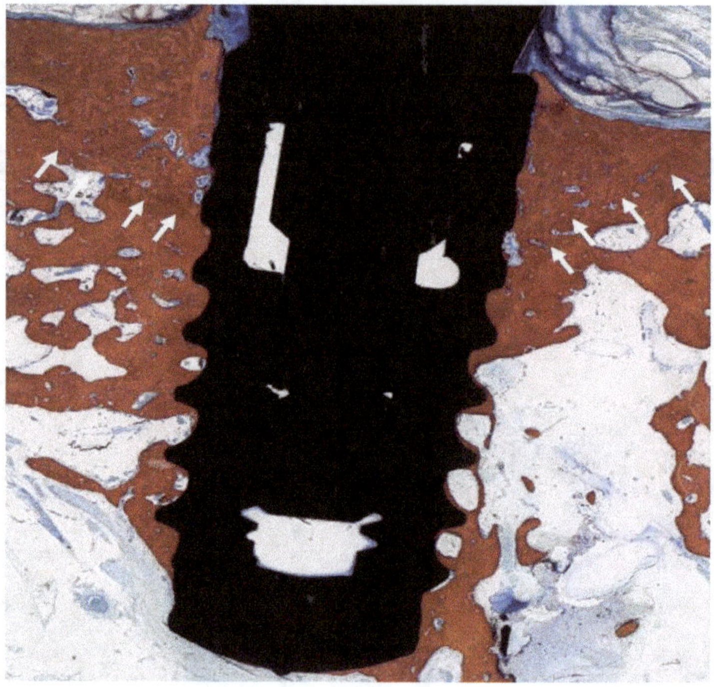

Figure 5. Histologic evaluation of healing after electrolytic cleaning (EC) (SLA® surface). The arrows indicate the bony crest before treatment. Complete coverage of the formerly exposed implant surface was achieved.

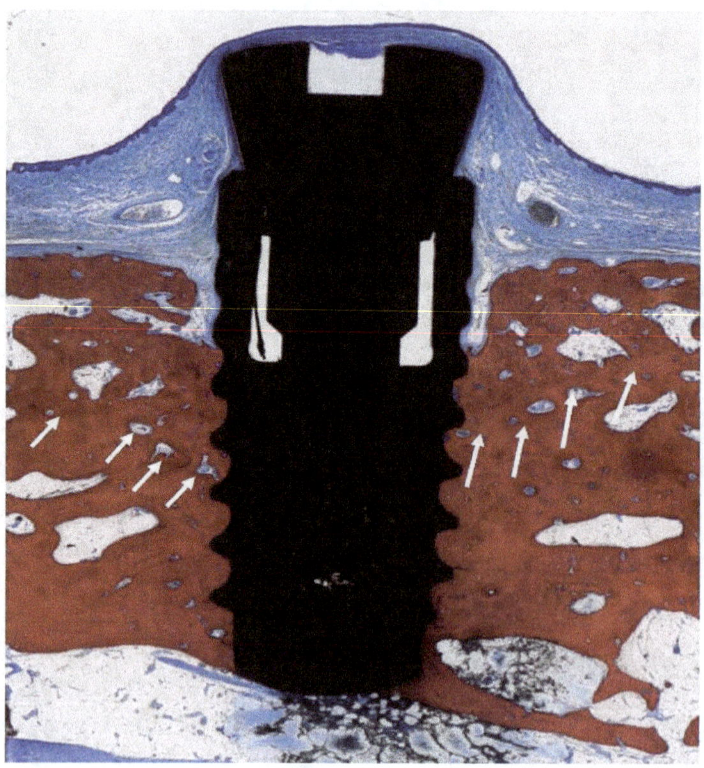

Figure 6. Histologic evaluation of healing after classical cleaning (CC) (SLA® surface). The arrows indicate the bony crest before treatment. Bone-to-implant contact was achieved but full regeneration could not be achieved in any implant.

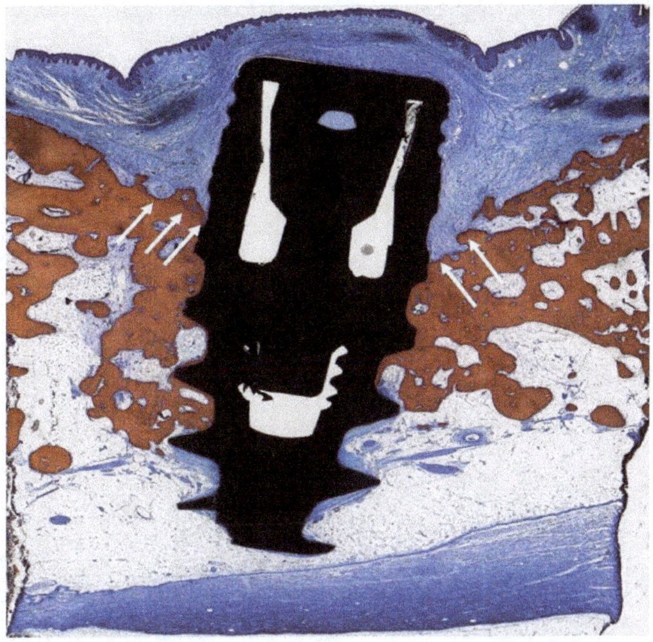

Figure 7. Histologic evaluation of healing after CC (TiUnite® surface). The arrows indicate the bony crest before treatment. A small amount of new bone-to-implant contact was achieved. No re-osseointegration could be achieved on major parts of the implant surface.

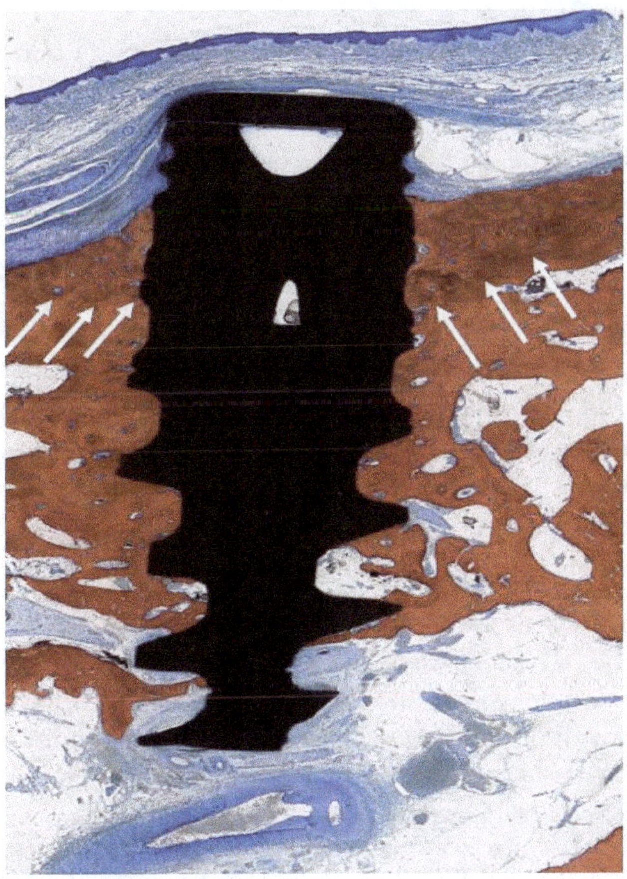

Figure 8. Histologic evaluation of healing after EC (TiUnite® surface). The arrows indicate the bony crest before treatment. Bone-to-implant contact was achieved as more crestal than the neighboring bone level.

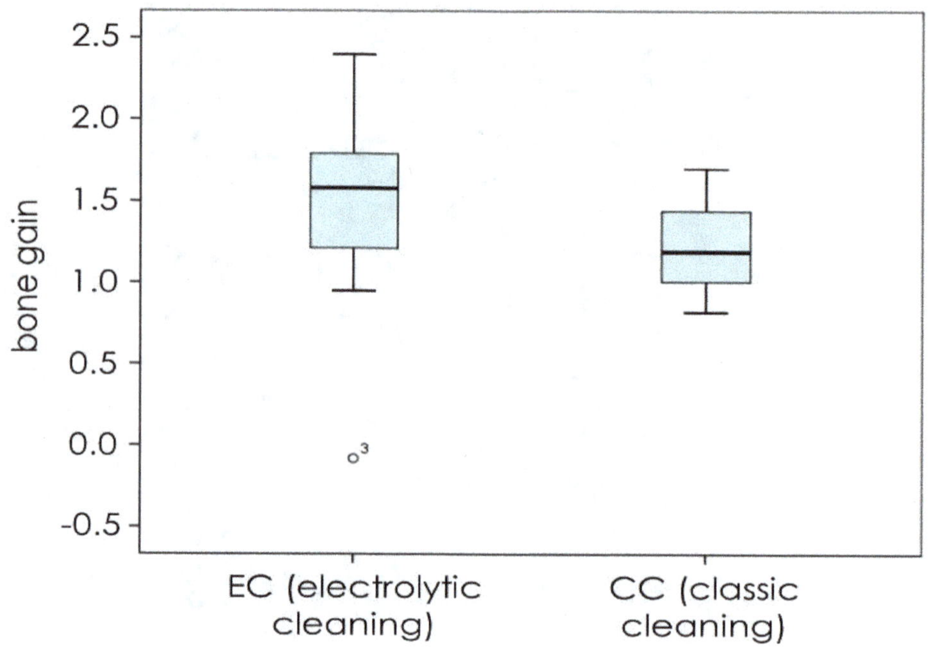

Figure 9. Bone gain for submerged implants at T5 in CC (8 implants) and EC (9 implants) groups display higher bone gain for the EC group.

4. Discussion

The results of this preclinical study may differ from results gained with the final devices used for this technique. Nevertheless, they may serve as proof of principle. As submerged healing was sought, the high number of exposures was an undesirable result. This may correlate with the fact that most of the defects were horizontal and required vertical augmentation. Furthermore, uneventful healing was not possible because of dogs biting on the surgical sites. Implants exposed to the platform cannot regenerate completely and were therefore excluded from statistical evaluation. This limits the meaningfulness of the study. Consequently, we were not able to prove the superiority of one of the treatment modalities in regenerating bone in contact with the implant surface because of the sample size.

Nevertheless, 17 implants were not exposed. When comparing bone regeneration in EC and CC in these cases, EC tended to be superior based on median, without reaching significance. Eight implants in the EC group achieved complete re-osseointegration, but none in the CC group. To the best of the authors' knowledge, complete regeneration has never before been described in the literature. This paper does not investigate the reasons for this observation. In the context of previous literature, it may be assumed that EC in contrast to CC removes the bacterial biofilm and other remnants to an extent that makes complete re-osseointegration possible [6,7]. The latter was proven through histology (Figures 5–8). Re-osseointegration is defined as new bone in direct contact with the formerly infected implant surface. Soft tissue thickness correlates to bone level. Thus bone regeneration to the platform cannot be expected in the case of exposure if the shoulder of the implant was visible [9]. If chewing forces were applied to the implant, complete regeneration also cannot be expected, even if the site stayed covered. Interestingly, complete regeneration was only possible in the EC group—even under these circumstances.

The regenerative potential of horizontal bone defects with no walls is worse than for contained, multi-walled defects [4,7]. In this animal study we observed massive horizontal bone loss and merging defects resulting in a severely resorbed ridge (Figure 3). In humans, an inter-implant distance of 3 mm is usually sufficient to maintain an interdental bone peak in the case of bone loss around implants [10]. We used an inter-implant distance of 6 mm and yet the defects still merged. This might be an indication that ligature-induced periimplantitis in a dog model behaves differently to periimplantitis in humans.

Considering our findings, dog models might be inappropriate for investigating the amount of bone generation. Fewer implants per ridge are suggested for future dog studies.

5. Conclusions

As a proof of concept, complete re-osseointegration was proven after electrolytic cleaning and augmentation.

Author Contributions: Conceptualization, M.S. and H.Z.; Data curation, M.S.; Formal analysis, M.S., L.N. and H.Z.; Funding acquisition M.S., U.B. and H.Z.; Investigation, M.S., L.N. and H.Z.; Methodology, M.S., U.B., F.R. and H.Z.; Project administration, M.S. and H.Z.; Resources, M.S. and H.Z.; Supervision, M.S. and H.Z.; Validation, M.S., L.N. and H.Z.; Visualization, M.S., L.N. and H.Z.; Writing—original draft, M.S.; Writing—review & editing, M.S., U.B., L.N., F.R., and H.Z. All authors have read and agreed to the published version of the manuscript.

References

1. Schwarz, F.; Herten, M.; Sager, M.; Bieling, K.; Sculean, A.; Becker, J. Comparison of naturally occurring and ligature-induced peri-implantitis bone defects in humans and dogs. *Clin. Oral Implants Res.* **2007**, *18*, 161–170. [CrossRef] [PubMed]
2. Seong, W.J.; Kotsakis, G.; Huh, J.-K.; Jeong, S.C.; Nam, K.Y.; Kim, J.R.; Heo, Y.C.; Kim, H.-C.; Zhang, L.; Evans, M.D.; et al. Clinical and microbiologic investigation of an expedited peri-implantitis dog model: An animal study. *BMC Oral Health* **2019**, *19*, 150. [CrossRef] [PubMed]
3. Schwarz, F.; Sculean, A.; Engebretson, S.P.; Becker, J.; Sager, M. Animal models for peri-implant mucositis and peri-implantitis. *Periodontol. 2000* **2015**, *68*, 168–181. [CrossRef] [PubMed]
4. Schwarz, F.; Sahm, N.; Schwarz, K.; Becker, J. Impact of defect configuration on the clinical outcome following surgical regenerative therapy of peri-implantitis. *J. Clin. Periodontol.* **2010**, *37*, 449–455. [CrossRef] [PubMed]
5. Renvert, S.; Polyzois, I.; Maguire, R. Re-osseointegration on previously contaminated surfaces: A systematic review. *Clin. Oral Implants Res.* **2009**, *20* (Suppl. 4), 216–227. [CrossRef] [PubMed]
6. Ratka, C.; Weigl, P.; Henrich, D.; Koch, F.; Schlee, M.; Zipprich, H. The Effect of In Vitro Electrolytic Cleaning on Biofilm-Contaminated Implant Surfaces. *J. Clin. Med.* **2019**, *8*, 1397. [CrossRef] [PubMed]
7. Schlee, M.; Rathe, F.; Brodbeck, U.; Ratka, C.; Zipprich, H. Treatment of periimplantitis-electrolytic cleaning versus mechanical and electrolytic cleaning—A randomized controlled clinical trial—6 month results. *J. Clin. Med.* **2019**, *8*, 1909. [CrossRef] [PubMed]
8. Jovanovic, S.A.; Kenney, E.B.; Carranza, F.A.; Donath, K. The regenerative potential of plaque-induced peri-implant bone defects treated by a submerged membrane technique: An experimental study. *Int. J. Oral Maxillofac Implants* **1993**, *8*, 13–18. [PubMed]
9. Linkevicius, T.; Puisys, A.; Linkeviciene, L.; Peciuliene, V.; Schlee, M. Crestal Bone Stability around Implants with Horizontally Matching Connection after Soft Tissue Thickening: A Prospective Clinical Trial. *Clin. Implant Dent. Relat. Res.* **2015**, *17*, 497–508. [CrossRef] [PubMed]
10. Tarnow, D.P.; Cho, S.C.; Wallace, S.S. The effect of inter-implant distance on the height of inter-implant bone crest. *J. Periodontol.* **2000**, *71*, 546–549. [CrossRef] [PubMed]

15

A Novel Osteotomy Preparation Technique to Preserve Implant Site Viability and Enhance Osteogenesis

Chih-Hao Chen [1,2,†], Benjamin R. Coyac [1,†], Masaki Arioka [1,3,†], Brian Leahy [1], U. Serdar Tulu [1], Maziar Aghvami [1], Stefan Holst [4,5], Waldemar Hoffmann [4], Antony Quarry [4], Oded Bahat [6], Benjamin Salmon [7,8], John B. Brunski [1] and Jill A. Helms [1,*]

1 Division of Plastic and Reconstructive Surgery, Department of Surgery, Stanford University School of Medicine, Stanford, CA 94305, USA; chchen5027@gmail.com (C.-H.C.); benjamin_coyac@hotmail.fr (B.R.C.); amasaki@stanford.edu (M.A.); bleahy94@gmail.com (B.L.); serdartulu@gmail.com (U.S.T.); maziara@stanford.edu (M.A.); brunsj6@stanford.edu (J.B.B.)

2 Craniofacial Research Center, Department of Plastic and Reconstructive Surgery, Chang Gung Memorial Hospital, Chang Gung University School of Medicine, Taoyuan 33305, Taiwan

3 Department of Clinical Pharmacology, Faculty of Medical Sciences, Kyushu University, Fukuoka 812-8582, Japan

4 Nobel Biocare Services AG P.O. Box, CH-8058 Zürich-Flughafen, Switzerland; stefan.holst@nobelbiocare.com (S.H.); waldemar.hoffmann@nobelbiocare.com (W.H.); antony.quarry@nobelbiocare.com (A.Q.)

5 Department of Prosthodontics, School of Dentistry, Johann-Wolfgang Goethe University, 60438 Frankfurt, Germany

6 Private Practice, Beverly Hills, CA 90210, USA; odedbahat@gmail.com

7 Paris Descartes-Sorbonne Paris Cité University, EA2496 Montrouge, France; benjamin.salmon@parisdescartes.fr

8 Dental Medicine Department, Bretonneau Hospital, HUPNVS, AP-HP, 75018 Paris, France

* Correspondence: jhelms@stanford.edu

† These authors contributed equally to this work.

Abstract: The preservation of bone viability at an osteotomy site is a critical variable for subsequent implant osseointegration. Recent biomechanical studies evaluating the consequences of site preparation led us to rethink the design of bone-cutting drills, especially those intended for implant site preparation. We present here a novel drill design that is designed to efficiently cut bone at a very low rotational velocity, obviating the need for irrigation as a coolant. The low-speed cutting produces little heat and, consequently, osteocyte viability is maintained. The lack of irrigation, coupled with the unique design of the cutting flutes, channels into the osteotomy autologous bone chips and osseous coagulum that have inherent osteogenic potential. Collectively, these features result in robust, new bone formation at rates significantly faster than those observed with conventional drilling protocols. These preclinical data have practical implications for the clinical preparation of osteotomies and alveolar bone reconstructive surgeries.

Keywords: osteogenesis; osteotomy; bone healing; bone chips; drilling tool design

1. Introduction

The medical and dental professions, with few exceptions, adapted commercially available tools for use that were developed for drilling other materials [1]. For example, bone-cutting tools, which are largely predicated on the design of metal-cutting instruments. Metal drills are end-cutting tools, e.g., only the tip of the drill is engaged in producing a hole, and the same is true for the vast majority of bone-cutting drills [2]. Metal drills and most bone drills are also designed to cut at a high rotational velocity, which means that the drill can be advanced with minimal axial thrust force [3]. Metal and bone drills generally have a relatively small rake angle, which means that particles generated by cutting are typically scattered from the site to avoid obstructing the drill. Metal drilling typically requires a lubricant that serves as a coolant [4]; in bone cutting, these functions are replaced by saline irrigation [5].

We studied the biological responses to osteotomy site preparation in multiple animal species [6–9] including humans [10], and these analyses, coupled with computational and finite element modeling [5], prompted us to reconsider the design of a bone-cutting tool, optimized for osteotomy site preparation. The resulting tool, called the OsseoShaper, is designed to limit osteocyte death caused by mechanical and thermal damage, and simultaneously retain osseous coagulum/bone chips generated by bone cutting. For this study, cutting tools were downscaled to accommodate the smaller size of the rat maxillae; however, the ratio of cutting-tool diameter and bone surface area was representative of what is used clinically. The purpose of this study was then to compare osteotomies produced by a downscaled OsseoShaper versus a conventional drill in terms of heat generation, osteocyte viability, bone remodeling, and onset of new bone formation.

2. Materials and Methods

2.1. Animals and Experimental Plan

Stanford APLAC approved all procedures (#13146), which conform to ARRIVE guidelines. In total, 18 female Wistar rats (Charles River Laboratories) were used in this study. All animals underwent ovariectomy (OVX) and bilateral maxillary first molar (M1) extraction when they were seven weeks old. Animals were then maintained for eight weeks, during which time the osteoporotic phenotype developed [11,12] and the extraction socket completed its healing [9]. All animals were then subjected to bilateral osteotomy site preparation in the healed M1 location. Animals were sacrificed at intervals of 0.5 days, three days, and seven days. Before surgery, general anesthesia was reached via intraperitoneal injection of ketamine (100 mg/kg) (Vedco, Inc., St. Joseph, MO, USA) and xylazine (10 mg/kg) (Akorn, Inc., Lake Forest, IL, USA), while analgesia was reached via subcutaneous injection of Buprenorphine SR (0.5 mg/kg). After surgery, rats recovered in a controlled, 37 °C environment, fed a soft food diet for the duration of the experiment and housed in groups of two. Weight changes were <10%. No adverse events (e.g., uncontrolled pain, infection, prolonged inflammation) were encountered.

2.2. Ovariectomy and Tooth Extraction

To align our experimental model with the average patient receiving a dental implant, e.g., >50 years old [13], seven-week-old female rats underwent OVX [14]. This produced in our animal model an osteopenic/osteoporotic phenotype, which is representative of patients over 50 years of age [15]. In brief, a dorsal midline incision was made between the mid-back and tail base. The peritoneal cavity was accessed through bilateral muscle layer incisions, the ovary was identified, and the connection between the fallopian tube and the uterine horn was suture-ligated. After bilateral removal of the ovaries, the wounds were closed layer by layer.

In parallel with the OVX, bilateral maxillary first molars (M1) were extracted. This further aligned our experimental model with patients, in which the majority of dental implants are placed in healed extraction sites [16]. In brief, micro-forceps were used to loosen and remove the tooth in toto. Bleeding was controlled by local compression. Healing of the extraction site was confirmed using histology and micro-computed tomographic (μCT) imaging. By post-extraction day 21 (PED21), the extraction site was fully healed, as shown by the fact that the bone volume/total volume (BV/TV) of the extraction site was equivalent to adjacent, pristine bone [10].

2.3. Osteotomy Site Preparation

To directly compare two surgical drilling tools for their ability to maintain osteotomy site viability, rats were anesthetized before a full thickness periosteal flap was elevated at the M1 tooth extraction site. A handpiece (KaVo Dental, Uxbridge, UK) with saline irrigation was used to produce a pilot 1.0-mm drill hole, followed by step-wise enlargement using progressively larger drill diameters (Table 1). In the OsseoShaper protocol, the same type of pilot drill was used to produce a pilot osteotomy; thereafter, a downscaled prototype of the OsseoShaper was used to enlarge the osteotomy to the same final maximum diameter as was achieved with the conventional surgical drill protocol. The mini OsseoShaper was used without irrigation. Drill speeds were adjusted to result in the same radial velocity for all drills and to compensate for slightly different diameters. Each osteotomy was made with a new drill. After osteotomy, tension-free primary closure of the periosteal flap was achieved using tissue glue (VetClose, Henry Schein, Dublin, OH, USA).

Table 1. Surgical drill parameters.

Company	External Diameter	Product Identifier
OsteoMed	1.0 mm	220-0065
OsteoMed	1.3 mm	220-0064
OsteoMed	1.6 mm	220-0116
Downscaled prototype of the OsseoShaper	1.0 mm (apex) 1.6 mm (crest)	Non-commercial prototype

2.4. Tissue Collection and Processing

Tissues were collected at post-osteotomy day (POD) 0.5 to evaluate micro-damage and programmed cell death caused by surgical drilling, as well as at POD3 and POD7, when new bone formation is initiated [7]. In brief, animals were euthanized; then, the entire maxillae were dissected free from other tissues and transferred to 4% paraformaldehyde (PFA) and stored at 4 °C overnight. After fixation, samples were decalcified in ethylenediaminetetraacetic acid (EDTA), embedded in paraffin, and sectioned at an 8-μm thickness for analyses. Tissue sections were deparaffinized in Citrisolv (Decon Labs, Inc., King of Prussia, PA, USA) and hydrated via a series of decreasing concentrations of ethanol before staining or other histological/cellular activity analyses.

2.5. Histology

For aniline blue staining, sections were treated with a saturated solution of picric acid followed by a 5% phosphotungstic acid solution and staining in 1% aniline blue. Slides were then dehydrated and mounted using Permount (Fisher Scientific, Hampton, NH, USA). For pentachrome staining, sections were pre-treated with 6% nitric acid and stained with toluidine blue solution for 5 min (0.5 g toluidine blue in 100 mL of distilled water at pH 1 to 1.5, adjusted with 0.5% HCl). Picrosirius red staining [17] was used to detect collagenous osteoid matrix. Tissues were stained with picrosirius red then viewed under polarized light. Tightly aligned fibrillary collagen molecules appear red compared to less organized collagen fibrils that show a color of shorter (green–yellow) wavelengths.

2.6. Quantification of Programmed Cell Death

Terminal deoxynucleotidyl transferase deoxyuridine triphosphate (dUTP) nick end labeling (TUNEL) staining (Roche Diagnostics GmbH, Mannheim, Germany) was performed according to the manufacturers' guidelines. Following deparaffinization and rehydration, paraffin sections were stained by incubating slides in permeabilization solution for 8 min, adding TUNEL reaction mixture, then incubating at 37 °C in the dark. Between these steps, paraffin sections were washed with phosphate-buffered saline (PBS). To quantify the extent of apoptotic osteocytes, TUNEL-stained tissue sections from 4–6 different samples were analyzed. Each section was photographed using a Leica digital image system at 20× magnification. The number of TUNEL-labeled osteocytes corresponding to apoptotic cells was determined, and the cells grouped according to their distance from the cut edge. The corresponding area for each group was then calculated. The number of apoptotic cells per unit area was calculated by dividing the number of apoptotic cells to the corresponding area (cell/mm^2).

2.7. *Tartrate-Resistant Acid Phosphatase (TRAP) Activity*

Identification of osteoclasts was done using TRAP staining. TRAP activity was observed using a leukocyte acid phosphatase staining kit (catalog #386A-1KT, Sigma-Aldrich, St. Louis, MO, USA). Tissue sections were processed according to the manufacturer's instructions. To quantify the TRAP activity, TRAP-stained tissue sections were photographed using a Leica digital image system at 10× magnification. The TRAP^{+ve} area corresponding to osteoclasts was determined within the radial zone extending 300 μm from the cutting edge. The TRAP^{+ve} ratio was calculated by dividing the TRAP^{+ve} pixels by the total pixels of the region of interest.

2.8. *Immunostaining*

To localize, within the osteotomies, cells that had initiated differentiation down an osteogenic lineage, immunostaining was performed using standard procedures [18]. In brief, following deparaffinization, endogenous peroxidase activity was quenched by 3% hydrogen peroxide for 5 min, and then washed in PBS. Slides were blocked with 5% goat serum (Vector S-1000) for 1 h at room temperature. The appropriate primary antibody was added and incubated overnight at 4 °C, then washed in PBS. The primary antibodies used in this study were Osterix (1:1200; ab22552, Abcam, Cambridge, MA, USA) and Cathepsin K (1:200; ab19027, Abcam, Cambridge, MA, USA). Samples were incubated with appropriate biotinylated secondary antibodies (Vector BA-x) for 30 min, then washed in PBS. An avidin/biotinylated enzyme complex (Kit ABC Peroxidase Standard Vectastain PK-4000, Vectorlabs, Burlingame, CA, USA) was added and incubated for 30 min, and a 3,3′-diaminobenzidine (DAB) substrate kit (Kit Vector Peroxidase substrate DAB SK-4100, Vectorlabs, Burlingame, CA, USA) was used to develop the color reaction. Phalloidin immunostaining was performed using Palloidin Control, DyLight 488 conjugate (1:300; PI21833, Invitrogen, Grand Island, NY, USA).

2.9. *Histomorphometric Analyses*

Histomorphometric measurements were performed using ImageJ software v.1.51 (NIH, Bethesda, MD, USA). To quantify the amount of new bone formation in the osteotomy site as a function of time, a minimum of four osteotomy sites were analyzed. For each osteotomy site, a minimum of six aniline blue-stained histologic sections that spanned the distance from the furcation to the apex were used to quantify new bone formation. Each section was photographed using a Leica digital image system at 20× magnification. To calculate the percentage of new bone formation, the number of aniline blue^{+ve} pixels within an osteotomy was measured and divided by the number of the total pixels in the same osteotomy area.

2.10. *Micro-Computed Tomography (μCT)*

Scanning and analyses followed published guidelines [19]. Three-dimensional μCT imaging was performed at various times after surgery. In brief, samples were fixed in 4% PFA at 4 °C overnight. Then, they were transferred to 70% ethanol solution for μCT scanning before the decalcification process. A μCT tomography data-acquisition system (VivaCT 40, Scanco, Brüttisellen, Switzerland) at 10.5-μm voxel size (70 kV, 115 μA, 300 ms of integration time) was used for scanning and reconstruction. Bone morphometry was performed using the acquisition system's analysis software (Scanco). Multiplanar reconstruction and volume rendering were carried out using Avizo (FEI, Hillsboro, OR, USA) and ImageJ v1.51 (NIH, Bethesda, MD, USA) software, before being imported into Adobe Photoshop and Illustrator (CC2017, Adobe, San Jose, CA, USA).

2.11. Calculation of Osteotomy Surface Roughness

To calculate the irregularity of the osteotomy walls, the Shape Filter plugin for ImageJ was employed [20]. Ten transverse sections were used to outline the contours of osteotomies using ImageJ. The contours were then converted to black-and-white images, and the plugin was used to obtain the convexity and solidity values. Convexity measured the surface roughness of a two-dimensional (2D) shape and was defined as H/P, where H was the perimeter of convex hull of the shape, and P was the perimeter of the contour. Solidity was defined as C/A, where C was the area occupied by the contour, and A was the area occupied by the convex hull of the contour. The perimeter of the contour was defined as the total length of the shape's perimeter. Shapes such as a square have equal lengths of convex hulls and perimeter of the contours, which results in a convexity = 1. A star, however, has a pentagon convex hull (consider the shape when surrounded by a rubber band) while the perimeter of the contour is the star shape itself. Since the perimeter of the star contour (P) is larger than the convex hull (H), its convexity (H/P) is <1 and, therefore, its surface is rougher compared to a same-sized pentagon.

2.12. Heat Transfer During Drilling

The temperature produced when cutting with a conventional protocol involving multiple drills was compared to site preparation with the mini OsseoShaper. Sawbones 35 (Pacific Research Laboratory, Vashon Island, DC, USA) was used. Drills and drilling protocols used are as listed in Table 1. Thermal radiation was measured immediately after drilling via an infrared camera (SEEK CompactPRO, Seek Thermal Application, Santa Barbara, CA, USA). The drilling protocol was repeated six times in new Sawbones. Means and standard deviations were reported.

The temperature distribution during drilling was also calculated in MATLAB using a finite difference method. Details of the heat transfer model are described in Reference [5]. The differences between the conventional drill and mini OsseoShaper models can be summarized as follows: in the conventional high-speed drilling, the heat flux was applied to the drill hole's boundary where the tip of the drill was located, and the tip was moved vertically. Below the drill tip, the value of the heat flux was set to zero, and irrigation was applied above the drill tip. In the OsseoShaper low-speed drilling, the heat flux was applied to the drill hole's boundary at and above the tip due to the tapered shape of the drill, such that the points of engagement between the drill and the bone increased over time as the drill was moved vertically.

2.13. Statistical Analyses

Results were presented in the form of means $\pm$ standard deviations, with N equal to the number of samples analyzed. Student's t-tests were performed. Significance was set at $p < 0.05$, and all statistical analyses were performed with SPSS software (IBM, Armonk, NY, USA).

3. Results

3.1. A New Surgical Drilling Tool That Cuts Efficiently at Very Low Speeds

Most osteotomies are produced through the stepwise enlargement of an initial pilot drill hole with sequentially larger diameter drills [21], all coupled with the use of copious irrigation [22]. We recapitulated that clinical scenario in a rat model, by producing osteotomies using surgical drills with progressively larger diameters. The final drill was 1.6 mm in diameter and was run at 1000 rpm with irrigation (Figure 1A). In osteotomies produced with the downscaled prototype of OsseoShaper, the same pilot drill hole was produced and then followed by a single drill, the OsseoShaper (Figure 1A). The OsseoShaper was run at 50 rpm without irrigation.

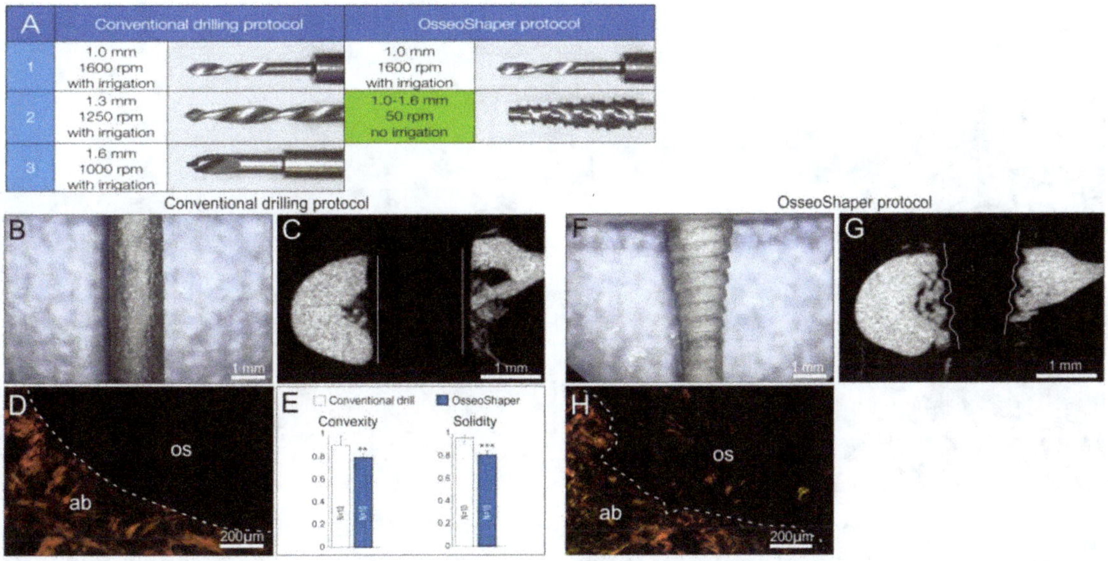

Figure 1. Osteotomy site preparation with OsseoShaper requires fewer steps and, unlike conventional drills, produces a rough surface. (**A**) All osteotomy site preparations began with the use of a 1.0-mm pilot drill run at 1600 rpm plus irrigation; afterward, the conventional osteotomy procedure used a 1.3-mm drill (1250 rpm plus irrigation) followed by a 1.6-mm drill (1000 rpm plus irrigation). The OsseoShaper protocol used the same 1.0-mm pilot drill at 1600 rpm plus irrigation, and was then followed by the OsseoShaper run at 50 rpm without irrigation. Using a conventional drill (**B**) in plexiglass demonstrates the shape and texture of a cut surfaces, and (**C**) in bone, µCT sections illustrate the parallel walls of the osteotomy. (**D**) Picrosirius red staining of a representative transverse tissue section demonstrates the resulting smooth cut surface. (**E**) Quantification of surface texture, as expressed by convexity and solidity, resulting from a conventional drilling protocol. Using an OsseoShaper (**F**) in plexiglass demonstrates a tapered shape with a threaded surface, (**G**) which is validated by µCT imaging. (**H**) Picrosirius red staining of a representative transverse tissue section demonstrates the textured cut surface and the retention of collagen containing osseous coagulum. Solid and dotted lines show the edge of the osteotomy. Two asterisks indicate $p < 0.01$. Three asterisks indicate $p < 0.001$. Scale bars (**B**,**C**,**F**,**G**) = 1 mm, and (**D**,**H**) = 200 µm. Abbreviations: ab, alveolar bone; os, osteotomy.

A conventional surgical drill is designed to cut only at its tip, which produces a smooth-walled osteotomy, visible both in plexiglass (Figure 1B) and µCT section of bone (Figure 1C). Analyses using picrosirius red staining revealed, under polarized light, the collagen organization at the cut edge when a conventional drill was employed (Figure 1D). Quantification of surface texture, as expressed by convexity and solidity, resulting from a conventional drilling protocol demonstrated the smoother cut edge (Figure 1E). By contrast, the OsseoShaper was designed with a cutting flute running its length; this resulted in a heteromorphic, textured osteotomy surface, visible both in plexiglass (Figure 1F) and in µCT (Figure 1G). Picrosirius red staining demonstrates the textured cut surface and the retention of collagen containing osseous coagulum (Figure 1H).

3.2. The OsseoShaper Allows the Retention of Viable, Autologous Bone Chips in the Osteotomy

Conventional drills have a rake angle that ranges from 0 to approximately 5°, the consequence of which is the production of small (<30 µm) bone particles. In addition, conventional drills are typically run at rotational velocities of 800 rpm or higher [23]. Finally, conventional drills are designed to rotate in the same direction, regardless of whether they are being advanced or withdrawn from the osteotomy. Collectively, these attributes result in minimal retention of particulate matter, as can be visualized when cutting Sawbone in vitro (Figure 2A). Coupled with irrigation, the majority of bone debris is typically removed from the osteotomy (Figure 2B).

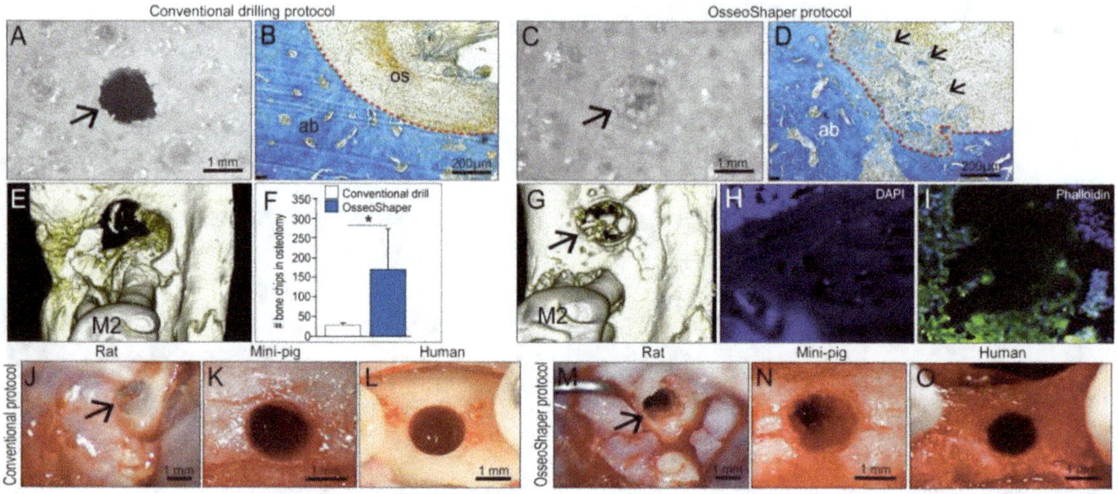

Figure 2. OsseoShaper-produced osteotomies retain more viable bone chips and osseous coagulum. Gross view of a hole produced in 0.32 g/cc Sawbone prepared with (**A**) a conventional drilling protocol versus (**C**) OsseoShaper. Representative transverse sections stained with aniline blue in the osteotomy sites using (**B**) a conventional drilling protocol and (**D**) OsseoShaper protocol. Micro-CT imaging of an osteotomy prepared with (**E**) a conventional drilling protocol versus (**G**) an OsseoShaper. (**F**) Quantification of bone chips in the osteotomy by μCT imaging ($N = 5$). Representative tissue sections of bone chips produced by the OsseoShaper using (**H**) 4′,6-diamidino-2-phenylindole (DAPI) and (**I**) phalloidin staining. Intra-operative view of an osteotomy prepared with conventional drills versus the OsseoShaper in rats (**J**,**M**), in mini-pigs (**K**,**N**), and in patients (**L**,**O**). Arrows indicate the osteotomy. Small arrows in (**D**) indicate the osteoid matrix. Dotted lines show the edge of the osteotomy. Asterisk indicates $p < 0.05$. Scale bars = 1 mm (**A**,**C**,**J**–**O**) and 200 μm (**B**,**E**). Abbreviations: as indicated previously.

By comparison, the rake angle on a mini OsseoShaper produces osseous coagulum and relatively large (~100 μm) bone chips; additionally, the OsseoShaper is designed to be reversed upon removal. These features result in the collection of bone chips in the cutting flutes, which are then transferred into the osteotomy while the tool is being withdrawn. These events can be visualized when cutting Sawbone (Figure 2C), and upon histologic examination of the osteotomy using aniline blue staining to detect osteoid matrix (Figure 2D).

Micro-CT imaging was used to quantify the volume of osseous coagulum and bone chips retained in the osteotomy. These analyses verified that OsseoShaper osteotomies retained significantly more osseous material than did conventionally prepared osteotomies (Figure 2E,F,G). A closer examination of the bone chips produced by the OsseoShaper using 4′,6-diamidino-2-phenylindole (DAPI; to detect viable cells) and phalloidin staining (to detect actin filaments) revealed that a subset of chips retained viable osteocytes within the osseous matrix (Figure 2H) and that the majority of chips were surrounded by viable cells (Figure 2I). Clinically, bone chips were only visible in the OsseoShaper-prepared osteotomy sites; this aspect was consistent among species, including rats, mini-pigs, and humans (Figure 2J–O).

3.3. The Mini OsseoShaper Preserves Peri-Implant Bone by Limiting Heat Transfer and Minimizing Thermal Apoptosis

A zone of osteocyte death is produced by conventional drilling [6,7,10]. For example, cutting at 1000 rpm with irrigation produced a ~250-μm-wide, circumferential distribution of $TUNEL^{+ve}$, apoptotic osteocytes (Figure 3A, quantified in C). By comparison, minimal osteocyte apoptosis was detected after OsseoShaper site preparation (Figure 3B, quantified in C).

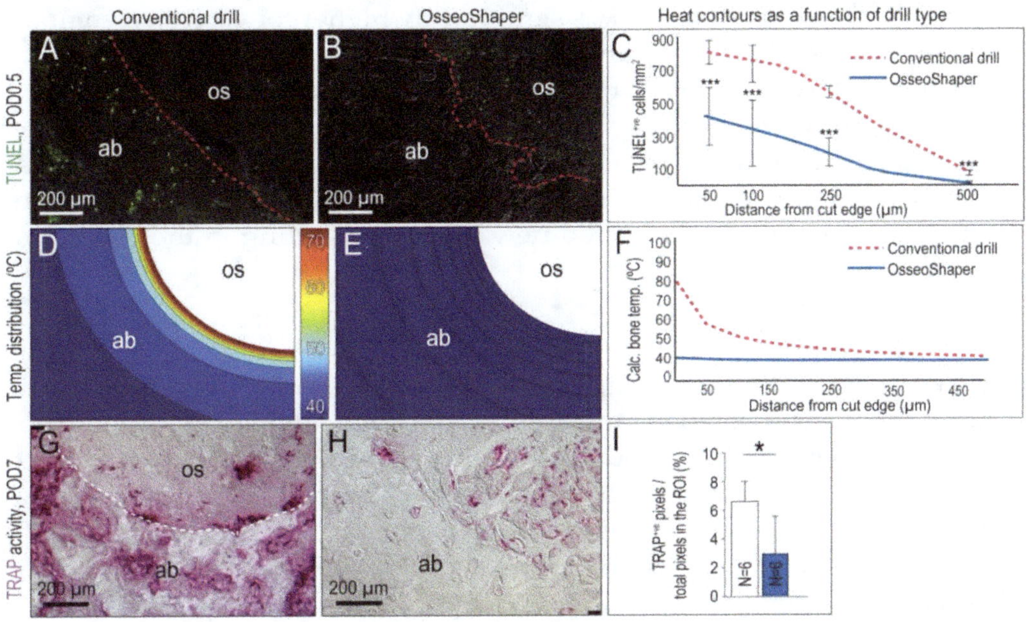

Figure 3. The OsseoShaper generates less heat, which results in a smaller zone of cell death and less tartrate-resistant acid phosphatase (TRAP)-mediated bone remodeling than conventional drills. (**A**) Representative tissue section from an osteotomy prepared using standard drills, where terminal deoxynucleotidyl transferase deoxyuridine triphosphate (dUTP) nick end labeling (TUNEL)$^{+ve}$ cells are apoptotic osteocytes. (**B**) Equivalent tissue section from an osteotomy prepared using the OsseoShaper, where the majority of apoptotic cells are detected in the osseous coagulum. (**C**) Distribution of TUNEL^{+ve} cells as a function of distance from cut edge of osteotomy. Computational models were used to map the distribution of heat in bone as a function of distance from the cut edge, in osteotomies produced using (**D**) conventional drills and (**E**) using the OsseoShaper. (**F**) Calculated temperatures in bone, expressed as a function of radial distance from conventional drills (dotted red line) and from the OsseoShaper (blue line) ($N = 6$). (**G**) Representative transverse tissue section from an osteotomy produced with conventional drills, analyzed on for TRAP activity on post-osteotomy day 7 (POD7). (**H**) TRAP activity on a representative transverse tissue section from an OsseoShaper-produced osteotomy. (**I**) Quantification of TRAP^{+ve} pixels/total pixels in the region of interest (ROI). A dotted line is used to indicate the cut edge of the osteotomy. Asterisk indicates $p < 0.05$. Scale bars = 200 µm. Abbreviations: as indicated previously.

A computational model was used to calculate peak temperatures produced by both types of cutting tools, taking into account the speed at which the drills were run, the density of the bone being cut, and, in the case of conventional drill protocols, the use of irrigation [5]. In the case of conventional protocols, a peak temperature of ~80 °C was generated at the cut edge, despite the use of copious irrigation (Figure 3D; quantified in F). Temperatures decreased as a function of distance from the cut edge but nevertheless, temperatures were >40 °C within a ~150-µm circumferential zone (Figure 3A and [6]).

By comparison, the mini OsseoShaper generated significantly lower (~40 °C) peak temperatures (Figure 3E; quantified in F). Even without the use of irrigation, calculated temperatures immediately adjacent to the cut edge remained in the physiologic range (Figure 3F), well below temperatures known to cause osteocytes necrosis, i.e., 45 °C [24].

An in vitro method supported our conclusion that drilling with the mini OsseoShaper produced less heat. Using Sawbones, site preparation was carried out following the same protocol as used for the site preparation in the rat maxilla (Figure 1A) and, immediately thereafter, the temperature of each drill was measured using an infrared camera (Figure S1, Supplementary Materials). The same method was used to measure heat radiating from the mini OsseoShaper. In the conventional protocol, the heat radiating from conventional drills was significantly higher for each step compared to the heat radiating from the mini OsseoShaper (Figure S1).

Osteocyte death is typically accompanied by peri-implant bone resorption [6,7]. In the case of osteotomies produced with conventional drills, the osteoclast marker TRAP was detected throughout the bone adjacent to the osteotomy edge, as well as in the osteotomy itself (Figure 3G). By contrast, mini OsseoShaper osteotomies exhibited minimal TRAP-mediated bone resorption (Figure 3H). The TRAP activity that was detected reflected new bone remodeling in the osteotomy (Figure 3H; quantified in I).

3.4. In Mini OsseoShaper Osteotomies, New Bone Formation Is Accelerated

The OsseoShaper was designed to retain osseous coagulum, e.g., mineralized particles including cortical and trabecular bone chips, blood, and stroma that have inherent osteogenic potential [25,26]. On POD3, evidence of this retained osseous coagulum was abundant; compared to conventionally prepared osteotomies, those prepared with the mini OsseoShaper were filled with aniline blue^{+ve} osteoid matrix (compare Figure 4A,B). This matrix served as a nidus for new bone formation and remodeling, as demonstrated by significantly higher Cathepsin K (Figure 4C,D; quantified in E) and Osterix (Figure 4F,G) expression in the mini OsseoShaper osteotomies. By POD7, mini OsseoShaper osteotomies were filled with new bone at a time point when conventionally prepared osteotomies had not yet started to repair (Figure 4H,I; quantified in J).

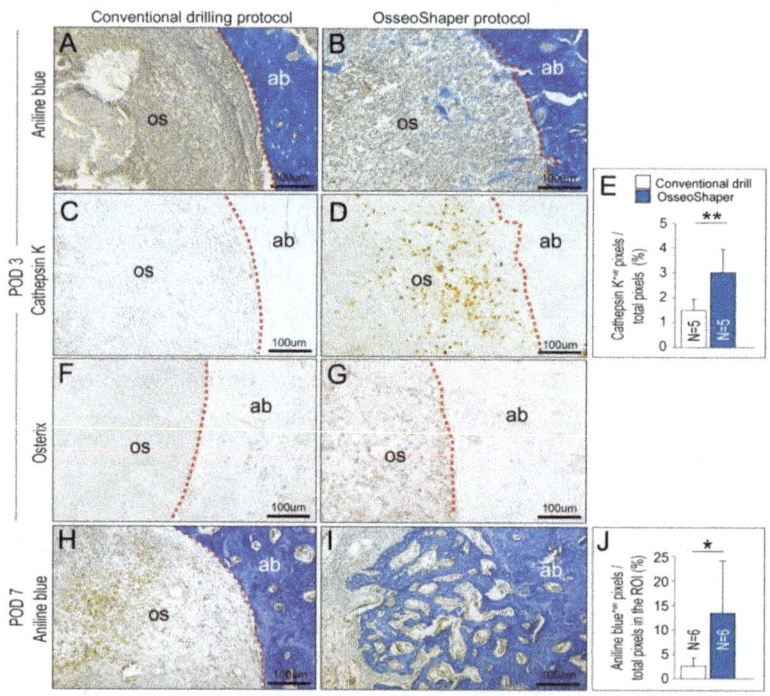

Figure 4. OsseoShaper drilling protocol promotes alveolar bone healing. Representative transverse tissue sections stained with aniline blue on post-osteotomy day 3 (POD3) following osteotomy site preparation with (**A**) conventional drills versus (**B**) the Nobel OsseoShaper. Note the presence of osseous coagulum in the osteotomy site prepared with the OsseoShaper. Adjacent tissue sections immunostained with Cathepsin K in the osteotomy sites of (**C**) conventional drills versus (**D**) the Nobel OsseoShaper. (**E**) Quantification of Cathepsin K^{+ve} pixels/total pixels in the osteotomy site. Adjacent tissue sections immunostained with Osterix in the osteotomy sites of (**F**) conventional drills versus (**G**) the OsseoShaper. (**H**) Tissue sections stained with aniline blue show minimal new bone formation in conventional drill group, while (**I**) osteotomies in the OsseoShaper group show more new bone formation on POD7. (**J**) Quantification of aniline blue^{+ve} pixels/total pixels in the osteotomy site. Dotted lines show the edge of the osteotomy. One asterisk indicates $p < 0.05$. Two asterisks indicate $p < 0.01$. Scale bars = 100 μm. Abbreviations: as indicated previously.

4. Discussion

Most reconstructive surgeries involve the cutting and removal of bone tissue [27] and, ideally, the goal is to resect a well-defined volume of bone and leave behind a cut edge that is favorable to early cell attachment and matrix deposition [28,29]. Clinicians universally agree that the preservation of cell viability is of utmost importance [30–32], and that high-speed rotating instruments can compromise this viability because they create thermal and mechanical trauma [33–37]. Irrigation can reduce some of the heat generated by high-speed rotatory surgical drills [22,38], but irrigation also removes bone chips, connective tissue stroma, blood, and stem-cell populations, collectively referred to as osseous coagulum, which have osteogenic potential [39–42].

The importance of preserving bone viability led to the development of a wide variety of new cutting tools for bone [43]. For example, gas and solid-state lasers use linear thermal absorption to ablate osteoid tissues and, while they are effective at removing the bone, they also generate heat and consequently show many of the same detrimental effects as drilling [44,45]. Plasma ablation lasers avoid some of these problems by creating energy pulses in very small (i.e., μm) zones that result in very high (several thousand Kelvin) temperatures over a very short (picosecond) duration. The result is limited thermal damage to the bone [46]; technical constraints, however, limit the use of these lasers in most clinical practices [47].

The OsseoShaper was designed to efficiently cut bone at a low (<50 rpm) velocity. This low-speed drilling results in less bone being cut per unit time and, therefore, less heat evolution per unit time (Figure 3). Less heat generation by the OsseoShaper translates into less of a temperature rise in the bone, which obviates the need for a coolant (Figure 3). The biological sequelae of lower heat generation by the mini OsseoShaper was shown by analyses for osteocyte apoptosis and osteoclast activity; because of the minimal temperature rise, few osteocytes underwent programmed cell death, which translated into less peri-implant bone resorption (Figure 3). Clinicians are fully aware that a viable osteotomy site is critical for new bone formation, and this point is perhaps best illustrated by the extent to which surgeons will go to reduce heat produced by rotary cutting tools. Here, we show that improved osteotomy site viability is indeed directly related to enhanced osteogenesis, which we believe will logically translate into a faster osseointegration of an implant placed into such osteotomies.

4.1. *A Unique Design That Enables Retention of Bone Chips and Osseous Coagulum in an Osteotomy Site*

Most drills produce bone chips and osseous coagulum, which has inherent osteogenic material that can stimulate new bone formation [25,26]. Most of this osteogenic material is flushed out of the site by irrigation [25], which is required to cool conventional drills. The rake angle of the OsseoShaper produces larger bone chips than conventional drilling protocols.

Most conventional drills rotate clockwise, whether advancing or withdrawing the tool and, coupled with the high rotational velocity, effectively disperse the bone chips and osseous coagulum. The OsseoShaper slowly rotates clockwise when advanced and is then reversed upon withdrawal; this design feature effectively retains bone chips and osseous coagulum in the osteotomy site (Figure 2). This feature was also visible in osteotomy site preparation performed in mini-pig and human individuals (Figure 2). Historic studies demonstrated that such bone chips that remain in situ are highly osteogenic [48].

Cutting flute placement affects the roughness of the osteotomy. Compared to the smooth-walled osteotomies produced by conventional drills, osteotomies produced by the OsseoShaper are textured (Figure 1). Some investigators speculated that a textured surface represents an optimal site for new bone deposition because it mimics the bone surface left behind after osteoclast-mediated remodeling [49].

Clinicians recognize that a bone graft from a patient has osteogenic potential and, therefore, a variety of methods were developed in an attempt to collect this autologous material [50]. Most, if not all, of these collection methods necessitate removal of the autologous bone chips from the body and storage ex vivo. In doing so, the bone graft material is potentially subjected to desiccation, temperature changes, e.g., deviations from 37 °C, and bacterial contamination. Use of the OsseoShaper negates these concerns; bone chips remain in situ and, in doing so, their viability is likely to be enhanced and/or preserved.

4.2. A Streamlined Protocol for Osteotomy Site Preparation

In conventional drilling protocols, a pilot hole is first produced; then, the osteotomy is gradually enlarged through the use of progressively larger diameter drills. A pilot hole is also created before use of the OsseoShaper, after which the final sized osteotomy is produced in a single step (Figure 1). In conventional drilling protocols, the use of multiple drills increases the chance of deviating from the intended axis of the osteotomy, which in turn impacts the axis of the implant placed into the osteotomy [51]. By reducing the number of surgical drills required to produce the final osteotomy, the alignment error is also effectively reduced [52], and subsequent implant placement will follow the axis of the last drill.

5. Conclusions

In our study, we present a new drill design that is meant to efficiently cut bone at a very low rotational speed, obviating the need for irrigation as a coolant and a lubricant. Osteocyte viability is maintained by the low-speed cutting that produces little heat. Autologous bone chips are generated and maintained on site thanks to the lack of irrigation, coupled with the unique design of the cutting flutes. This osseous coagulum has inherent osteogenic capacities. Collectively, a robust formation of new bone is observed with the new drill design, at rates significantly faster than those observed with conventional drilling protocols. These data have practical applications for clinical implant site preparation and alveolar bone reconstruction.

Author Contributions: Conceptualization, S.H. and A.Q.; methodology, J.A.H. and J.B.B.; data generation, C.-H.C., B.R.C., M.A. (Masaki Arioka), B.L., U.S.T., M.A. (Maziar Aghvami), B.S., W.H., A.Q., and O.B.; writing—original draft preparation, C.-H.C., B.R.C., M.A. (Masaki Arioka), J.B.B., and J.A.H.; writing—review and editing, C.-H.C., B.R.C., M.A. (Masaki Arioka), J.B.B., W.H., and J.A.H. All authors read and approved the manuscript.

Acknowledgments: Special thanks to Audrey Schmitt, DDS, MSc (periodontist, private practice, Rouen, France) for providing surgical photographs from a conventional osteotomy site preparation. J.A.H. and J.B.B. are paid consultants for Nobel Biocare.

References

1. Jackson, C.J.; Ghosh, S.K.; Johnson, W. On the evolution of drill-bit shapes. *J. Mech. Work Technol.* **1989**, *18*, 231–267. [CrossRef]
2. Pandey, R.K.; Panda, S.S. Drilling of bone: A comprehensive review. *J. Clin. Orthop. Trauma* **2013**, *4*, 15–30. [CrossRef] [PubMed]
3. Abouzgia, M.B.; James, D.F. Measurements of shaft speed while drilling through bone. *J. Oral. Maxillofac. Surg.* **1995**, *53*, 1308–1315, Discussion in **1995**, *53*, 1315–1316. [CrossRef]
4. Yan, P.; Rong, Y.M.; Wang, G. The effect of cutting fluids applied in metal cutting process. *Proc. Inst. Mech. Eng. B* **2016**, *230*, 19–37. [CrossRef]
5. Aghvami, M.; Brunski, J.B.; Serdar Tulu, U.; Chen, C.H.; Helms, J.A. A Thermal and Biological Analysis of Bone Drilling. *J. Biomech. Eng.* **2018**, *140*. [CrossRef]
6. Cha, J.Y.; Pereira, M.D.; Smith, A.A.; Houschyar, K.S.; Yin, X.; Mouraret, S.; Brunski, J.B.; Helms, J.A. Multiscale analyses of the bone-implant interface. *J. Dent. Res.* **2015**, *94*, 482–490. [CrossRef] [PubMed]
7. Wang, L.; Aghvami, M.; Brunski, J.; Helms, J. Biophysical regulation of osteotomy healing: An animal study. *Clin. Implant Dent. Relat. Res.* **2017**, *19*, 590–599. [CrossRef] [PubMed]
8. Pei, X.; Wang, L.; Chen, C.; Yuan, X.; Wan, Q.; Helms, J.A. Contribution of the PDL to osteotomy repair and implant osseointegration. *J. Dent. Res.* **2017**, *96*, 909–916. [CrossRef]
9. Li, J.; Yin, X.; Huang, L.; Mouraret, S.; Brunski, J.B.; Cordova, L.; Salmon, B.; Helms, J.A. Relationships among bone quality, implant osseointegration, and Wnt signaling. *J. Dent. Res.* **2017**, *96*, 822–831. [CrossRef]
10. Chen, C.H.; Pei, X.; Tulu, U.S.; Aghvami, M.; Chen, C.T.; Gaudilliere, D.; Arioka, M.; Maghazeh Moghim, M.; Bahat, O.; Kolinski, M.; et al. A comparative assessment of implant site viability in humans and rats. *J. Dent. Res.* **2018**, *97*, 451–459. [CrossRef]

11. Chen, C.H.; Wang, L.; Serdar Tulu, U.; Arioka, M.; Moghim, M.M.; Salmon, B.; Chen, C.T.; Hoffmann, W.; Gilgenbach, J.; Brunski, J.B.; et al. An osteopenic/osteoporotic phenotype delays alveolar bone repair. *Bone* **2018**, *112*, 212–219. [CrossRef] [PubMed]
12. Arioka, M.; Zhang, X.; Li, Z.; Tulu, U.S.; Liu, Y.; Wang, L.; Yuan, X.; Helms, J.A. Osteoporotic changes in the periodontium impair alveolar bone healing. *J. Dent. Res.* **2019**. [CrossRef]
13. Mangano, F.; Mortellaro, C.; Mangano, N.; Mangano, C. Is low serum vitamin d associated with early dental implant failure? A retrospective evaluation on 1625 implants placed in 822 patients. *Mediators Inflamm.* **2016**. [CrossRef] [PubMed]
14. Kalu, D.N. The ovariectomized rat model of postmenopausal bone loss. *Bone Miner.* **1991**, *15*, 175–191. [CrossRef]
15. Cummings, S.R.; Melton, L.J. Epidemiology and outcomes of osteoporotic fractures. *Lancet* **2002**, *359*, 1761–1767. [CrossRef]
16. Chen, S.T.; Beagle, J.; Jensen, S.S.; Chiapasco, M.; Darby, I. Consensus statements and recommended clinical procedures regarding surgical techniques. *Int. J. Oral Maxillofac. Implants* **2009**, *24*, 272–278.
17. Yin, X.; Li, J.; Chen, T.; Mouraret, S.; Dhamdhere, G.; Brunski, J.B.; Zou, S.; Helms, J.A. Rescuing failed oral implants via Wnt activation. *J. Clin. Periodontol.* **2015**. [CrossRef] [PubMed]
18. Minear, S.; Leucht, P.; Jiang, J.; Liu, B.; Zeng, A.; Fuerer, C.; Nusse, R.; Helms, J.A. Wnt proteins promote bone regeneration. *Sci. Transl. Med.* **2010**, *2*. [CrossRef]
19. Bouxsein, M.L.; Boyd, S.K.; Christiansen, B.A.; Guldberg, R.E.; Jepsen, K.J.; Muller, R. Guidelines for assessment of bone microstructure in rodents using micro-computed tomography. *J. Bone Miner. Res.* **2010**, *25*, 1468–1486. [CrossRef]
20. Wagner, T.; Lipinski, H.G. IJBlob: An ImageJ library for connected component analysis and shape analysis. *J. Open Res. Softw.* **2013**, *1*, 6–8.8
21. Wang, L.; Wu, Y.; Perez, K.C.; Hyman, S.; Brunski, J.B.; Tulu, U.; Bao, C.; Salmon, B.; Helms, J.A. Effects of Condensation on Peri-implant Bone Density and Remodeling. *J. Dent. Res.* **2017**, *96*, 413–420. [CrossRef] [PubMed]
22. Isler, S.C.; Cansiz, E.; Tanyel, C.; Soluk, M.; Selvi, F.; Cebi, Z. The effect of irrigation temperature on bone healing. *Int. J. Med. Sci.* **2011**, *8*, 704–708. [CrossRef] [PubMed]
23. Almeida, K.P.; Delgado-Ruiz, R.; Carneiro, L.G.; Leiva, A.B.; Calvo-Guirado, J.L.; Gomez-Moreno, G.; Malmstrom, H.; Romanos, G.E. Influence of Drilling Speed on Stability of Tapered Dental Implants: An Ex Vivo Experimental Study. *Int. J. Oral Maxillofac. Implants* **2016**, *31*, 795–798. [CrossRef] [PubMed]
24. Dolan, E.B.; Haugh, M.G.; Tallon, D.; Casey, C.; McNamara, L.M. Heat-shock-induced cellular responses to temperature elevations occurring during orthopaedic cutting. *J. R. Soc. Interface* **2012**, *9*, 3503–3513. [CrossRef] [PubMed]
25. Robinson, R.E. The osseous coagulum for bone induction technique. A review. *J. Calif. Dent. Assoc.* **1970**, *46*, 18–27. [PubMed]
26. Robinson, E. Osseous coagulum for bone induction. *J. Periodontol.* **1969**, *40*, 503–510. [CrossRef]
27. Preston, C.F.; Fulkerson, E.W.; Meislin, R.; Di Cesare, P.E. Osteotomy about the knee: Applications, techniques, and results. *J. Knee Surg.* **2005**, *18*, 258–272. [CrossRef]
28. Yeniyol, S.; Jimbo, R.; Marin, C.; Tovar, N.; Janal, M.N.; Coelho, P.G. The effect of drilling speed on early bone healing to oral implants. *Oral Surg. Oral Med. Oral Pathol. Oral Radiol.* **2013**, *116*, 550–555. [CrossRef]
29. Giro, G.; Marin, C.; Granato, R.; Bonfante, E.A.; Suzuki, M.; Janal, M.N.; Coelho, P.G. Effect of drilling technique on the early integration of plateau root form endosteal implants: an experimental study in dogs. *J. Oral Maxillofac. Surg.* **2011**, *69*, 2158–2163. [CrossRef]
30. Miron, R.J.; Gruber, R.; Hedbom, E.; Saulacic, N.; Zhang, Y.; Sculean, A.; Bosshardt, D.D.; Buser, D. Impact of bone harvesting techniques on cell viability and the release of growth factors of autografts. *Clin. Implant Dent. Relat. Res.* **2013**, *15*, 481–489. [CrossRef]
31. Maus, U.; Andereya, S.; Gravius, S.; Siebert, C.H.; Schippmann, T.; Ohnsorge, J.A.; Niedhart, C. How to store autologous bone graft perioperatively: an in vitro study. *Arch. Orthop. Trauma Surg.* **2008**, *128*, 1007–1011. [CrossRef] [PubMed]
32. Laursen, M.; Christensen, F.B.; Bunger, C.; Lind, M. Optimal handling of fresh cancellous bone graft: different peroperative storing techniques evaluated by in vitro osteoblast-like cell metabolism. *Acta Orthop. Scand.* **2003**, *74*, 490–496. [CrossRef] [PubMed]
33. Davidson, S.R.; James, D.F. Drilling in bone: Modeling heat generation and temperature distribution. *J. Biomech. Eng.* **2003**, *125*, 305–314. [CrossRef] [PubMed]

34. Eriksson, A.R.; Albrektsson, T. Temperature threshold levels for heat-induced bone tissue injury: A vital-microscopic study in the rabbit. *J. Prosthet. Dent.* **1983**, *50*, 101–107. [CrossRef]
35. Lundskog, J. Heat and bone tissue. An experimental investigation of the thermal properties of bone and threshold levels for thermal injury. *Scand. J. Plast. Reconstr. Surg.* **1972**, *9*, 1–80. [PubMed]
36. Eriksson, A.; Albrektsson, T.; Grane, B.; McQueen, D. Thermal injury to bone. A vital-microscopic description of heat effects. *Int. J. Oral Surg.* **1982**, *11*, 115–121. [CrossRef]
37. Matthews, L.S.; Hirsch, C. Temperatures measured in human cortical bone when drilling. *J. Bone Joint. Surg. Am.* **1972**, *54*, 297–308. [CrossRef] [PubMed]
38. Tawy, G.F.; Rowe, P.J.; Riches, P.E. Thermal damage done to bone by burring and sawing with and without irrigation in knee arthroplasty. *J. Arthroplasty* **2016**, *31*, 1102–1108. [CrossRef]
39. Gazdag, A.R.; Lane, J.M.; Glaser, D.; Forster, R.A. Alternatives to autogenous bone graft: Efficacy and indications. *J. Am. Acad Orthop. Surg.* **1995**, *3*, 1–8. [CrossRef]
40. Khan, S.N.; Cammisa, F.P., Jr.; Sandhu, H.S.; Diwan, A.D.; Girardi, F.P.; Lane, J.M. The biology of bone grafting. *J. Am. Acad Orthop. Surg.* **2005**, *13*, 77–86. [CrossRef]
41. Burchardt, H. Biology of bone transplantation. *Orthop. Clin. North Am.* **1987**, *18*, 187–196. [PubMed]
42. Chen, T.; Li, J.; Cordova, L.A.; Liu, B.; Mouraret, S.; Sun, Q.; Salmon, B.; Helms, J. A WNT protein therapeutic improves the bone-forming capacity of autografts from aged animals. *Sci. Rep.* **2018**, *8*, 119. [CrossRef] [PubMed]
43. Bertollo, N.; Walsh, W.R. Drilling of bone: Practicality, limitations and complications associated with surgical drill-bits. *Biomech. Appl.* **2011**. [CrossRef]
44. Lustmann, J.; Ulmansky, M.; Fuxbrunner, A.; Lewis, A. Photoacoustic injury and bone healing following 193nm excimer laser ablation. *Lasers Surg. Med.* **1992**, *12*, 390–396. [CrossRef] [PubMed]
45. Vogel, A.; Venugopalan, V. Mechanisms of pulsed laser ablation of biological tissues. *Chem. Rev.* **2003**, *103*, 577–644. [CrossRef] [PubMed]
46. Leucht, P.; Lam, K.; Kim, J.B.; Mackanos, M.A.; Simanovskii, D.M.; Longaker, M.T.; Contag, C.H.; Schwettman, H.A.; Helms, J.A. Accelerated bone repair after plasma laser corticotomies. *Ann. Surg.* **2007**, *246*, 140–150. [CrossRef] [PubMed]
47. Romanos, G.E.; Gupta, B.; Yunker, M.; Romanos, E.B.; Malmstrom, H. Lasers use in dental implantology. *Implant Dent.* **2013**, *22*, 282–288. [CrossRef] [PubMed]
48. Rivault, A.F.; Toto, P.D.; Levy, S.; Gargiulo, A.W. Autogenous bone grafts: osseous coagulum and osseous retrograde procedures in primates. *J. Periodontol.* **1971**, *42*, 787–796. [CrossRef]
49. Bell, S.; Ajami, E.; Davies, J.E. An improved mechanical testing method to assess bone-implant anchorage. *J. Vis. Exp.* **2014**. [CrossRef]
50. Young, M.P.; Worthington, H.V.; Lloyd, R.E.; Drucker, D.B.; Sloan, P.; Carter, D.H. Bone collected during dental implant surgery: A clinical and histological study. *Clin. Oral Implants Res.* **2002**, *13*, 298–303. [CrossRef]
51. Schneider, D.; Marquardt, P.; Zwahlen, M.; Jung, R.E. A systematic review on the accuracy and the clinical outcome of computer-guided template-based implant dentistry. *Clin. Oral Implants Res.* **2009**, *20* (Suppl. 4), 73–86. [CrossRef] [PubMed]
52. Horwitz, J.; Zuabi, O.; Machtei, E.E. Accuracy of a computerized tomography-guided template-assisted implant placement system: an in vitro study. *Clin. Oral Implants Res.* **2009**, *20*, 1156–1162. [CrossRef] [PubMed]

16

The Effect of In Vitro Electrolytic Cleaning on Biofilm-Contaminated Implant Surfaces

Christoph Ratka [1,†], Paul Weigl [1,†], Dirk Henrich [2], Felix Koch [3], Markus Schlee [3] and Holger Zipprich [1,*]

1 Department of Prosthodontics, Goethe University, 60590 Frankfurt am Main, Germany
2 Department of Trauma, Hand & Reconstructive Surgery, Goethe University, 60590 Frankfurt am Main, Germany
3 Private Practice, and Department of Maxillofacial Surgery, Goethe University, 60590 Frankfurt am Main, Germany
* Correspondence: zipprich@em.uni-frankfurt.de
† These authors contributed equally to this work.

Abstract: Purpose: Bacterial biofilms are a major problem in the treatment of infected dental and orthopedic implants. The purpose of this study is to investigate the cleaning effect of an electrolytic approach (EC) compared to a powder-spray system (PSS) on titanium surfaces. Materials and Methods: The tested implants (different surfaces and alloys) were collated into six groups and treated ether with EC or PSS. After a mature biofilm was established, the implants were treated, immersed in a nutritional solution, and streaked on Columbia agar. Colony-forming units (CFUs) were counted after breeding and testing (EC), and control (PSS) groups were compared using a paired sample *t*-test. Results: No bacterial growth was observed in the EC groups. After thinning to 1:1,000,000, 258.1 ± 19.9 (group 2), 264.4 ± 36.5 (group 4), and 245.3 ± 40.7 (group 6) CFUs could be counted in the PSS groups. The difference between the electrolytic approach (test groups 1, 3, and 5) and PSS (control groups 2, 4, and 6) was statistically extremely significant (p-value $< 2.2 \times 10^{-16}$). Conclusion: Only EC inactivated the bacterial biofilm, and PSS left reproducible bacteria behind. Within the limits of this in vitro test, clinical relevance could be demonstrated.

Keywords: dental implant; biofilm; infection; perio-prosthetic joint infection; periimplantitis; electrolytic cleaning

1. Introduction

Growing numbers of inserted dental implants correlate to an increasing number of infected implants [1]. Periimplantitis (PI) is defined as an inflammatory process affecting both periimplant soft and hard tissue. Craterlike bone defects, ongoing bone loss, pus, and bleeding on probing (BoP) are clinical parameters that have to be present to justify the diagnosis of PI [2,3]. PI correlates to bacterial biofilms growing on implants or abutments [4]. In view of the various definitions of PI and the lack of agreement in the dental community about an acceptable threshold of bone loss, there is no consensus on when pathology starts and how PI can be diagnosed precisely. Hence, there is no consensus about prevalence data [5–7]. A proper treatment modality is lacking [8]. Whether the bacterial biofilm is the single causal factor or only correlates to PI [9] is still a matter of discussion. This debate about etiology is not merely an academic question, but may influence the success rate of therapy, because of possible differences in specimen susceptibility and uncorrectable surgical or mechanical obstacles. In any event, biofilm needs to be removed to prevent progression of disease, or to treat PI successfully. As implant surfaces exposed to the oral cavity are immediately colonized by bacteria, the surfaces need to be re-osseointegrated for good long-term results [10].

Infection of plates or other orthopedic devices, or endoprostheses caused by polymicrobial biofilms, is a major challenge. The average infection rate of implants in the shoulder, knee, and hip is less than 2% in most treatment centers [11,12]. A recent meta-analysis demonstrates an overall cumulative incidence of endoprosthetic joint infection across all studies of 0.78% [13]. It has been reported that, in the United States, more than 1 million implants placed in shoulders, knees, and hips need to be replaced every year due to infections [14]. A systematic review showed a reinfection rate of 7.6% (95% CI 3.4–13.1) of hip and knee replacements [15]. Polymicrobial biofilm on orthopedic implants shows high resistance to immune defense, and will result in local inhibition of granulocyte activity around the implant. This effect is referred to as frustrated phagocytosis, which leads to degranulation, reduced ingestion ability, and production of oxygen radicals in the granulocytes [16]. The standard treatment protocol for infected orthopedic implants is replacement in a one- or two-stage procedure, with a success rate of 80–90% [17,18]. Even early infections within the first 30 days after implantation that are treated by aggressive debridement and long-time antibiotics yield success rates of only 71% [19,20].

In most cases, all treatment modalities fail to cure infected implants, requiring replacement of the implant or causing at least an inadequate failure rate and immense costs. Therefore, it is necessary to search for another approach to decontaminate infected implants.

Several ablative methods to remove biofilms, such as mechanical debridement with curettes, brushes, lasers, cotton pellets, cold plasma, or air-powder sprays, combined or not combined with disinfecting or antibiotic agents, have been discussed. Re-osseointegration of formerly infected dental implant surfaces was reported in animal studies for between 39% and 46% of the surface [21]. There is no evidence of whether and to what percentage re-osseointegration occurs clinically. A recent review of the literature demonstrated the equality of all published methods, and no method seemed able to achieve stable results over time [22]. Follow-up revealed recurrence of the disease in up to 100% for some methods after one year [8]. A powder-spray system (PSS) is commonly used to clean implant surfaces. Erythritol (size 14 μm) or glycine (size 25 μm) particles are accelerated by air pressure (2 bar). When the particles impact at an angle of 30–60° at an ideal working distance of 3–5 mm, the kinetic energy of the powder removes biofilm, according to the manufacturer's manual. Several animal studies investigating re-osseointegration after cleaning with a PSS proved incomplete re-osseointegration [21]. Improvement of periimplant parameters, such as BoP, probing depth, and pus was clinically proven after the PSS, but re-osseointegration was not proven. Furthermore, the PSS failed to demonstrate superiority over any other treatment modality [23–25]. Possible reasons for this incomplete cleaning efficacy might be craterlike bone defects, with limited access and thus an improper working angle and distance of the device, the macro- and micro-design of implant surface, and oversized particles for much smaller bacteria hidden in the microstructure of textured implants. In an in vitro test, implants contaminated with *E. coli* were treated with a continuous current of 0–10 mA. Two implants were loaded as either cathode or anode, resulting in reduced numbers of bacteria on both implants. On anodic implants, a current of more than 75 mA caused complete killing of the bacteria [26]. Zipprich et al. loaded the implant as a cathode, and a platinum-coated titanium acted as the anode [27]. In this in vitro trial, the implants were exposed to a sodium-iodine solution buffered by lactic acid to avoid alkalization of the salt solution [27]. Hydrolytic splitting of water produces hydrogen cations as long as the implants are loaded. These hydrogen cations penetrate the biofilm, and after an electron has been taken from the implant surface, hydrogen forms between the implant surface and the biofilm. The hydrogen bubbles remove the biofilm. While all the other discussed methods for removing a biofilm are ablative, the electrolytic approach presented here works under the biofilm, directly on the implant surface, regardless of surface characteristics or alloy. Our results support the finding that the potassium iodine solution allows a higher current than the previously published sodium chloride solution [27]. This results in higher hydrogen production and a possible direct bactericidal effect. A cooperating working group examined the exact working mode of this method and proved its effectiveness in killing bacteria [28]. The current gold standard in dentistry is to remove biofilm with a PSS. These positive preliminary results for an electrolytic approach (EC) encouraged the authors to compare the cleaning effect of air-powder-water spray as an accepted method of cleaning contaminated implant surfaces with the new electrolytic approach in vitro.

2. Materials and Methods

2.1. Null Hypothesis

The null hypothesis is that the electrolytic approach works equally as well as PSS cleaning.

2.2. Preparation of Test Implant and Grouping

For the study, test implants were designed and produced by the authors to be as close as possible to clinical reality in implant and orthopedic surgery. The test specimens were made of grade 4 and 5 titanium, and consisted of a test and a carrier part (Figure 1). The design of the test part was similar to a standard, parallel-threaded dental implant (Ø 4.0 mm/L = 11.0 mm pitch = 0.6 mm) with different surface modifications. The carrier part was machined to serve as the electricity conductor and to fix the test specimen in the experimental set-up without influencing the area of interest of the test area. Furthermore, the test and carrier part could be separated at a predetermined breaking point to avoid bacterial contamination of the test area during handling.

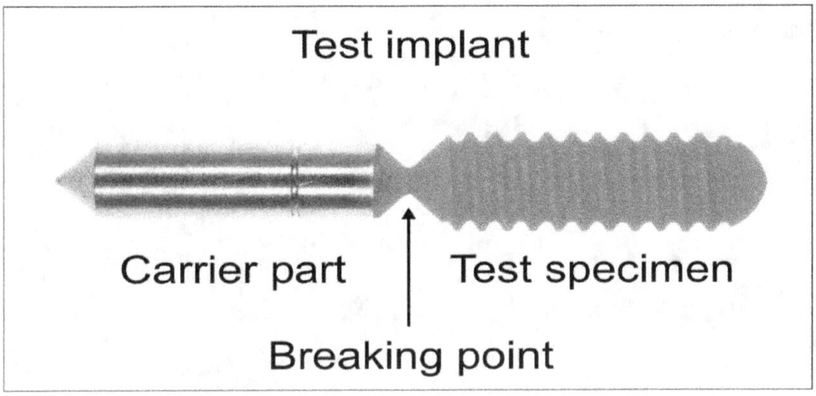

Figure 1. The structure of test implants.

Six groups of implants (n = 12 per group, 72 in total) were investigated. Ten per group were treated (60 in total), while two served as negative controls and were not treated (12 in total):

Group 1: titanium grade 4 + sandblasting and acid-etching + electrolytic cleaning;

Group 2: titanium grade 4 + sandblasting and acid-etching + air-powder-water spray cleaning;

Group 3: titanium grade 5 + sandblasting and acid-etching + electrolytic cleaning;

Group 4: titanium grade 5 + sandblasting and acid-etching + air-powder-water spray cleaning;

Group 5: titanium grade 4 + anodic oxidation + electrolytic cleaning;

Group 6: titanium grade 4 + anodic oxidation + air-powder-water spray cleaning.

Groups 1, 3, and 5 (test group) were treated with an electrolytic treatment, and groups 2, 4, and 6 (control group) were treated with a PSS.

2.3. Saliva Collection

In order to ensure a diversity of microorganisms, saliva was collected from three volunteers (different ages, 2 male, 1 female, healthy, no medication or drugs). The collected saliva (3 mL) was pooled, centrifuged to spin down any large debris and cells (2600 g for 10 min), and the liquid supernatant was mixed with 0.5 L nutrition solution culture (Bacto Tryptic Soy Broth, Becton Dickenson, Heidelberg, Germany), and incubated under 37 °C on the rocking device for 48 h, as previously described [29]. The solution was then filled into tubes (1.5 mL, Eppendorf Safe-Lock Tubes, Eppendorf, Hamburg, Germany) and frozen at −18 °C to provide identical samples for all further tests.

2.4. Establishing the Biofilm

To breed the biofilm on the implants, the required bacterial samples were thawed and bred with 300 mL nutrition solution in a beaker at 37 °C for 24 h. The carrier parts of the sterilized implants were masked to reduce bacterial contamination and fixed on a base plate. The experimental set-up was then immersed in the beaker with the culture medium to initiate formation of the biofilm. The beaker was placed in the rocking incubator for 14 days at a temperature of 37 °C. Previous tests with daily checks with a scanning electron micrograph (SEM) had demonstrated that 14 days were necessary to achieve a mature, multilayer biofilm (Figure 2). Every two days, the bacterial culture medium was replaced with freshly prepared nutritional solution.

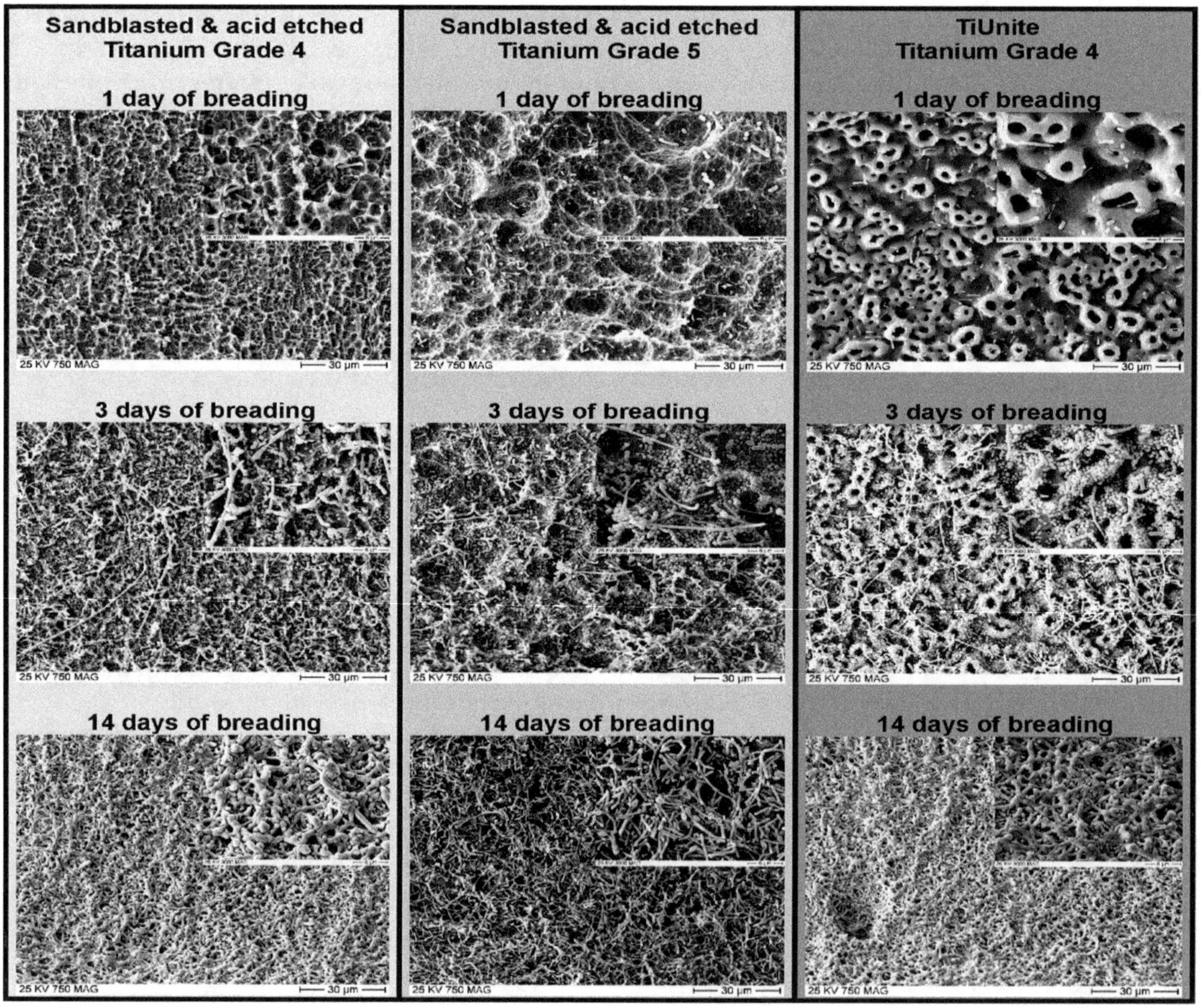

Figure 2. Progredient formation of biofilms on different surfaces.

2.5. Electrolytic Cleaning (Test Group)

The implants in groups 1, 3, and 5 were cleaned by an electrolytic process. Figure 3 shows the construction of the electrolytic chamber. After demasking of the biofilm-coated test implant with a customized ejector, the implant was mounted on the bottom of the electrolytic chamber with a customized connector. The test implant served as the cathode. The connector had an inner titanium sleeve (titanium grade 4) covered by an insulating polyetheretherketone (PEEK) carrier. The inner titanium sleeve was connected to the electric source, and the PEEK carrier masked the carrier part of the test implant for only three quarters. This design was chosen to guarantee that it was possible to separate the test specimen using a customized tool, without touching the PEEK carrier, which was not been cleaned during the electrolytic procedure. The connector was mounted in a polytetrafluoroethylene (PTFE) socket to ensure stability of the electrolytic chamber.

After the cathode was fixed, the glass cylinder of the chamber was mounted, and 35 mL of electrolyte (sodium iodide (200 g/L), potassium iodide (200 g/L), L(+)-lactic acid (20 g/L), and water (800 g/L)) was poured into the chamber. Fresh electrolyte was used for each test.

The anode (titanium grade 4) was coated with platinum to prevent passivation of its surface. The anode was fixed in a hollow PTFE tube to ensure direct contact of the platinum-plated part with the electrolyte (∅ 5.0 mm/L = 4.0 mm). After the other end of the PTFE tube had been mounted in the cap of the chamber, the anode and cathode were connected to a voltage source (PeakTech 6060, PeakTech, Ahrensburg, Germany).

A voltage of 6 V was applied for 5 minutes, resulting in a current of up to 1100 mA.

After the cleaning process was finished, the cap of the chamber was removed, and the used electrolyte was poured into a beaker. The biofilm floated as a visible layer on the fluid in the beaker, and was pipetted with some fluid to prove the vitality of the collected bacteria (waste from electrolytic cleaning).

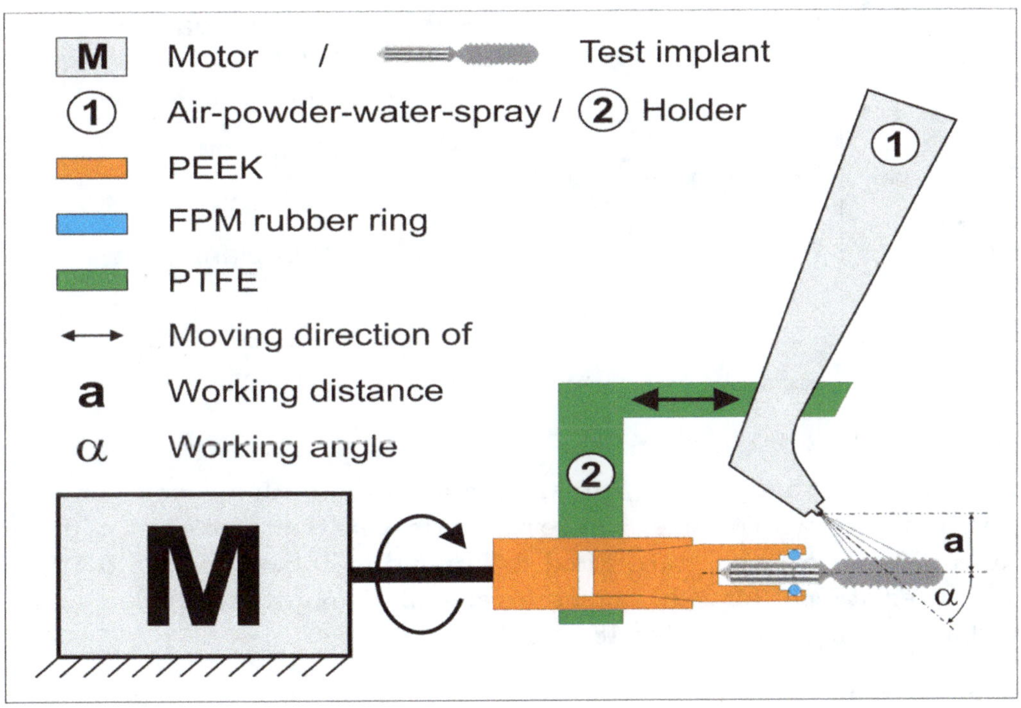

Figure 3. The assembly of the powder-water spray device. PEEK = polyetheretherketone, FPM = fluorine rubber, PTFE = polytetrafluorothgylene.

2.6. Air-Powder-Water Spray (PSS) Cleaning (Control Group)

The implants in groups 2, 4, and 6 were treated by a PSS (BA 8000, Mectron GmbH, Cologne, Germany). To ensure a reproducible and comparable cleaning effect, a test apparatus was assembled, as shown in Figure 4. The aim was to reproduce the working angle and distance according to the manufacturer´s operating manual (45° and 10 mm). The test implants were mounted on a sterile PEEK carrier (Figure 4, in orange), which masked three quarters of the carrier part and was then fixed in a PTFE connecting bar (Figure 4). The holder provided the same working angle and distance for all the tested implants. The holder and its fixed handpiece were moved manually along the implant axis while the test implant rotated, being driven by a motor around its axis (40 rpm) to ensure proper and repeatable cleaning of the implants (Figure 4). Sterile water (Aqua ad injectabilia, Braun, Melsungen, Germany) and aminoacetic acid powder (glycine powder, Mectron GmbH, Cologne, Germany) were used with an air pressure of 2 bar being applied for 60 s. The waste liquid produced during the cleaning process was collected in a beaker to prove the vitality of the removed biofilm (waste from air-powder-water cleaning).

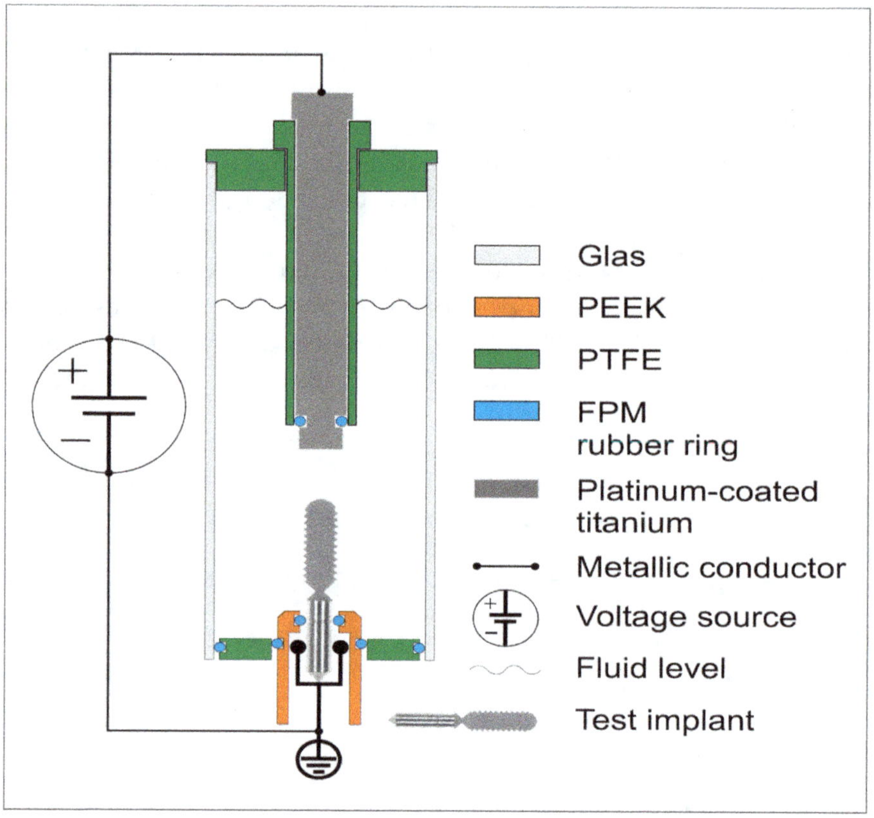

Figure 4. The structure of the electrolytic chamber.

2.7. Rinsing and Test Sample Incubation

After cleaning, the test and control implants were rinsed with air-water spray for 5 seconds (distance of 5 cm) and dried with oil-free air. The test parts were then broken off at the predetermined breaking point in a sterile manner, transferred to Eppendorf tubes filled with 1.5 mL nutritional solution, and incubated at 37 °C for 24 h. Ehrensberger et al. demonstrated that no additional colonies grew when incubation time was extended 18 h. [30]

2.8. Analysis of the Bacterial Growth

The solution in each Eppendorf tube was pipetted, transferred and streaked with an L-spatula on blood agar (Columbia Blood Agar-VWR, BDH Chemicals, Leuven, Belgium). The plate was incubated at 37 °C for 24 h.

The rest of the contents of the Eppendorf tube was gradually diluted in six steps to 1:1,000,000. Each step was also spread on a blood agar plate and treated as described above. In total, seven dilution steps were bred (210 in test group, 210 in control group, 420 in total).

The change in the plate condition was photographed after 24 h. The number of colony-forming units (CFUs) were counted using the software ImageJ (version 1.51u, National Institutes of Health,

Bethesda, MD, USA). The difference between the two Poisson rates has been applied to evaluate the difference in bacterial growth.

2.9. *Sterility of the Experimental Set-Up (Positive Control)*

To prove the sterility of the different experimental set-ups, the air-powder-water spray was directed to blood agar plates (two per group, six in total). The sterility of the nutritional solution was proved by breeding it at 37 °C for 24 h, and then spreading it on a blood agar plate. The agar plates were incubated at 37 °C for 24 h, and then CFUs were counted.

2.10. *Quality of Biofilm (Negative Control)*

To prove the quality of the biofilm, two test implants from each group (12 in total) served as the negative control and were not cleaned. After biofilm formation, the nutritional solution was rinsed away with sterile water. One implant per group (six in total) was rinsed with sterile water (Aqua ad injectabilia, Braun, Melsungen, Germany) and dried in air for 24 h. The usual fixation in ethanol was not done, to avoid washing-out of the matrix. The samples were gold-coated and examined using a Philips SE XL30 (LaB6 cathode) scanning electron micrograph (SEM) with 20 kV power and a spot size 4 to check biofilm formation and quality. One implant per group (six in total) was incubated in an Eppendorf tube with 1.5 mL nutritional solution and bred at 37 °C for 24 h. In anticipation of floating bacteria, the nutritional solution was spread on blood agar and bred at 37 °C for 24 h. Colony forming units (CFUs) were then counted (Figure 5).

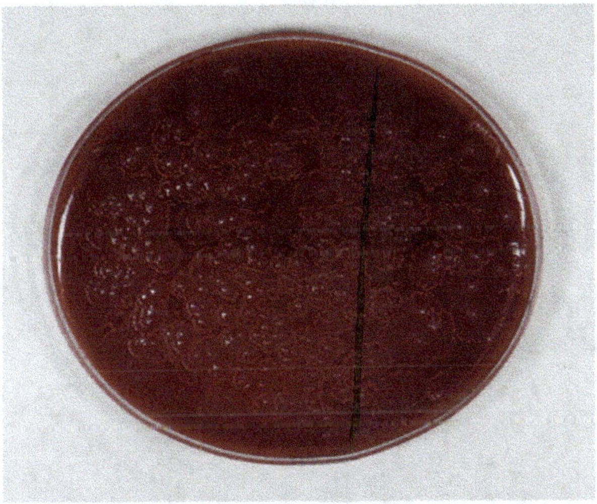

Figure 5. Bacterial growth with the nutritional solution of the negative control (not treated). Dilution grade 1:1,000,000.

2.11. *Vitality of Bacteria after Cleaning*

To prove the vitality, the waste from both cleaning methods (electrolytic and PSS) was spread on blood agar and bred at 37 °C for 24 h. Then CFUs were counted.

2.12. *Counting Colonies*

The number of colonies that had grown on the blood agar plates were manually counted using the ImageJ (version 1.51u) software.

2.13. *Statistics*

The number of colonies that had grown on the blood agar plates after a dilution to 1:1,000,000 where manually counted and processed by the ImageJ (version 1.51u) software.

Continuous variables are reported as mean ± standard deviation. All groups were tested for normality by the Shapiro-Wilk test. Comparisons between the two cleaning methods were performed with the paired sample *t*-test. Comparisons between the surface and material groups for AirFlow were performed with the Kruskal-Wallis test.

A two-sided *p*-value of $\leq$0.05 was considered statistically significant. Statistical analysis was performed with R (R Foundation for Statistical Computing, Vienna, Austria).

3. Results

3.1. *Quality of Biofilm (Negative Control)*

The formation of a mature layer of biofilm completely covering the surface of all six tested implants was demonstrated upon checking by scanning electron micrograph (SEM). Six implants were not treated, but were incubated as described. CFUs could not be counted because the blood agar plate was totally covered with a closed layer of bacteria.

3.2. *Colony-Forming Unit Count*

In groups 1, 3, and 5 (test groups, electrolytic cleaning), 210 blood agar plates were evaluated. Not a single CFU could be counted on any blood agar plate. Neither dilution (Figure 6) nor alloy nor surface had any influence on this observation.

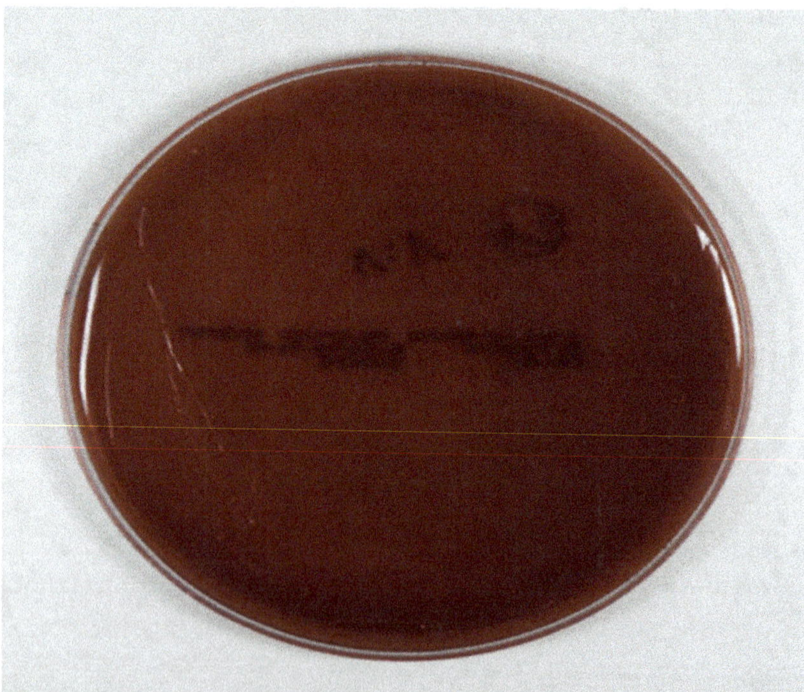

Figure 6. Bacterial growth after electrolytic cleaning. Dilution grade 1:1.

The cultivation of the waste liquid collected from the electrolytic cleaning process also showed no bacterial growth.

In the control groups (2, 4, and 6; PSS; 210 agar plates), the growth of bacteria was observed on every agar plate with any dilution grade (Figure 7), irrespective of dilution, alloy, or surface. CFU counting was not possible in the first five steps of dilution (from 1:1 to 1:100,000), because the bacteria grew over the whole agar plate. CFU counting was possible at a dilution of 1:1,000,000. In all PSS groups, more than 200 CFUs were documented (group 2 = 258.1 ± 19.9, group 4 = 264.4 ± 36.5, group 6 = 245.3 ± 40.7) (Table 1). The cultivation of the collected waste liquid always showed bacterial growth.

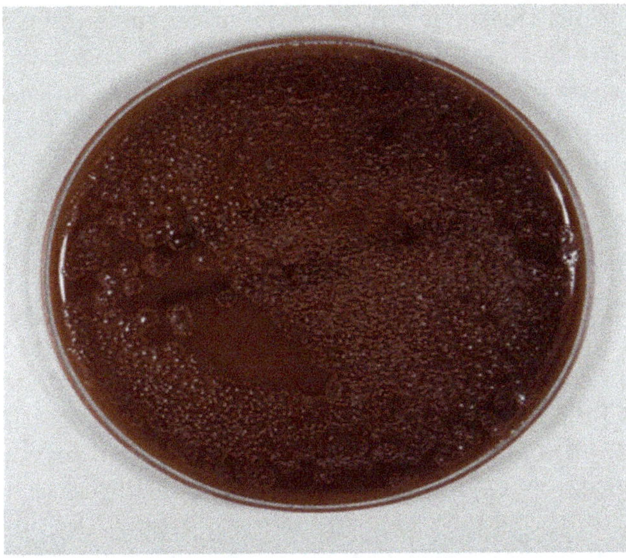

Figure 7. Bacterial growth after air-powder-water spray cleaning. Dilution grade 1: 1,000,000.

Table 1. Colony-forming unit (CFU) counts per grade of titanium, surface, dilution, and cleaning method.

Cleaning Method	**Electrolytic**	**PPS**	**Electrolytic**	**PPS**	**Electrolytic**	**PPS**
Material & Surface	Group 1: Ti Grade 4 + SAE	Group 2: Ti Grade 4 + SAE	Group 3: Ti Grade 5 + SAE	Group 4: Ti Grade 5 + SAE	Group 5: Ti Grade 4 + AO	Group 6: Ti Grade 4 + AO
Dilution	∅ CFU	∅ CFU	∅ CFU	∅ CFU	∅ CFU	∅ CFU
1:1	0	na	0	na	0	na
1:10	0	na	0	na	0	na
1:100	0	na	0	na	0	na
1:1000	0	na	0	na	0	na
1:10,000	0	na	0	na	0	na
1:100,000	0	na	0	na	0	na
1:1,000,000	0	258.1 ± 19.9	0	264.4 ±36.5	0	245.3 ± 40.7

The difference between the electrolytic approach (test groups 1, 3, and 5) and PSS (control groups 2, 4, and 6) was statistically extremely significant (p-value $< 2.2 \times 10^{-16}$). In control groups 2, 4, and 6 (PSS), no difference in cleaning efficacy could be detected (p-value = 0.3465) when comparing the different implant materials and surfaces. In test groups 1, 3, and 5 (electrolytic approach), no colony-forming units (CFUs) were detected. Therefore, there were no differences between the different implant materials and surfaces.

3.3. *Sterility of Experimental Set-Up (Positive Control)*

No sign of bacterial growth was observed on the blood agar after PSS was sprayed directly onto blood agar plates. No sign of bacterial growth was observed on the blood agar after the nutritional solution was bred. This indicates that the air powder-water spray system and the prepared nutritional solution were free from bacterial contamination.

4. Discussion

The application of voltage to reduce bacterial load has been described several times in the literature. Ehrensberger et al. [30] evaluated the influence of cathodic voltage-controlled electrical stimulation (CVCES) to eradicate methicillin-resistant *S. aureus* (MRSA) from titanium surfaces in vitro and in Long-Evans rats. The application of −1.8 V for 1 h reduced MRSA CFU counts by 87% in bone and 88% in titanium, compared to the open-circuit potential in vitro, and by 97% in titanium in vivo. No histological changes were detected in the rat model. CVCES increased the interfacial capacitance (from 18.93 to 98.25 μF/cm^2) and decreased the polarization resistance (from 868.25 to 108 Ω/cm^2). Because of the negative charge of the titanium surface and the negative surface charge of *S. aureus*, attachment of the biofilm may be influenced. Furthermore, it has been discussed that the electric field on polarized electrodes generates anions by electrolytic splitting, which disrupts and pushes away the biofilm [24,31,32]. The major reaction at the cathode is the reduction of water or the reduction of oxygen:

Reaction 1: $2H_2O + 2e^- \rightarrow H_2 + OH^-$

Reaction 2: $O_2 + 4^- + 2H_2O \rightarrow 4\ OH^-$

Blenkinsopp et al. proposed an altered transport of ions within the biofilm [33]. Portinga et al. demonstrated an extended attachment of bacteria to the biofilm after donation of their free electrons to the matrix. Free electrons on the cathode might disturb this adherence [31,34], To summarize, the antimicrobial effects seem to be related to voltage-dependent surface properties of the titanium.

Several authors [26,35,36] have reported that loading two contaminated dental implants (one as anode and the other as cathode) in NaCl as electrolyte significantly reduces the number of bacteria. The downside of the published method is that toxic chloric and hypochlorous acid are reaction products, and the pH in the periimplant area decreased or increased significantly.

Zipprich et al. [27] introduced an electrolytic approach to remove biofilm from explanted implants by using a mixture of sodium iodide, potassium iodide, and water buffered by L(+)-lactic acid. Schneider et al. [28] investigated the underlying mechanism of this method of electrolytic cleaning. Several disinfecting agents, such as triiodide and hydrogen peroxide, were generated on the implant surface loaded as the cathode. The authors proved in an in vitro test that the major effect in removing the biofilm was the generation of hydrogen on the implant surface, which pushed away the biofilm mechanically. Based on these findings, the authors decided to prove the effectiveness and efficiency of this approach in this in vitro test. It is very difficult to perform a controlled in vitro study on a "real" biofilm in real periimplantitis cases, because its three-dimensional structure is destroyed while the implant is removed, and anaerobic bacteria would not survive this process. The nutritional and biological conditions of an in vivo biofilm will differ from biofilms used in this in vitro test. Such samples may harbor different mixtures of bacteria. This pitfall compromises all in vitro studies done on periimplant biofilms. On the other hand, it was demonstrated that microbiota associated with periimplantitis are quite variable and inconsistent [4].

Different methods of growing biofilms have been published. Most of the articles used single-species biofilms with very little relation to real periimplant biofilms. *S. aureus* is a colony-forming bacterium associated with infected dental or orthopedic implants, and was bred for several days on titanium surfaces [30,37]. Mohn used *E. coli*, which is not associated with periimplantitis [26]. Other authors harvested intraoral subgingival plaque and exposed titanium plates in a nutritional solution for seven days [38]. John et al. cultivated biofilms by exposing titanium plates fixed on splints for 48 hours in the oral cavity of two specimens [39]. In preparation for this study, we were not able to reproduce the claims of these authors to achieve a mature biofilm covering the complete implant surface in the published timeline, when using a model with intraoral bacteria. It took 14 days to achieve a multilayer mature biofilm covering the whole implant surface (Figure 2).

To imitate micro- and macrostructure, we decided to use lifelike test implants. To carry such implants in the mouth for several days to accumulate bacteria would be unacceptable for humans. Consequently, we had to develop a realistic extraoral model to breed a biofilm. A single-species model was used, and did not form a complete monolayer of bacteria nor a multilayer biofilm. To achieve the most realistic diversity of microorganisms, the saliva was collected and pooled from three volunteers, bred extra-orally, and frozen to ensure the same biota for all the tests. In preparation for this study, we found out that it takes 14 days to achieve the expected quality and thickness of biofilm. In vitro, it could have been demonstrated that a cold plasma device can clean heling abutments more effectively than conventional cleaning [40].

No published method was able to remove all bacteria from implant surfaces in the clinical setting. Moreover, bacteria will re-colonize implant surfaces exposed to the oral cavity within a matter of hours [10]. The theory that elimination of the biofilm will cure periimplantitis is an attractive one [4]. Clinically, it may be necessary to remove the bacteria and extracellular matrix in a way that will allow re-osseointegration of formerly infected surfaces.

We were able to demonstrate that no bacteria could be cultivated in the nutritional solution and powder used for a PSS, thus proving the sterility of the experimental set-up. The vitality of the bred biofilm was proved visually by SEM and by CFU counting after its cultivation on blood agar plates. As different titanium alloys and surface modifications are used in dental and orthopedic surgery, we tested titanium grades 4 and 5, as well as acid-etched, sandblasted, and anodized implant surfaces. Their effectiveness in the removal of bacteria was compared to a standard method (PSS).

The results were unequivocally clear. It was not possible to breed bacteria after the implants had been cleaned by the electrolytic approach. Every implant cleaned by the air-powder-water spray contained so many bacteria that all the blood agar plates were totally overgrown with a lawn of bacteria. A single CFU could only be counted after dilution to 1:1,000,000. The waste collected while using the PSS contained vital bacteria, and breeding them on blood agar plates demonstrated their vitality.

In conclusion, the air-powder-water spray does not sufficiently remove the biofilm. This might explain why, in a recent review, a re-osseointegration rate of only 39%–46% was possible in animal models [21]. Considering the angle of threads, the micro-texture of the implants combined with oversized particles, and craterlike bone defects, it is more possible to follow the manufacturer´s manual (working distance of 3–5 mm and an angle of 30–60°) and to clean the microstructure properly. The electrolytic approach sterilized all the tested implants, irrespective of alloy or surface. No vital bacteria were detectable. For this reason, the null hypothesis had to be rejected.

The electrolytic approach seems to be a promising method for treating infected dental and orthopedic implants.

5. Conclusions

In this study, it was proven that electrolytic cleaning of lifelike dental implants contaminated with vital oral biofilms sterilizes the implant surfaces. One of the gold-standard methods of cleaning by air-powder-water spray failed to achieve an adequate result. Clinical testing is necessary to prove the clinical impact of these findings in dentistry and orthopedic surgery.

Author Contributions: Conceptualization, C.R., P.W., D.H., F.K. and H.Z.; methodology, C.R., P.W., D.H., F.K., M.S and H.Z.; software, C.R.; validation, C.R., P.W., D.H., F.K., M.S. and H.Z.; formal analysis, C.R., M.S. and H.Z.; investigation, C.R., D.H. and H.Z.; resources, H.Z.; data curation, C.R., P.W., M.S. and H.Z.; writing—original draft preparation, C.R., M.S. and H.Z.; writing—review and editing, C.R., P.W., D.H., F.K., M.S. and H.Z.; visualization, C.R., P.W., M.S. and H.Z.; supervision, C.R. and H.Z.; project administration, C.R and H.Z.; funding acquisition, M.S., H.Z.

Acknowledgments: The authors Schlee and Zipprich declare themselves as holding patents on the described technology, and to have financial interests. We appreciate Ümniye Balaban from the Institute for Biostatistics and Mathematical Modeling Center of Health Sciences, Hospital and Department of Medicine of the Goethe University for her support with the statistics. We appreciate Charlotte zur Megede and Jana Weiler for support in collecting the data.

References

1. Sendyk, D.I.; Chrcanovic, B.R.; Albrektsson, T.; Wennerberg, A.; Zindel Deboni, M.C. Does Surgical Experience Influence Implant Survival Rate? A Systematic Review and Meta-Analysis. *Int. J. Prosthodont.* **2017**, *30* 341–347. [CrossRef]
2. Lang, N.P.; Berglundh, T. Periimplant diseases: Where are we now?—Consensus of the Seventh European Workshop on Periodontology. *J. Clin. Periodontol.* **2011**, *38*, 178–181. [CrossRef]

3. Berglundh, T.; Armitage, G.; Araújo, M.G.; Avila-Ortiz, G.; Blanco, J.; Camargo, P.M.; Chen, S.; Cochran, D.; Derks, J.; Figuero, E.; et al. Peri-implant diseases and conditions: Consensus report of workgroup 4 of the 2017 World Workshop on the Classification of Periodontal and Peri-Implant Diseases and Conditions. *J. Periodontol.* **2018**, *89*, S313–S318. [CrossRef]
4. Mombelli, A.; Décaillet, F. The characteristics of biofilms in peri-implant disease. *J. Clin. Periodontol.* **2011**, *38*, 203–213. [CrossRef]
5. Mombelli, A.; Müller, N.; Cionca, N. The epidemiology of peri-implantitis. *Clin. Oral Implants Res.* **2012**, *23*, 67–76. [CrossRef]
6. Derks, J.; Tomasi, C. Peri-implant health and disease. A systematic review of current epidemiology. *J. Clin. Periodontol.* **2015**, *42*, S158–S171. [CrossRef]
7. Coli, P.; Christiaens, V.; Sennerby, L.; de Bruyn, H. Reliability of periodontal diagnostic tools for monitoring peri-implant health and disease. *Periodontology 2000* **2017**, *73*, 203–217. [CrossRef]
8. Esposito, M.; Grusovin, M.G.; Worthington, H.V. Treatment of peri-implantitis: What interventions are effective? A Cochrane systematic review. *Eur. J. Oral Implant.* **2012**, *5*, S21–S41.
9. Canullo, L.; Montegrotto Group for the Study of Peri-implant Disease; Schlee, M.; Wagner, W.; Covani, U. International Brainstorming Meeting on Etiologic and Risk Factors of Peri-implantitis, Montegrotto (Padua, Italy), August 2014. *Int. J. Oral Maxillofac. Implants* **2015**, *30*, 1093–1104. [CrossRef]
10. Fürst, M.M.; Salvi, G.E.; Lang, N.P.; Persson, G.R. Bacterial colonization immediately after installation on oral titanium implants. *Clin. Oral Implants Res.* **2007**, *18*, 501–508. [CrossRef]
11. Zoubos, A.B.; Galanakos, S.P.; Soucacos, P.N. Orthopedics and biofilm—What do we know? A review. *Med. Sci. Monit.* **2012**, *18*, RA89–RA96. [CrossRef]
12. Cargill, J.S.; Upton, M. Low concentrations of vancomycin stimulate biofilm formation in some clinical isolates of Staphylococcus epidermidis. *J. Clin. Pathol.* **2009**, *62*, 1112–1116. [CrossRef]
13. Hexter, A.T.; Hislop, S.M.; Blunn, G.W.; Liddle, A.D. The effect of bearing surface on risk of periprosthetic joint infection in total hip arthroplasty: A systematic review and meta-analysis. *Bone Joint J.* **2018**, *100-B*, 134–142. [CrossRef]
14. Gilson, M.; Gossec, L.; Mariette, X.; Gherissi, D.; Guyot, M.H.; Berthelot, J.M.; et al. NIH consensus conference: Total hip replacement. NIH Consensus Development Panel on Total Hip Replacement. *JAMA* **1995**, *273*, 1950–1956.
15. Rowan, F.E.; Donaldson, M.J.; Pietrzak, J.R.; Haddad, F.S. The Role of One-Stage Exchange for Prosthetic Joint Infection. *Curr. Rev. Musculoskelet. Med.* **2018**, *11*, 370–379. [CrossRef]
16. Zimmerli, W.; Sendi, P. Pathogenesis of implant-associated infection: the role of the host. *Semin. Immunopathol.* **2011**, *33*, 295–306. [CrossRef]
17. Biring, G.S.; Kostamo, T.; Garbuz, D.S.; Masri, B.A.; Duncan, C.P. Two-stage revision arthroplasty of the hip for infection using an interim articulated Prostalac hip spacer: A 10- to 15-year follow-up study. *J. Bone Joint Surg. Br.* **2009**, *91*, 1431–1437. [CrossRef]
18. Sia, I.G.; Berbari, E.F.; Karchmer, A.W. Prosthetic Joint Infections. *Infect. Dis. Clin. North Am.* **2005**, *19*, 885–914. [CrossRef]
19. Byren, I.; Bejon, P.; Atkins, B.L.; Angus, B.; Masters, S.; McLardy-Smith, P.; Gundle, R.; Berendt, A. One hundred and twelve infected arthroplasties treated with 'DAIR' (debridement, antibiotics and implant retention): antibiotic duration and outcome. *J. Antimicrob. Chemother.* **2009**, *63*, 1264–1271. [CrossRef]
20. Helou, O.C.; Berbari, E.F.; Lahr, B.D.; Eckel-Passow, J.E.; Razonable, R.R.; Sia, I.G.; Virk, A.; Walker, R.C.; Steckelberg, J.M.; Wilson, W.R.; et al. Efficacy and safety of rifampin containing regimen for staphylococcal prosthetic joint infections treated with debridement and retention. *Eur. J. Clin. Microbiol. Infect. Dis.* **2010**, *29*, 961–967. [CrossRef]
21. Tastepe, C.S.; Van Waas, R.; Liu, Y.; Wismeijer, D. Air powder abrasive treatment as an implant surface cleaning method: A literature review. *Int. J. Oral Maxillofac. Implants* **2012**, *27*, 1461–1473.
22. Claffey, N.; Clarke, E.; Polyzois, I.; Renvert, S. Surgical treatment of peri-implantitis. *J. Clin. Periodontol.* **2008**, *35*, 316–332. [CrossRef]
23. De Almeida, J.M.; Matheus, H.R.; Rodrigues Gusman, D.J.; Faleiros, P.L.; Januário de Araújo, N.; Noronha Novaes, V.C. Effectiveness of Mechanical Debridement Combined With Adjunctive Therapies for Nonsurgical Treatment of Periimplantitis: A Systematic Review. *Implant Dent.* **2017**, *26*, 137–144. [CrossRef]

24. Del Pozo, J.L.; Rouse, M.S.; Mandrekar, J.N.; Steckelberg, J.M.; Patel, R. The electricidal effect: Reduction of Staphylococcus and pseudomonas biofilms by prolonged exposure to low-intensity electrical current. *Antimicrob. Agents Chemother.* **2009**, *53*, 41–45. [CrossRef]
25. Schwarz, F.; Becker, K.; Sager, M. Efficacy of professionally administered plaque removal with or without adjunctive measures for the treatment of peri-implant mucositis. A systematic review and meta-analysis. *J. Clin. Periodontol.* **2015**, *42*, 202–213. [CrossRef]
26. Mohn, D.; Zehnder, M.; Stark, W.J.; Imfeld, T. Electrochemical Disinfection of Dental Implants—A Proof of Concept. *PLoS ONE* **2011**, *6*, e16157. [CrossRef]
27. Zipprich, H.; Ratka, C.; Schlee, M.; Brodbeck, U.; Lauer, H.C.; Seitz, O. Periimplantitistherapie: Durchbruch mit neuer Reinigungsmethode. *Dentalmagazin* **2013**, *31*, 14–17.
28. Schneider, S.; Rudolph, M.; Bause, V.; Terfort, A. Electrochemical removal of biofilms from titanium dental implant surfaces. *Bioelectrochemistry* **2018**, *121*, 84–94. [CrossRef]
29. Tian, Y.; He, X.; Torralba, M.; Yooseph, S.; Nelson, K.E.; Lux, R.; McLean, J.S.; Yu, G.; Shi, W. Using DGGE profiling ro develop a novel culture medium suitable for oral microbial communities. *Mol. Oral Microbiol.* **2010**, *25*, 357–367. [CrossRef]
30. Ehrensberger, M.T.; Tobias, M.E.; Nodzo, S.R.; Hansen, L.A.; Luke-Marshall, N.R.; Cole, R.F.; Wild, L.M.; Campagnari, A.A. Cathodic voltage-controlled electrical stimulation of titanium implants as treatment for methicillin-resistant Staphylococcus aureus periprosthetic infections. *Biomaterials* **2015**, *41*, 97–105. [CrossRef]
31. Poortinga, A.T.; Smit, J.; Van Der Mei, H.C.; Busscher, H.J. Electric field induced desorption of bacteria from a conditioning film covered substratum. *Biotechnol. Bioeng.* **2001**, *76*, 395–399. [CrossRef]
32. Van Der Borden, A.; Van Der Mei, H.; Busscher, H. Electric block current induced detachment from surgical stainless steel and decreased viability of Staphylococcus epidermidis. *Biomaterials* **2005**, *26*, 6731–6735. [CrossRef]
33. A Blenkinsopp, S.; Khoury, A.E.; Costerton, J.W. Electrical enhancement of biocide efficacy against Pseudomonas aeruginosa biofilms. *Appl. Environ. Microbiol.* **1992**, *58*, 3770–3773.
34. Poortinga, A.; Bos, R.; Busscher, H. Measurement of charge transfer during bacterial adhesion to an indium tin oxide surface in a parallel plate flow chamber. *J. Microbiol. Methods* **1999**, *38*, 183–189. [CrossRef]
35. Sahrmann, P.; Zehnder, M.; Mohn, D.; Meier, A.; Imfeld, T.; Thurnheer, T. Effect of low direct current on anaerobic multispecies biofilm adhering to a titanium implant surface. *Clin. Implant Dent. Relat. Res.* **2014**, *16*, 552–556. [CrossRef]
36. Sandvik, E.L.; McLeod, B.R.; Parker, A.E.; Stewart, P.S. Direct Electric Current Treatment under Physiologic Saline Conditions Kills Staphylococcus epidermidis Biofilms via Electrolytic Generation of Hypochlorous Acid. *PLoS ONE* **2013**, *8*, e55118. [CrossRef]
37. Salvi, G.E.; Fürst, M.M.; Lang, N.P.; Persson, G.R. One-year bacterial colonization patterns of Staphylococcus aureus and other bacteria at implants and adjacent teeth. *Clin. Oral Implants Res.* **2008**, *19*, 242–248. [CrossRef]
38. Koban, I.; Holtfreter, B.; Hübner, N.-O.; Matthes, R.; Sietmann, R.; Kindel, E.; Weltmann, K.-D.; Welk, A.; Kramer, A.; Kocher, T. Antimicrobial efficacy of non-thermal plasma in comparison to chlorhexidine against dental biofilms on titanium discs in vitro - proof of principle experiment. *J. Clin. Periodontol.* **2011**, *38*, 956–965. [CrossRef]
39. John, G.; Schwarz, F.; Becker, J. Taurolidine as an effective and biocompatible additive for plaque-removing techniques on implant surfaces. *Clin. Oral Investig.* **2015**, *19*, 1069–1077. [CrossRef]
40. Stacchi, C.; Berton, F.; Porrelli, D.; Lombardi, T. Reuse of Implant Healing Abutments: Comparative Evaluation of the Efficacy of Two Cleaning Procedures. *Int. J. Prosthodont.* **2018**, *31*, 161–162. [CrossRef]

17

Heat Generation at the Implant–Bone Interface by Insertion of Ceramic and Titanium Implants

Holger Zipprich [1,*,†], Paul Weigl [1,†], Eugenie König [2], Alexandra Toderas [3], Ümniye Balaban [4] and Christoph Ratka [1]

1. Department of Prosthodontics, Faculty of Oral and Dental Medicine at Goethe University, 60590 Frankfurt am Main, Germany; weigl@em.uni-frankfurt.de (P.W.); c.ratka@gmx.de (C.R.)
2. Private Practice, 60385 Frankfurt am Main, Germany; koenig-@hotmail.de
3. Private Practice, 60313 Frankfurt am Main, Germany; toderasalexandra@gmail.com
4. Institute of Biostatistics and Mathematical Modelling at Goethe University, 60590 Frankfurt am Main, Germany; balaban@med.uni-frankfurt.de

* Correspondence: zipprich@em.uni-frankfurt.de

† Holger Zipprich and Paul Weigl contributed equally to this study.

Abstract: Purpose: The aim of this study is to record material- and surface-dependent heat dissipation during the process of inserting implants into native animal bone. Materials and Methods: Implants made of titanium and zirconium that were identical in macrodesign were inserted under controlled conditions into a bovine rib tempered to 37 °C. The resulting surface temperature was measured on two bone windows by an infrared camera. The results of the six experimental groups, ceramic machined (1), sandblasted (2), and sandblasted and acid-etched surfaces (3) versus titanium implants with the corresponding surfaces (4, 5, and 6) were statistically tested. Results: The average temperature increase, 3 mm subcrestally at ceramic implants, differed with high statistical significance ($p = 7.163 \times 10^{-9}$, resulting from group-adjusted linear mixed-effects model) from titanium. The surface texture of ceramic implants shows a statistical difference between group 3 (15.44 ± 3.63 °C) and group 1 (19.94 ± 3.28 °C) or group 2 (19.39 ± 5.73 °C) surfaces. Within the titanium implants, the temperature changes were similar for all surfaces. Conclusion: Within the limits of an in vitro study, the high temperature rises at ceramic versus titanium implants should be limited by a very slow insertion velocity.

Keywords: zirconia; dental implant; insertion; bone–implant interface; heat; bone damage; early loss

---

1. Introduction

Although titanium and its alloys have been used successfully in dental implantology for more than five decades, there is increasing demand for a nonmetallic alternative.

The alternative material should, of course, retain the good properties of titanium and, if possible, even improve it and eliminate the disadvantages. These primarily include the color, which can cause a greyish discoloration of the peri-implant soft tissue in the esthetic area, leading to the patient's perception that the replaced tooth root is made of metal. Patients particularly prioritize high simulation quality for materials used to replace lost tissue. This has led to a similar development in restorative dentistry, although inlays and onlays made of gold alloy or crowns and bridges with a metal framework have had excellent long-term clinical results. Nevertheless, their importance is increasingly diminishing because they are being replaced by all-ceramic restorations, as patients perceive ceramic to simulate tooth hardness much better than metal. Even metal crowns and bridge frameworks that are nonvisible, because they are fully veneered, have increasingly been replaced by high-strength ceramic versions. This trend, which exists in restorative dentistry, now seems to be repeated in oral implantology:

an artificial tooth root made of ceramic simulates the replaced tissue better than titanium. In other words, in terms of the choice of materials, patients always opt for, or clinicians always tend to use, ceramics for replacing tooth tissue.

A major disadvantage of ceramic implants is their early loss that occurs in clinical trials and is observable in daily practice, which is usually associated with no clinically apparent inflammation. This phenomenon, described as aseptic loosening, is caused by a lack of osseointegration [1] or linked to reactivation of the inflammatory immune system [2]. Different forms of bone injury caused by osteotomy can be eliminated because identical osteotomy protocols are used clinically to create the bone cavity for titanium and ceramic implants. Only during implant insertion can it be assumed that there is a higher risk of overheating with ceramics than with titanium because of their different thermal conductivities. Overheating leads to increased damage or destruction of the bone directly on the implant surface.

The aim of this study is to record the material-dependent heat dissipation during the process of inserting implants into native animal bone in an in vitro setup. In addition, the influence of different implant surface treatments is evaluated. Implants made of titanium and zirconium that were identical in macrodesign were used for this purpose.

2. Materials and Methods

2.1. Implant Specimen and Surface Treatments

Y-TZP (Yttria–Tetragonal Zirconia Polycrystal) two-piece zirconia implants (5 × 14 mm) from the BPI system (BPI Biological and Physical GmbH & Co. KG, Sindelfingen, Germany) served in their packed original state as the specimen for machined ceramic implants. These cylindrical screw implants were designed with four apical cutting grooves and had a self-cutting property (Figure 1).

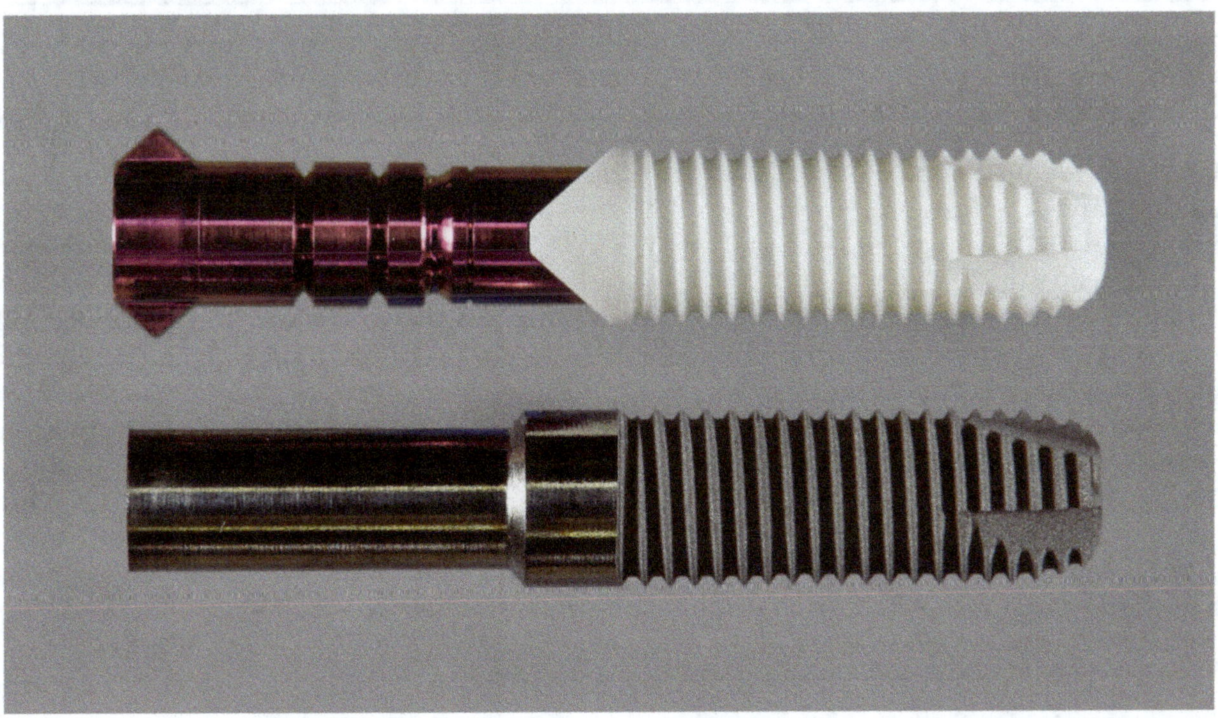

Figure 1. Implants made of zirconia and titanium with identical macrodesigns of the endosteal part coupled with the metallic insertion device.

However, the implants made of titanium from the same manufacturer differed in macrodesign from the above-mentioned ceramic implants. Therefore, the endosteal parts of the BPI ceramic implants were re-engineered to match endosteal titanium grade 4 machined parts. To simplify the re-engineering, the titanium implants were not manufactured as a two-piece (implant and abutment separable) but as a one-piece implant system (Figure 1).

In addition to the influence of the implant materials on heat generation at the implant–bone interface during the insertion process, the effect of an implant surface modification was also investigated. The topography of each surface type was scanned under a scanning electron microscope (SEM S-4500, Hitachi, Tokyo, Japan) (Figure 2). The roughness (Sa) of the implant surface in each group was measured according to ISO-25178 by a laser-scanning microscope (KEYENCE, VK-X100, Osaka, Japan).

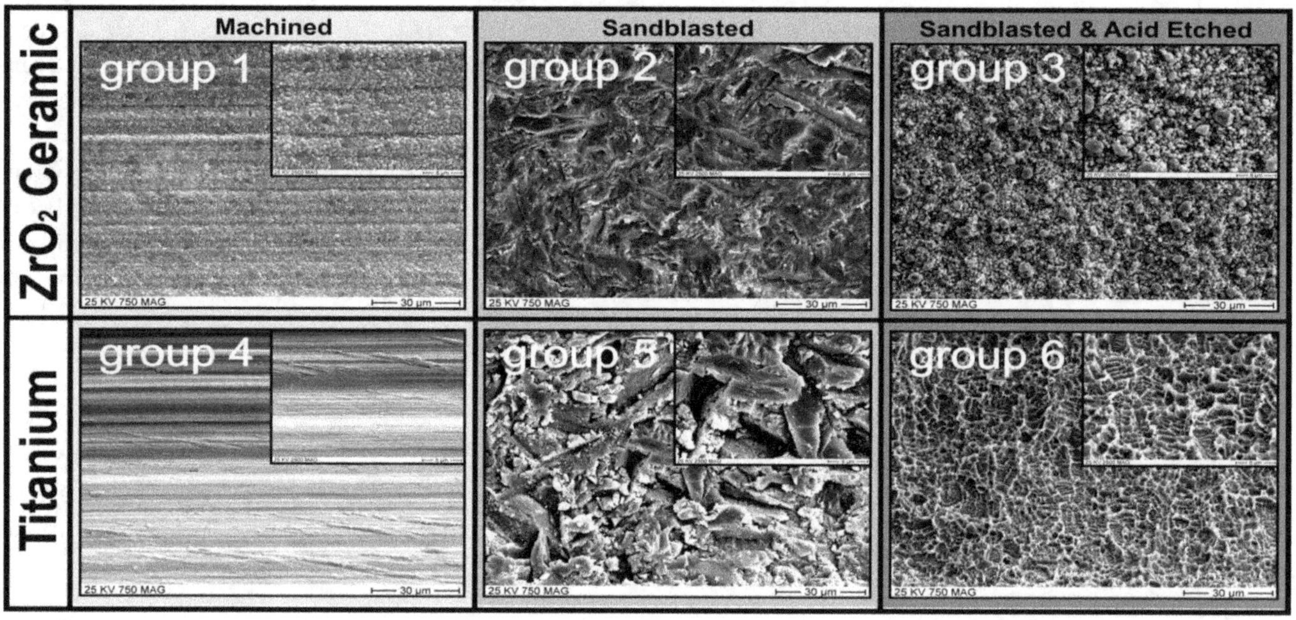

Figure 2. SEM images showing results of the different implant surface treatments. **Groups 1** and **4**: nontreated machined surfaces; **Groups 2** and **5**: sandblasted surfaces (corundum mesh size = 110 µm, working pressure = 6 bar); **Groups 3** and **6**: sandblasted and acid-etched surfaces (result: hydrophilic).

Based on two different methods of surface treatment, 6 groups of implant specimens were produced:

Groups 1 and 4: nontreated, machined, Y-TZP, two-piece zirconia (group 1) and one-piece titanium implants (group 4). The machined surface is shown in Figure 2 (Groups 1 and 4). The diameter of both implants was 5.00 mm.

Groups 2 and 5: once testing with group 1 and 4 implant specimens was finished, each implant was cleaned by water steam jet and 70% ethanol. The implant was additionally given a microstructure by sandblasting with corundum (mesh size = 110 µm, working pressure = 6 bar) at an automatic turning speed of 100 rpm until the diameter of the implants was reduced to 4.95 mm. The SEM images in Figure 2 (Groups 2 and 5) show the result of the surface treatment.

Groups 3 and 6: Once testing with group 2 and 5 implant specimens was finished, each implant was cleaned again by water steam jet and ethanol (70%). The sandblasted surface was then acid-etched to produce a nanostructure showing hydrophilic properties. The result of the acid-etching process is shown in Figure 2 (Groups 3 and 6). The diameter of the implants was further reduced to 4.90 mm.

2.2. Measurement of Heat Generation and Dissipation

The temperature at the bone–implant interface during insertion was dynamically measured by an infrared camera PI160 (PI16048T900, Optris, Berlin, Germany). The infrared camera took real-time images at a frequency of 120 Hz with an uncooled microbolometer focal plane array (FPA) detector with 160 × 120 pixels. The sensor had a spectral range from 7.5 to 13 µm and was equipped with a wide-angle lens with a field of view (FOV) of 48° × 37°. The thermal sensitivity with respect to the relative accuracy of the camera was 0.1 °C, and the minimum measuring distance was 20 mm. The absolute accuracy of the measurement was 2 °C. The temperature data from the camera were transmitted to the computer as thermal images, evaluated using Optris PI Connect software, and transferred to a spreadsheet for statistical analysis.

2.3. Bone Segments

It has been reported that the macroscopic structure of cortex and cancellous bone in the bovine rib is similar to that in the human jaw, and the bone density dependent on its position could be comparable to classes I–IV according to Lekholm & Zarb or D2–D4 according to the Mish classification in the human jaw [3–6]. The distal part of the bovine rib was used and classified as D2/D3 bone. Therefore, 14 ribs were used in this study to simulate the condition in the human jaw. Bone density measurements have not been made because the friction when inserting cylindrical implants arises mainly on the hard cortex bone [7,8] if a sufficiently high torque has been generated there (40 to 60 Ncm in this study). Therefore, when selecting the bone segments, particular care was taken to ensure that the cortical layer thickness was somewhat the same for all bovine bony ribs [7].

2.4. Experimental Settings

In each experiment, the implant was connected to the screwing unit, ensuring a stable rotational speed during insertion of the implant. In the screwing unit, the driving force was produced by a pneumatic cylinder (C85N10-75, ISO air cylinder series C85, SMC Pneumatik GmbH, Egelsbach, Germany). Then, the motor (DC-servo drive series 3564K024B CS, Faulhaber GmbH & Co KG, Schöneich, Germany) connected to a gearbox (series 30/1, 134:1, Faulhaber GmbH & Co KG, Schöneich, Germany) transmitted the force to the torque sensor (DR-20-2Nm; Lorenz Messtechnik GmbH, Alfdorf, Germany) and the collet holder. The implant was connected to the collet holder by a round-headed Allen key (3 mm) to allow rotation. The Allen key was loosely fitted to the mounting post of the implant so that insertion of the implant could remain centered in the prepared bone cavity guided by implant threads and a cone-shaped apex.

The screwing unit could be driven forward or backward axially, and its movement was recorded by a linear inductive distance sensor (LVP 100, Micro-Epsilon Messtechnik GmbH & Co. KG, Ortenburg, Germany). To simulate the environment of surrounding tissues, the bone segment and the implant were covered in a preheated polycarbonate thermo box (37 °C) to prevent heat dissipation. The infrared camera was fixed to the cover of the thermo box. The complete experimental settings are shown in Figure 3.

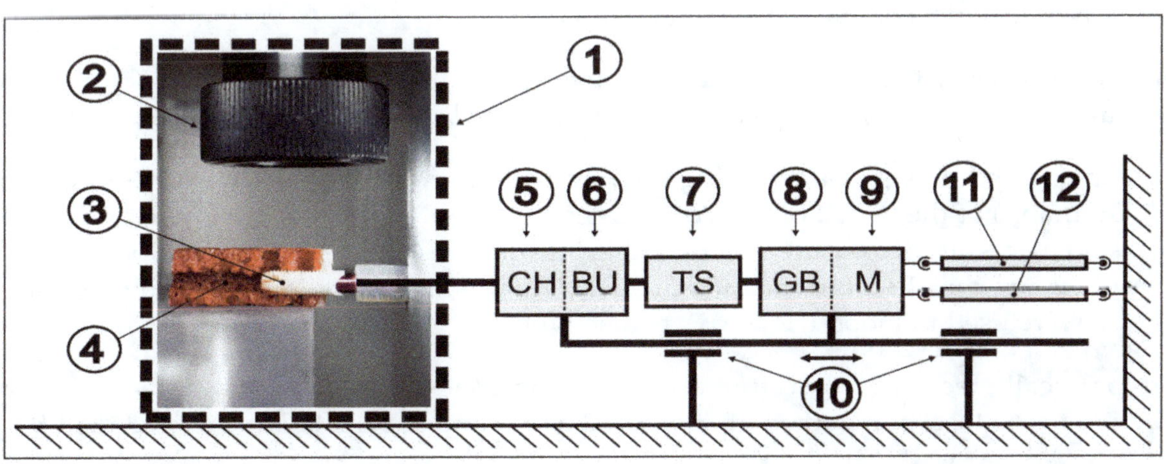

Figure 3. Diagram of the experimental setting. (**1**) Thermo box; (**2**) lens of infrared camera; (**3**) fully inserted ceramic implant; (**4**) transection of the rib segment; (**5**) collet holder (CH); (**6**) bearing unit (BU); (**7**) torque sensor (TS); (**8**) gearbox (GB); (**9**) motor (M); (**10**) linear bearing; (**11**) pneumatic cylinder; (**12**) distance sensor.

2.5. Experimental Protocol

Fourteen of the zirconia implants (groups 1–3) were included in the whole experiment, and each implant underwent 3 loops as a result of the surface treatments applied. After each implant had been assigned to one bovine rib, each bovine rib ($BR_{(1)}$–$BR_{(14)}$) was cut into 3 sequential rib segments ($RS1_{BR(1)}$–$RS3_{BR(1)}$ to $RS1_{BR(14)}$–$RS3_{BR(14)}$). Each implant (I1–I14) would undergo one type of surface modification (machined (m), sandblasted (sb), sandblasted and acid-etched (ae)) before each test program (TP1–TP3). The test sequence of the samples and the corresponding rib segments were organized as follows:

Each implant was inserted into one new rib segment after each surface modification. First, all machined implants ($I1_{(m)}$–$I14_{(m)}$) were inserted into 14 rib segments ($RS1_{BR(1)-BR(14)}$). Then, after sandblasting, implants ($I1_{(sb)}$–$I14_{(sb)}$) were inserted into rib segments ($RS2_{BR(1)-BR(14)}$). Finally, after acid-etched treatment, implants ($I1_{(ae)}$–$I14_{(ae)}$) were inserted into rib segments ($RS3_{BR(1)-BR(14)}$). Surface modification usually took several days. In order to maintain the bone in the same fresh condition in all the tests, bone segments were frozen beforehand in Ringer's solution at −10 °C and were defrosted immediately prior to the experiment.

The titanium implants underwent identical protocols. Since they were made especially for this study, a higher number of pieces was available at the beginning of the trial. Therefore, with torques outside the interval of 40 to 60 Ncm, new Ti implants were used to repeat the insertion test so that 15 measurements per group could be realized (Table 1). The selected torque window was clinically sufficient for immediate restoration of ceramic implants (>35 Ncm), which are often still used as one-piece implants. Furthermore, smaller torques do not produce sufficiently high temperatures by friction between the implant surface and the hard cortical bone [8] to be able to detect the effect of different thermal conductivities between titanium and ceramic at the bone–implant interface.

Contrary to Ti implants, for this study only 14 ceramic implants were available from the manufacturer. Therefore, when the torque was too low or too high, bone penetration tests with the respective surface structure were no longer repeated in order to mechanically protect the connection of the implant driver with the ceramic implant. In addition, cleaning the surfaces of bone remnants would have been a process in which, above all, the roughened ceramic surfaces could have been structurally changed; thus, the equality of specimens could no longer be ensured. Because of this limitation of available ceramic implants, only 8 measurements in group 1, 11 measurements in group 2, and 11 measurements in group 3 could be realized (Table 1).

When one test started, the selected bone segment would be defrosted in Ringer's solution at 37 °C and stored at the same temperature in the oven to simulate the human condition.

The implant bed was prepared using a twist drill (Type N, 118° DIN 338 R-N, Gühring KG, Albstadt, Germany) at the speed of 800 rpm. Since the bone was already wetted, additional water cooling was not necessary. To ensure a comparable insertion resistance in the three loops, the diameter of each implant site matched the implant diameter, that is, twist drills with diameters of 4.3, 4.25, and 4.20 mm were used in loops 1, 2, and 3, respectively.

To dynamically record temperature directly at the bone–implant interface, two bone windows perpendicular to the insertion path were made at 3 and 9 mm subcrestally by a twist drill (Figure 4).

Table 1. Temperature increase of the 6 groups.

Group	Analyzed (40–60 Ncm)/Inserted	Material	Surface Treatment	Surface Roughness Sa (µm)	Compacta Thickness (mm)	Insertion Torque (Ncm)	Temperature Increase BW-1 (°C)	ΔT > 10 °C BW-1		ΔT > 13 °C BW-1		ΔT > 18 °C BW-1		Temperature Increase BW-2 (°C)
								No.	Time (s)	No.	Time (s)	No.	Time (s)	
1	8/14	ZrO_2	M	0.93 ± 0.16	2.51 ± 0.25	52.61 ± 5.10	19.94 ± 3.28	8/8	39.06	8/8	25.10	5/8	11.36	7.50 ± 2.64 °C
2	11/14	ZrO_2	S	1.86 ± 0.38	2.75 ± 0.47	48.97 ± 6.43	19.39 ± 5.73	11/11	28.10	10/11	16.93	6/11	7.98	6.14 ± 2.40 °C
3	11/14	ZrO_2	SAE	2.14 ± 0.62	2.61 ± 0.39	48.79 ± 5.19	15.44 ± 3.63	10/11	20.37	8/11	10.19	3/11	0.43	6.07 ± 3.11 °C
4	15/22	Ti Grade 4	M	0.37 ± 0.04	2.46 ± 0.12	50.10 ± 8.69	9.33 ± 4.18	7/15	22.49	3/15	19.07	1/15	20.40	6.03 ± 3.69 °C
5	15/20	Ti Grade 4	S	2.15 ± 0.24	2.46 ± 0.12	50.99 ± 7.97	9.20 ± 3.31	6/15	23.05	2/15	15.65	-	-	4.33 ± 3.26 °C
6	15/21	Ti Grade 4	SAE	1.89 ± 0.18	2.42 ± 0.09	50.72 ± 7.22	7.68 ± 2.68	2/15	17.45	-	-	-	-	4.41 ± 2.47 °C

M = machined, S = sandblasted, SAE = sandblasted and acid etched, BW = bone window.

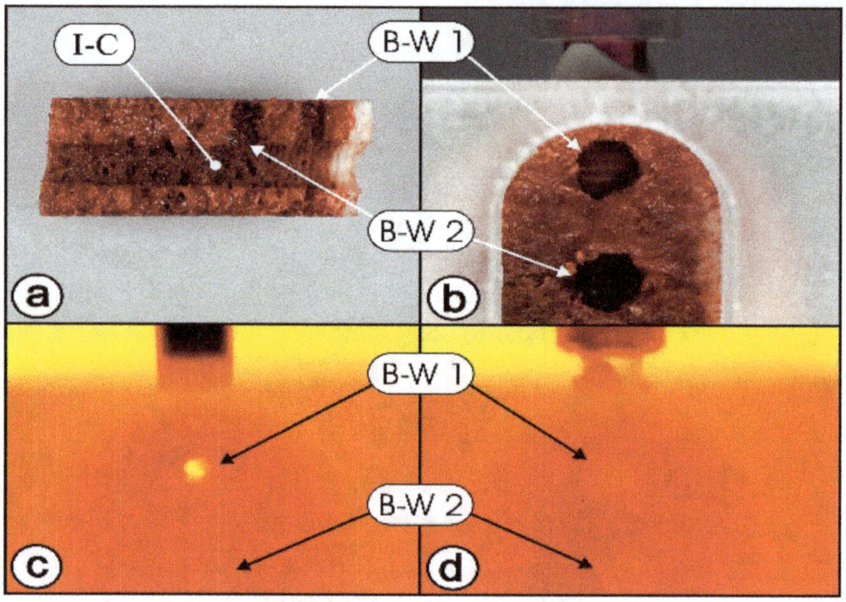

Figure 4. Dynamic temperature record at the bone–implant interface. (**a**) Transection of a rib segment; (**b**) overview of a rib segment; (**c**) infrared image at T3 in Figure 5; (**d**) infrared image at T7 in Figure 5. I-C = Implant Cavity 1; B-W 1 = Bone Window 1; B-W 2 = Bone Window 2.

A

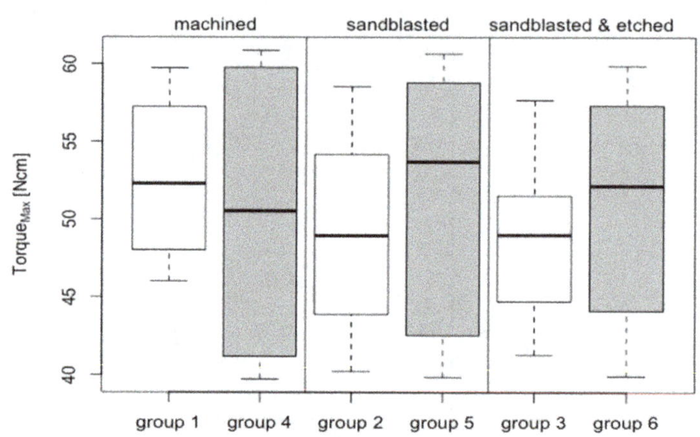

B

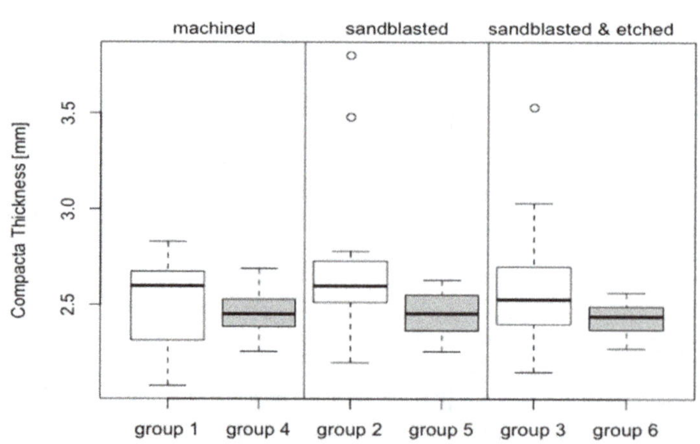

Figure 5. *Cont.*

C

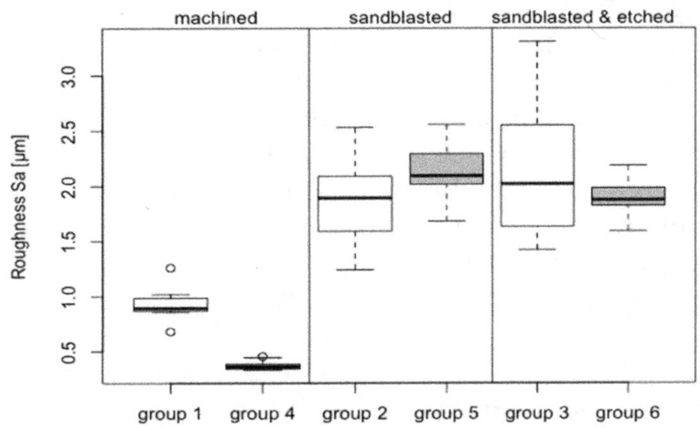

Figure 5. Box plots comparing (**A**) insertion torque, (**B**) cortical bone thickness, and (**C**) roughness.

Before each test, the bone was brought to a temperature of 37 °C inside an oven with saturated humidity. After the bone segment was immobilized, the implant was prewetted in Ringer's solution used to simulate human blood, and then it was driven with a starting pressure of 5 N and a constant rotational speed of 25 rpm to a depth of 12 mm inside the bone. Meanwhile, the infrared camera continuously recorded the temperature through each bone window (2b & T7 in Figure 5), and the difference between the maximum and the starting temperature (37 °C) during insertion would be calculated (ΔT). The change of torque was recorded by torque sensors (DR-20, Lorenz Messtechnik GmbH, Alfdorf, Germany) with the frequency of 100 Hz. Data from groups in which the insertion torque was above 60 Ncm or below 40 Ncm were excluded from the analysis.

After each experiment, the thickness of cortical bone at the insertion point was measured with a caliper gauge. When the temperature, measured at the position 3 mm subcrestally, exceeded 47 °C (ΔT >10 °C) [9], 50 °C (>13 °C) [10], or 55 °C (>18 °C) [11], the corresponding exposure time was calculated.

2.6. Statistical Analysis

Continuous variables are represented as mean ± standard deviation for each group. Comparisons were performed using the Mann–Whitney *U* test, *t*-test, or paired *t*-test. Comparisons with more than 2 groups were analyzed by ANOVA or the Kruskal–Wallis test, depending on Gaussian distribution. Additionally, comparisons using adjusted linear mixed-effects models (LMEs) were performed. Gaussian distributions of data were assessed with the Shapiro–Wilk test. The level of significance in post hoc tests was corrected for multiple testing. The level of significance was set at $\alpha = 0.05$, and all tests were two-sided. Statistical analysis was performed using R 3.6.1 with the packages multicomp 1.4-10, nlme 3.1-140, and plotrix 3.6-3. R, and the packages used are available from CRAN at http://CRAN.R-project.org/.

3. Results

3.1. Group-Related Parameters of Specimens and in Vitro Setup

To ensure that temperature change assessments were comparable with each other, only the implants with insertion torque between 40 and 60 Ncm were included in the analysis. Six machined and three sandblasted implants (groups 1 and 2, respectively) that exceeded an insertion torque of 60 Ncm, and three sandblasted etched implants (group 3) that had an insertion torque under 40 Ncm, were excluded from the analysis. From groups 4 to 6, all 15 specimens were analyzed. The resulting insertion torque was comparable for all 6 groups (group 1: 52.61 ± 5.10 Ncm; group 2: 48.97 ± 6.43

Ncm; group 3: 48.79 ± 5.19 Ncm; group 4: 50.10 ± 8.69 Ncm; group 5: 50.99 ± 7.97 Ncm; group 6: 50.72 ± 7.22 Ncm; $p > 0.05$; Figure 5a.).

The thickness of the cortical plate of the bovine bone rib was similar between the 6 groups (group 1: 2.51 ± 0.25 mm; group 2: 2.75 ± 0.47 mm; group 3: 2.61 ± 0.39 mm; group 4: 2.46 ± 0.12 mm; group 5: 2.46 ± 0.12 mm; group 6: 2.42 ± 0.09 mm; $p > 0.05$; Figure 5b).

The average roughness (Sa) of the machined implants (group 1: 0.93 ± 0.16 μm; group 4: 0.37 ± 0.04) was, as expected, significantly lower than that of sandblasted implants (group 2: 1.86 ± 0.38 μm; group 5: 2.15 ± 0.24 μm; all comparisons have p-values < 0.001) and sandblasted and acid-etched implants (group 3: 2.14 ± 0.62 μm; group 6: 1.89 ± 0.18 μm; all comparisons have p-values < 0.001; Figure 5c). The difference in surface roughness between ceramic and titanium implants after sandblasting (group 2 vs. group 5) and after sandblasting and acid-etching (groups 3 vs. 6) was not statistically significant ($p > 0.05$). The roughness between the machined surfaces (groups 1 and 4) was not statistically significant ($p > 0.05$). In paired comparisons of the surface treatments, the machined and the sandblasted groups showed significant differences (groups 1 and 4 $p = 1.213 \times 10^{-4}$; groups 2 and 5 $p = 0.025756$). The sandblasted and acid-etched groups (groups 3 and 6) showed no significant differences ($p > 0.05$).

3.2. *Maximum Temperature Increase*

3.2.1. Bone Window 1

In bone window 1 (located 3 mm subcrestally), the average temperature increase at the zirconia implants had a high statistically significant difference to that of titanium implants ($p = 7.163 \times 10^{-9}$, resulting from group-adjusted linear mixed-effects models).

Within the zirconia implants (groups 1: 19.94 °C ± 3.28 °C; 2: 19.39 °C ± 5.73 °C; 3: 15.44 °C ± 3.63 °C) there were significant differences between groups 2 and 3 ($p = 0.04426$) and groups 1 and 3 ($p = 0.007525$; Figure 6). By contrast, there was no significant difference between the comparison of groups 1 and 2 ($p > 0.05$).

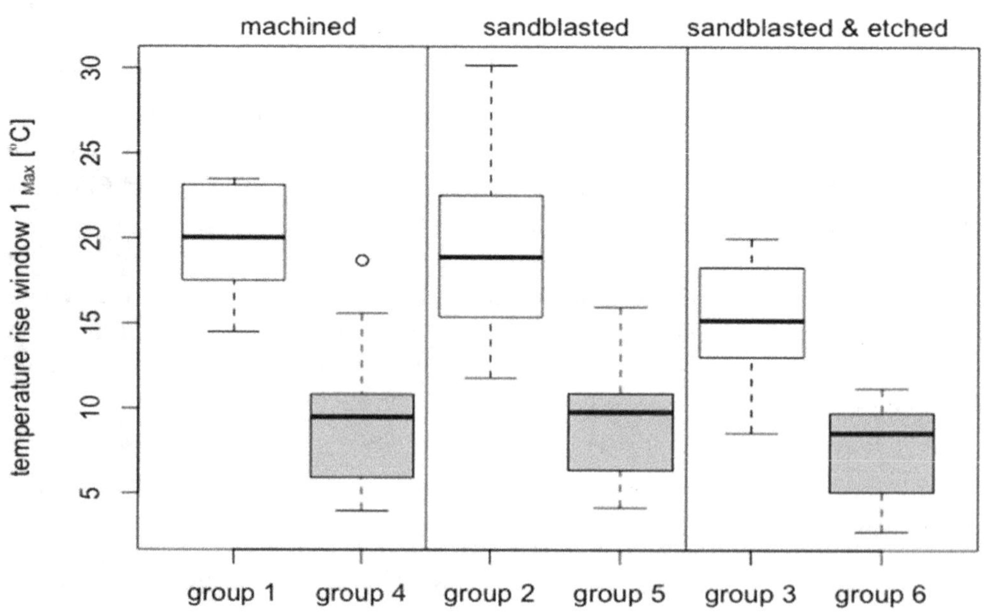

Figure 6. Box plots showing rise of temperature at bone window 1—results of all 6 groups.

Within the titanium implants (group 4: 9.33 °C ± 4.18 °C; group 5: 9.20 °C ± 3.31 °C; group 6: 7.68 °C ± 2.68 °C), the temperature changes were similar for all groups ($p > 0.05$).

In paired comparisons of the different materials with the identical surface treatments, all groups showed highly significant differences (groups 1 and 4 $p = 3.728 \times 10^{-11}$; groups 2 and 5 $p = 7.721 \times 10^{-6}$; groups 3 and 6 $p = 1.725 \times 10^{-6}$ Figure 6).

3.2.2. Bone Window 2

In bone window 2 (located 9 mm subcrestally), the average temperature increase at the zirconia implants had a high statistically significant difference than that of titanium implants ($p = 7.182 \times 10^{-12}$, resulting from group-adjusted linear mixed-effects models).

Within the zirconia implants (group 1: 7.50 °C ± 2.64 °C; group 2: 6.14 °C ± 2.40 °C; group 3: 6.07 °C ± 3.11 °C), the temperature changes were similar for all groups ($p > 0.05$).

Within the titanium implants (group 4: 6.03 °C ± 3.69 °C; group 5: 4.33 °C ± 3.26 °C; group 6: 4.41 °C ± 2.47 °C), the temperature changes were similar for all groups ($p > 0.05$).

3.3. Overheating Exposure Time

3.3.1. Bone Window 1

$\Delta T > 10$ °C

In bone window 1, the average exposure times under $\Delta T > 10$ °C at the zirconia implants were 39.06 s for machined (all 8 of 8 in group 1), 28.10 s for sandblasted (11 of 11 in group 2), and then decreased to 20.37 s for sandblasted etched implants (10 of 11 in group 3). The average exposure times under $\Delta T > 10$ °C at the titanium implants were 22.49 s for machined (7 of 15 in group 4), 23.05 s for sandblasted (6 of 15 in group 5), and then decreased to 17.45 s for sandblasted etched implants (2 of 15 in group 6). None of the tested implants experienced a temperature increase of more than 10 °C over a period of more than 60 s.

$\Delta T > 13$ °C

The average exposure time under $\Delta T > 13$ °C for ceramic implants was 25.10 s in group 1, 16.93 s in group 2, and 10.19 s in group 3. Three machined implants (group 1: 42.2, 36.1, and 32.1 s) and two sandblasted implants (group 2: 34.6 and 33.2 s) experienced more than 30 s temperature increase of over 13 °C. No sandblasted and acid-etched implants (group 3) experienced such a temperature change for longer than 30 s.

The average exposure time under $\Delta T > 13$ °C for titanium implants was 19.03 s at 3 of 15 implants in group 4 (group 4: 19.8, 21.8, and 15.6 s). Two machined implants experienced more than 13 °C temperature increase (group 5: 13.9 and 17.4 s) No sandblasted and acid-etched implants (group 6) experienced a temperature increase of 13 °C or more.

$\Delta T > 18$ °C

The average exposure time under $\Delta T > 18$ °C for ceramic implants was 11.36 s at 5 of 8 implants in group 1, 7.98 s at 6 of 11 implants in group 2, and 0.43 s at 3 of 11 implants in group 3. Two machined ceramic implants (group 1: 25.4 and 14.2 s) and two sandblasted ceramic implants (group 2: 19.0 and 16.7 s) experienced a temperature increase of more than 18 °C for more than 14 s. No sandblasted and acid-etched implants (group 3) experienced a temperature change greater than 18 °C for more than 14 s.

Only one titanium implant (group 4) exceeded 18.70 °C and had an exposure time of 20.40 s for $\Delta T > 18$ °C.

3.3.2. Bone Window 2

In bone window 2, the temperature increase never exceeded values > 10 °C.

3.4. Material-Dependent Thermal Energy Propagation

Figure 7 shows the image captured by the infrared camera during the process of inserting titanium and ceramic implants, both with sandblasted and acid-etched surfaces. Prior to the insertion process—meaning the implants were completely outside of the bone cavity—there was very little temperature difference between the titanium implant (33.2 °C) and the ceramic implant (31.2 °C). Bone window 1 shows the nearly regulated temperature of the thermo box (Figure 3) encapsulating the in vitro setup (37.5 °C; 37.2 °C).

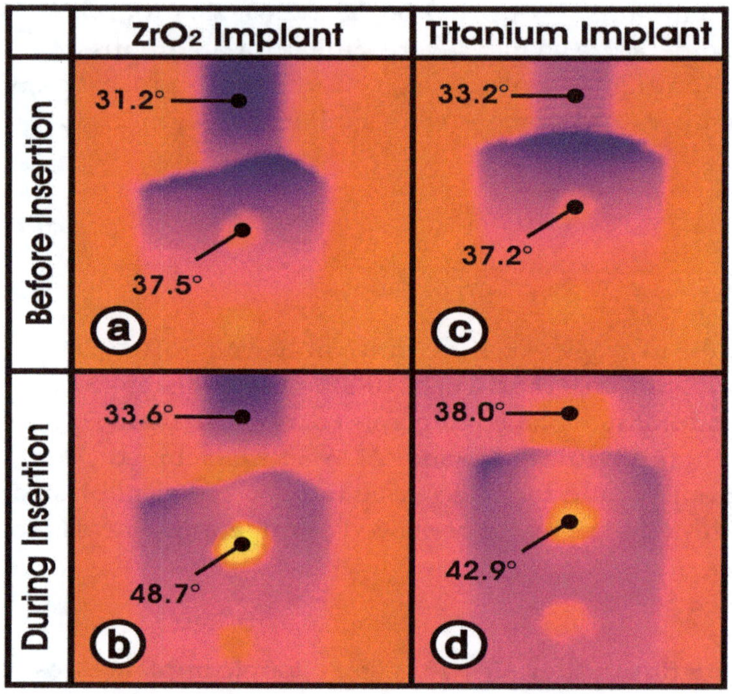

Figure 7. Material-dependent heat dissipation. (**a**) ceramic implant before insertion; (**b**) ceramic implant during insertion; (**c**) titanium implant before insertion; (**d**) titanium implant during insertion.

At the moment of maximum temperature development during implant insertion, the ceramic implant was heated to 48.7 °C below the cortical bone (bone window 1) and to 33.6 °C outside the bone. In contrast, the titanium implant showed 42.9 °C within bone window 1 and 38.0 °C outside the bone. Thus, at the same distance, the titanium implant had a 3 times lower temperature gradient than the ceramic implant during the insertion process ($\Delta T_{ceramic}$ = 15.1 °C vs. $\Delta T_{titanium}$ = 4.9 °C).

The summary of all results is shown in Table 1.

4. Discussion

The aim of the in vitro study was to dynamically detect heat development at the bone–implant interface during the entire process of inserting a cylindrical screw implant into bone. For this purpose, an in vitro setup was developed, which achieves the highest possible quality of simulation of the clinical conditions and uses of test specimens, which differ in only one parameter, as far as possible.

4.1. Identical Specimen

It was important for good reproducibility of the temperature values at the implant surface that the implant specimens had an identical endosteal macrodesign and were identically manufactured (Figures 1 and 2). The measured surface roughness (Figure 5b) did not differ significantly between the ceramic (ZrO_2) and titanium implant materials in the sandblasted and sandblasted-etched surfaces. Only on the machined implants was the titanium surface statistically significantly smoother.

Repetition of the test series with the same implants after each additional surface treatment allowed for a nearly identical macrodesign with a different microdesign. Only removal of material by subtractive surface treatment caused a reduction in implant diameter. However, this was recorded by measurement and taken into account in the osteotomy protocol. In other words, the last cutter for bone preparation was also correspondingly smaller in diameter.

4.2. In Vitro Setup

Several published articles reporting on heat development when screwing an implant into the bone cavity have used bovine bone [12], in particular the bovine rib [9,10,13–16]. Bone segments with a cortical thickness of around 2.5 mm were chosen in order to mimic the known thickness of the human mandible (1.0–2.5 mm) [17–19] and to ensure the almost same amount of friction between bone and implant surfaces [7,8]. The temperature rise was generated in the ceramic implant mainly in the cortex bone (see bone window No. 1). In cancellous bone, however, there were no statistically significant differences in the temperature increase. This reinforces the assumed mechanism of temperature generation: in the case of a sufficiently high torque (40–60 Nm) and a conventional screw thread, most of the friction is generated between hard bone and the implant surface. Only special aggressive threads—for example, in Nobel Active in spongy bone, a mechanism other than friction—can generate high torque or primary stability—compression of trabeculae. Therefore, in the selection of the bone ribs, particular attention was paid to a comparable layer thickness of the cortex [7]. Since the spongy part of the rib in the present macrodesign of the examined implants (cylindrical, conventional screw thread) hardly generates any friction or heating, determination of the bone mineral density was omitted. Therefore, a high variation in the bone density in the spongy region of the rib probably has no influence on the measurement results in bone window 2.

Although blood circulation was absent in this case, the remaining conditions such as the chemical composition, density, humidity, structure, as well as mechanical and thermal properties were similar to those of the human bone. By contrast, artificial bone models cannot properly simulate the human bone because there are huge differences in thermal conductivity and heat capacity [20].

The anatomical structure—cortical bone and the underlying cancellous bone—are suitable for simulation of a toothless, healed alveolar bone. In order to keep the high anatomical variance of bovine ribs reasonably small in this investigation, the ribs were frozen after a test run so that measurements could at least be done on the identical bovine rib after the respective surface treatment of the implants for the second and third test runs.

An infrared camera (Figure 3) measured the temperature during the insertion process. In contrast to this investigation, Markovic et al. [21] captured the temperature at the surface of a bone segment. The two bone windows in this study allowed temperature to be measured directly on the implant surface. As a result, system-related measurement distortions due to differently positioned temperature probes in peri-implant bone could be avoided [9,10,13–16].

The above factors resulted in a relatively small variation of the temperature values per experimental group (Figures 6 and 7). Thus, the goal of good reproducibility of the measurement conditions was achieved in the experimental setup used. In addition, the direct measurement of the surface temperature of the implants makes the nonsimulated, cooling effect of a well-perfused bone marrow smaller than with probes placed in the peri-implant bone [9,10,13–16]. Furthermore, the low thermal conductivity of bone (approximately 1/100 of titanium) can lead to thermal isolation of the sensors. The temperature-controlled thermo box (Figure 3(1)) additionally contributed to the good reproducibility of the measured temperature values (Figure 7).

In the selection of bovine ribs, care was taken to ensure that the layer thickness of the cortical bone did not differ a great deal (Figure 5b). It is apparent that, in a cylindrical implant, the heat generated by friction is primarily generated by the hard cortical bone and only slightly by the soft cancellous bone located below. The torques achieved during the insertion process were another indicator of identical experimental conditions: trial implants were hardly distinguishable in macro- and microdesigns and comparable layer thicknesses of the cortical bone (Figure 5a). In this study, the experimental parameters were chosen to simulate a high insertion torque (40–60 Ncm). It was above the average level suggested by most manufacturers (35 or 45 Ncm); nevertheless, this range was still below the maximum endurance for the ceramic implants.

In the case of rare outliers in insertion torques, the temperature readings were not included in the evaluation, but the complete measurement was repeated with the respective implant.

The remaining parameters (ambient temperature, rpm and feed at insertion, and dimension of the bone cavity) were kept reproducible and constant with conventional control circuits in the experimental setup (Figure 3).

4.3. Temperature Increase at Bone Window 1

The implant surface temperatures just below the cortical bone were highly significantly different between the ceramic and titanium implants. Statistical evaluation was performed using a group-adjusted linear mixed-effects model.

The increased temperature of the ceramic implant was due to its poor thermal conductivity. It was 2.5 W/mK and, thus, nearly ten times lower than titanium (22 W/mK). The thermal energy generated at the bone–implant interface during insertion dissipated poorly over the ceramic implant at locations further away. The thermal energy remained at the place of its formation and led to a higher temperature. This phenomenon is visible in Figure 7 from the infrared camera image. During the insertion process, the ceramic implant outside the bone (33.6 °C) heated up significantly less than the titanium implant (38.0 °C) under nearly identical experimental conditions. This means that much more heat (48.7 °C) was created in the bone at window 1 on the ceramic implant surface than in the titanium implant (42.9 °C). The increase in temperature, due to the greatly reduced thermal conductivity of ceramics, can hardly be reduced by intensive water cooling because the water has no access to the implant–bone interface during screwing-in of the implant [8], and the poor heat conduction of ceramics only cools the implant, which is not yet in the bone. It is obvious that only an extremely slow insertion of the implant can reduce the heating of the cortex bone [7,8,12,22].

Analysis of the temperature in bone window 1 (Figure 6) for all six experimental groups again showed a statistically significant increase in temperature at the ceramic implant compared to the titanium implant, regardless of the surface structure. However, the increase in temperature of ceramic implants with sandblasted and acid-etched surfaces (15.44 °C) was statistically significantly smaller than that with the machined (19.94 °C) or purely sandblasted (19.39 °C) ceramic surface. This effect of surface modification could possibly occur as a result of the high porosity of the sandblasted and acid-etched surface of ZrO_2 implants (Figure 2). In particular, it shows nanoscopic pores smaller than 500 nm. This type of pore is too small to be reflected in the roughness average (Sa) but can be filled with blood and other tissue fluids, which in turn can function as heat storage and a cooling fluid. In other words, the blood and tissue fluid on the surface are heated. The heat capacity of water is 4.182 kJ/kg/K, which is more than 10 times higher than that of zirconia at 0.4 kJ/kg/K, and the density of zirconia is 6.08 g/cm^3, which is 6 times higher than that of water. Thus, in order to increase the temperature of blood or tissue fluid on the blasted and acid-etched surface by 1 °C, a 1.72 times higher heat energy would be required than in the ZrO_2 surfaces without fluids captured in nanoscopic pores—like machined (group 1) or sandblasted surfaces (group 2), where the latter results in a higher temperature increase at the implant–bone interfaces (Figure 6).

Another explanation of the result is based on a tribological effect [23]. Improved lubrication by the fluid trapped in the nanoscopic pores produces reduced heat development as it rotates through the cortical bone.

However, the temperature increase in the titanium implants is independent of their surface condition (Figure 6). This result might be related to good thermal conductivity, which allows rapid cooling of the titanium surface in bone window 1. In the bone window itself, there is no friction caused by close-fitting peri-implant bone.

4.4. Temperature Increase at Bone Window 2

The temperatures at the implant surface occurring in cancellous bone were different between the ceramic and titanium implants. Statistical evaluation was performed using a group-adjusted linear mixed-effects model.

The inter-group comparison (Figure 8) shows no statistically significant differences in temperature increase with respect to the test parameters of implant material and surface texture. Owing to low rigidity and the tissue structure interspersed with fat, the cancellous bone causes considerably less friction at the implant–bone interface than at the stiff and hard cortical bone. Therefore, the different thermal conductivities of the ceramic and titanium implants probably play a minor role in the temperature increase in bone window 2.

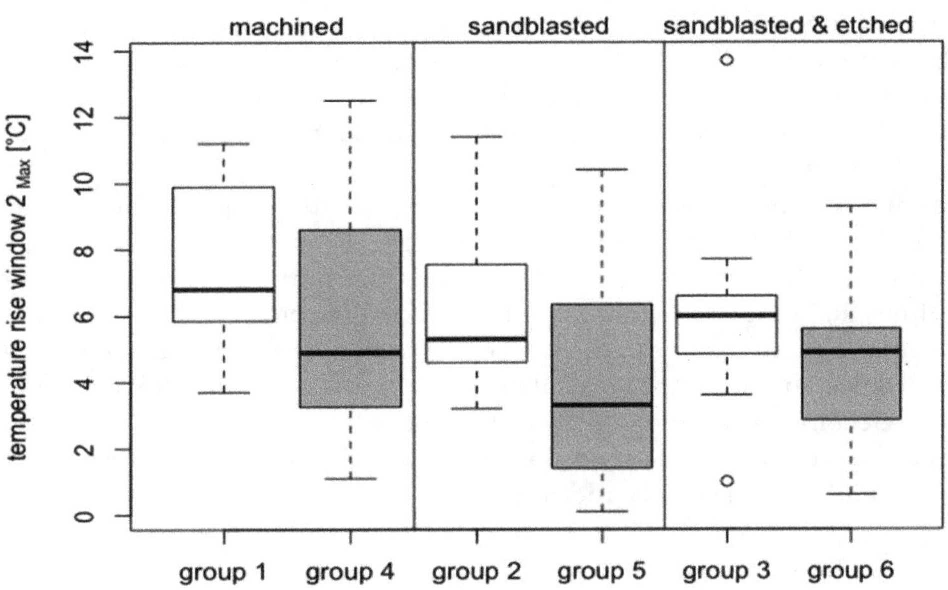

Figure 8. Box plots showing rise of temperature at bone window 2—results of all 6 groups.

4.5. Differences in Bone Window 1 versus Bone Window 2

In this study, the bone windows for heat measurement were prepared 3 and 9 mm subcrestally in order to measure the change of the bone–implant interfacial temperature during implant insertion at the positions near the cortex and inside the implant cavity, respectively. As expected, the interfacial increase of temperature near the cortex was higher than that deep in the cancellous bone, regardless of the surface modification. In the study by Sener et al., the highest temperature in the process of preparing the implant bed was also observed in the superficial part of the implant cavity, and the heat decreased in the direction of the implant apex [17].

The different structure of cortical and cancellous bone as well as the higher frictional coefficient of hard cortical bone can lead to different frictional effects on the bone–implant surface; furthermore, the bone region at window 1 is exposed to friction for a longer time than the region of window 2 near the apex of the implant cavity. These factors, combined with the different thermal conductivities of the cortical and cancellous bone, result in more heat energy produced and accumulated in the cortical part during implant insertion.

Previously published studies showed different temperature increases during insertion of a titanium implant (0.55–9.81 °C) [12,21,24,25]. This might be due to temperatures being measured at the outer surface of the bone segment [24] or at a distance of 0.5–1 mm from the implant [12,21,25]. In addition, Sumer et al. [9] found more heat was generated with ceramic drills than with stainless steel drills at the superficial part of the drilling cavity.

4.6. Heat Caused Damage to Peri-implant Bone

The damage to the bone caused by overheating is related to the time it is exposed to the heating [26–28]. The higher the bone–implant interfacial temperature, the shorter the time it takes for bone damage to appear [26]. Eriksson and Albrektsson claim that bone damage occurs when the bone–implant interfacial temperature reaches at least 47 °C for 1 min [27]. As a result, the primary stability of the implants would decrease, and implants might loosen shortly after loading [28]. Furthermore, it was shown by Lundskog [26] that osteocytes underwent necrosis as soon as the bone was exposed to 50 °C for more than 30 s. Schmelzeisen et al. [28] showed that a temperature between 50 and 60 °C caused irreversible damage to osteocytes for an exposure time of 8 to 20 s. Based on that study, the median values of 55 °C and 14 s were applied as critical parameters in the current study. The interfacial temperature of ceramic implants measured near the cortical plate (bone window 1) were 56.94 °C on machined, 56.39 °C on sandblasted, and 52.43 °C on sandblasted-etched implants, with the starting temperature of 37 °C. Thus, the potential for bone damage induced by overheating was present on each surface. However, the heat and the relative exposure time decreased with the sandblasted and acid-etched surfaces, suggesting that the risk of bone damage could be reduced with proper surface modification.

Nevertheless, the results of this in vitro study might not fully represent the reality under clinical conditions [11,29]. The difference resulting from blood circulation and the thermal conductivity between nonlive and live tissues can influence the change in interfacial temperature [26]. Since the blood flow is six times higher in cancellous bone than in cortical bone, and blood can absorb part of the heat produced during implant insertion, the interfacial temperature increase in the cancellous bone is supposed to be smaller than that in the cortical bone. In view of this fact, the authors did not expect a significant cooling effect inside a patient's cortical bone.

Based on this study, the heat produced during the implant insertion process mainly depends on the implant material and less on surface modification.

5. Conclusions

The results of this in vitro study show a temperature rise that is dangerous for the peri-implant cortical bone when a ceramic implant is inserted. Despite limited transferability to the clinical situation, the authors recommend a very slow insertion velocity for ceramic implants to avoid early implant losses.

Author Contributions: Conceptualization, H.Z., P.W. and E.K.; Data curation, H.Z.; Formal analysis, H.Z., E.K., U.B. and C.R.; Funding acquisition, H.Z.; Investigation, H.Z., E.K., A.T. and C.R.; Methodology, H.Z., E.K. and A.T.; Project administration, H.Z., P.W. and C.R.; Resources, H.Z.; Software, H.Z.; Supervision, H.Z., P.W. and C.R.; Validation, H.ZFig., P.W., E.K., A.T. and C.R.; Visualization, H.Z., P.W. and C.R.; Writing—original draft, H.Z., P.W., E.K. and C.R.; Writing—review & editing, H.Z., P.W., E.K., A.T., U.B. and C.R.

Acknowledgments: This research did not receive any specific grant from funding agencies in the public, commercial, or not-for-profit sectors.

References

1. Cionca, N.; Müller, N.; Mombelli, A. Two-piece zirconia implants supporting all-ceramic crowns: A prospective clinical study. *Clin. Oral Implant. Res.* **2015**, *26*, 413–418. [CrossRef] [PubMed]
2. Albrektsson, T.; Jemt, T.; Mölne, J.; Tengvall, P.; Wennerberg, A. On inflammation-immunological balance theory-A critical apprehension of disease concepts around implants: Mucositis and marginal bone loss may represent normal conditions and not necessarily a state of disease. *Clin. Implant Dent. Relat. Res.* **2019**, *21*, 183–189. [CrossRef] [PubMed]
3. Lachmann, S.; Jager, B.; Axmann, D.; Gomez-Roman, G.; Groten, M.; Weber, H. Resonance frequency analysis and damping capacity assessment. Part I: An in vitro study on measurement reliability and a method of comparison in the determination of primary dental implant stability. *Clin. Oral Implant. Res.* **2006**, *17*, 75–79. [CrossRef]

4. Garcia-Vives, N.; Andres-Garcia, R.; Rios-Santos, V.; Fernandez-Palacin, A.; Bullon-Fernandez, P.; Herrero-Climent, M.; Herrero-Climent, F. In vitro evaluation of the type of implant bed preparation with osteotomes in bone type IV and its influence on the stability of two implant systems. *Med. Oral Patol. Oral Cir. Bucal* **2009**, *14*, 455–460.
5. Moon, S.H.; Um, H.S.; Lee, J.K.; Chang, B.S.; Lee, M.K. The effect of implant shape and bone preparation on primary stability. *J. Periodontal Implant Sci.* **2010**, *40*, 239–243. [CrossRef] [PubMed]
6. Baker, J.A.; Vora, S.; Bairam, L.; Kim, H.I.; Davis, E.L.; Andreana, S. Piezoelectric vs. conventional implant site preparation: Ex vivo implant primary stability. *Clin. Oral Implant. Res.* **2012**, *23*, 433–437. [CrossRef]
7. Matsuoka, M.; Motoyoshi, M.; Sakaguchi, M.; Shinohara, A.; Shigeede, T.; Saito, Y.; Matsuda, M.; Shimizu, N. Friction heat during self-drilling of an orthodontic miniscrew. *Int. J. Oral Maxillofac. Surg.* **2011**, *40*, 191–194. [CrossRef]
8. Aghvami, M.; Brunski, J.B.; Tulu, U.S.; Chen, C.H.; Helms, J.A. A Thermal and Biological Analysis of Bone Drilling. *J. Biomech. Eng.* **2018**, *140*, 101010. [CrossRef]
9. Sumer, M.; Misir, A.F.; Telcioglu, N.T.; Guler, A.U.; Yenisey, M. Comparison of heat generation during implant drilling using stainless steel and ceramic drills. *J. Oral Maxillofac. Surg.* **2011**, *69*, 1350–1354. [CrossRef]
10. Biyikli, S.; Modest, M.F.; Tarr, R. Measurements of thermal properties for human femora. *J. Biomed. Mater. Res.* **1986**, *20*, 1335–1345. [CrossRef] [PubMed]
11. Trisi, P.; Berardini, M.; Falco, A.; Vulpiani, M.P.; Masciotra, L. Effect of 50 to 60°C heating on osseointegration of dental implants in dense bone: An in vivo histological study. *Implant Dent.* **2014**, *23*, 516–521. [CrossRef] [PubMed]
12. Flanagan, D. Heat generated during seating of dental implant fixtures. *J. Oral Implantol.* **2014**, *40*, 174–181. [CrossRef] [PubMed]
13. Matthews, L.S.; Hirsch, C. Temperatures measured in human cortical bone when drilling. *J. Bone Jt. Surg.* **1972**, *54*, 297–308. [CrossRef] [PubMed]
14. Matthews, L.S.; Green, C.A.; Goldstein, S.A. The thermal effects of skeletal fixation-pin insertion in bone. *J. Bone Jt. Surg.* **1984**, *66*, 1077–1083. [CrossRef] [PubMed]
15. Bachus, K.N.; Rondina, M.T.; Hutchinson, D.T. The effects of drilling force on cortical temperatures and their duration: An in vitro study. *Med. Eng. Phys.* **2000**, *22*, 685–691. [CrossRef]
16. Oh, H.J.; Wikesjo, U.M.; Kang, H.S.; Ku, Y.; Eom, T.G.; Koo, K.T. Effect of implant drill characteristics on heat generation in osteotomy sites: A pilot study. *Clin. Oral Implant. Res.* **2011**, *22*, 722–726. [CrossRef]
17. Sener, B.C.; Dergin, G.; Gursoy, B.; Kelesoglu, E.; Slih, I. Effects of irrigation temperature on heat control in vitro at different drilling depths. *Clin. Oral Implant. Res.* **2009**, *20*, 294–298. [CrossRef] [PubMed]
18. Schmelzeisen, H. Thermische Schäden bei der Osteosynthese. *OP-Journal* **1992**, *8*, 26–29. (In German)
19. Eriksson, A.R.; Albrektsson, T.; Albrektsson, B. Heat caused by drilling cortical bone. Temperature measured in vivo in patients and animals. *Acta. Orthop. Scand.* **1984**, *55*, 629–631. [CrossRef]
20. Kunze, K.G.; Hofstetter, H.; Posalaky, I.; Winkler, B. Veränderung der Knochendurchblutung nach Osteotomien und Osteosynthesen. *Unfallchirurgie* **1981**, *7*, 169–180. (In German) [CrossRef]
21. Markovic, A.; Misic, T.; Milicic, B.; Calvo-Guirado, J.L.; Aleksic, Z.; Dinic, A. Heat generation during implant placement in low-density bone: Effect of surgical technique, insertion torque and implant macro design. *Clin. Oral Implant. Res.* **2013**, *24*, 798–805. [CrossRef]
22. Stocchero, M.; Jinno, Y.; Toia, M.; Ahmad, M.; Papia, E.; Yamaguchi, S.; Becktor, J.P. Intraosseous Temperature Change during Installation of Dental Implants with Two Different Surfaces and Different Drilling Protocols: An In Vivo Study in Sheep. *J. Clin. Med.* **2019**, *8*, 1198. [CrossRef] [PubMed]
23. Ludema, K.C.; Ajayi, L. *Friction, Wear, Lubrication: A Textbook in Tribology*, 2nd ed.; CRS Press: Boca Raton, FL, USA, 2018; ISBN 9781482210170.
24. Markovic, A.; Misic, T.; Mancic, D.; Jovanovic, I.; Scepanovic, M.; Jezdic, Z. Real-time thermographic analysis of low-density bone during implant placement: A randomized parallel-group clinical study comparing lateral condensation with bone drilling surgical technique. *Clin. Oral Implant. Res.* **2014**, *25*, 910–918. [CrossRef]
25. Sumer, M.; Keskiner, I.; Mercan, U.; Misir, F.; Cankaya, S. Assessment of heat generation during implant insertion. *J. Prosthet. Dent.* **2014**, *112*, 522–525. [CrossRef] [PubMed]

26. Lundskog, J. Heat and bone tissue. An experimental investigation of the thermal properties of bone and threshold levels for thermal injury. *Scand. J. Plast. Reconstr. Surg.* **1972**, *9*, 1–80. [PubMed]
27. Eriksson, A.R.; Albrektsson, T. Temperature threshold levels for heat-induced bone tissue injury: A vital-microscopic study in the rabbit. *J. Prosthet. Dent.* **1983**, *50*, 101–107. [CrossRef]
28. Schmelzeisen, H. *Der Bohrvorgang in der Kortikalis: Mechanik, Thermometrie, Morphologie*; Springer: Berlin/Heidelberg, Germany, 1990. (In German)
29. Trisi, P.; Berardini, M.; Falco, A.; Vulpiani, M.P. Effect of temperature on the dental implant osseointegration development in low-density bone: An in vivo histological evaluation. *Implant Dent.* **2015**, *24*, 96–100. [CrossRef] [PubMed]

Permissions

All chapters in this book were first published by MDPI; hereby published with permission under the Creative Commons Attribution License or equivalent. Every chapter published in this book has been scrutinized by our experts. Their significance has been extensively debated. The topics covered herein carry significant findings which will fuel the growth of the discipline. They may even be implemented as practical applications or may be referred to as a beginning point for another development.

The contributors of this book come from diverse backgrounds, making this book a truly international effort. This book will bring forth new frontiers with its revolutionizing research information and detailed analysis of the nascent developments around the world.

We would like to thank all the contributing authors for lending their expertise to make the book truly unique. They have played a crucial role in the development of this book. Without their invaluable contributions this book wouldn't have been possible. They have made vital efforts to compile up to date information on the varied aspects of this subject to make this book a valuable addition to the collection of many professionals and students.

This book was conceptualized with the vision of imparting up-to-date information and advanced data in this field. To ensure the same, a matchless editorial board was set up. Every individual on the board went through rigorous rounds of assessment to prove their worth. After which they invested a large part of their time researching and compiling the most relevant data for our readers.

The editorial board has been involved in producing this book since its inception. They have spent rigorous hours researching and exploring the diverse topics which have resulted in the successful publishing of this book. They have passed on their knowledge of decades through this book. To expedite this challenging task, the publisher supported the team at every step. A small team of assistant editors was also appointed to further simplify the editing procedure and attain best results for the readers.

Apart from the editorial board, the designing team has also invested a significant amount of their time in understanding the subject and creating the most relevant covers. They scrutinized every image to scout for the most suitable representation of the subject and create an appropriate cover for the book.

The publishing team has been an ardent support to the editorial, designing and production team. Their endless efforts to recruit the best for this project, has resulted in the accomplishment of this book. They are a veteran in the field of academics and their pool of knowledge is as vast as their experience in printing. Their expertise and guidance has proved useful at every step. Their uncompromising quality standards have made this book an exceptional effort. Their encouragement from time to time has been an inspiration for everyone.

The publisher and the editorial board hope that this book will prove to be a valuable piece of knowledge for researchers, students, practitioners and scholars across the globe.

List of Contributors

Ying-Sui Sun
School of Dental Technology, Taipei Medical University, Taipei 11031, Taiwan
Department of Dentistry, National Yang-Ming University, Taipei 11221, Taiwan

Yu-An Lin
Institute of Oral Biology, National Yang-Ming University, Taipei 11221, Taiwan

Her-Hsiung Huang
Department of Dentistry, National Yang-Ming University, Taipei 11221, Taiwan
Institute of Oral Biology, National Yang-Ming University, Taipei 11221, Taiwan
Department of Bioinformatics and Medical Engineering, Asia University, Taichung 41354, Taiwan
Department of Medical Research, China Medical University Hospital, China Medical University, Taichung 40402, Taiwan
Department of Stomatology, Taipei Veterans General Hospital, Taipei 11217, Taiwan
Department of Education and Research, Taipei City Hospital, Taipei 10341, Taiwan

Felice Lorusso, Sammy Noumbissi and Antonio Scarano
Department of Medical, Oral and Biotechnological Sciences, University of Chieti-Pescara, Via dei Vestini, 31, 66100 Chieti, Italy
Zirconia Implant Research Group (Z.I.R.G), International Academy of Ceramic Implantology, Silver Spring, MD 20910, USA

Inchingolo Francesco
Department of Interdisciplinary Medicine, University of Bari Aldo Moro, 70121 Bari, Italy

Biagio Rapone
Department of Basic Medical Sciences, Neurosciences and Sense Organs, University of Bari Aldo Moro, 70121 Bari, Italy

Ahmad G. A. Khater
Faculty of Oral and Dental Medicine, Ahram Canadian University, 6th of October City, 8655 Giza, Egypt

Ming-Jun Li, Pei-Ching Kung, Yuan-Wei Chang and Nien-Ti Tsou
Department of Materials Science and Engineering, National Chiao Tung University, Hsin-chu 30010, Taiwan

Enrique Fernández-Bodereau
Department of Fixed Prosthodontics, Faculty of Dentistry, Universidad Nacional de Córdoba, Córdoba 5000, Argentine

Viviana Yolanda Flores
Department of Oral Biology, Faculty of Dentistry, Universidad Nacional de Córdoba, Córdoba 5000, Argentine

Rafael Arcesio Delgado-Ruiz
Department of Prosthodontics, School of Dental Dental Medicine, Stony Brook, NY 1103, USA

Juan Manuel Aragoneses
Department of Dental Research in Universidad Federico Henríquez y Carvajal (UFHEC), Santo Domingo 10107, Dominicana Republic

José Luis Calvo-Guirado
Department of Oral and Implant Surgery, Faculty of Health Sciences, Universidad Católica San Antonio de Murcia (UCAM), Murcia 30002, Spain

Sergio Alexandre Gehrke
Biotecnos Research Center, 11100 Montevideo, Uruguay
Master Postgraduate Program in Biotechnology of UCAM, 11100 Montevideo, Uruguay

Mauro Bercianos and Jorge Gonzalo Aguerrondo
Postgraduate Program in Biotechnology of UCAM, 11100 Montevideo, Uruguay

Juan Carlos Prados-Frutos
Department of Medicine and Surgery, Rey Juan Carlos University, Alcorcón, 28922 Madrid, Spain

Pei-Ching Kung, Shih-Shun Chien and Nien-Ti Tsou
Department of Materials Science and Engineering, National Chiao Tung University, Ta Hsueh Road, Hsinchu 300, Taiwan

Jung-Ju Kim, Jeong Chan Kim and Jun-Beom Lee
Department of Periodontology, Seoul National University School of Dentistry, Seoul 03080, Korea

Jae-Hyun Lee
Department of Prosthodontics, One-Stop Specialty Center, Seoul National University Dental Hospital, Seoul 03080, Korea

Chang-Bin Cho and In-Sung Luke Yeo
Department of Prosthodontics, Seoul National University School of Dentistry, and Dental Research Institute, 101 Daehak-Ro, Jongno-Gu, Seoul 03080, Korea

Sung Youn Jung, Cho Yeon Park, Hyun Ki Kang and Byung-Moo Min
Department of Oral Biochemistry and Program in Cancer and Developmental Biology, Seoul National University School of Dentistry, and Dental Research Institute, 101 Daehak-Ro, Jongno-Gu, Seoul 03080, Korea

Maria Menini, Paolo Pesce, Domenico Baldi and Paolo Pera
Division of Implant Prosthodontics, Department of Surgical Sciences, University of Genoa, 16132 Genoa, Italy

Gabriela Coronel Vargas
Department of Health Sciences, University of Genoa, 16126 Genoa, Italy

Alberto Izzotti
Department of Health Sciences, University of Genoa, 16126 Genoa, Italy
IRCCS Ospedale Policlinico San Martino, 16132 Genoa, Italy

David Reinedahl, Carina B. Johansson, Petra Hammarström Johansson and Ann Wennerberg
Department of Prosthodontics, Institute of Odontology, Sahlgrenska Academy, University of Gothenburg, Gothenburg 405 30, Sweden

Silvia Galli
Department of Prosthodontics, Faculty of Odontology, Malmö University, Malmö 205 06, Sweden

Tomas Albrektsson
Department of Prosthodontics, Faculty of Odontology, Malmö University, Malmö 205 06, Sweden
Department of Biomaterials, Institute of Clinical Sciences, Sahlgrenska Academy, University of Gothenburg, Gothenburg 40530, Sweden

Dirk U. Duddeck
Department of Prosthodontics, Geriatric Dentistry and Craniomandibular Disorders, University Charité Berlin, 14197 Berlin, Germany
CleanImplant Foundation, Research Department, 10117 Berlin, Germany

Oded Bahat
Private Practice, Beverly Hills, CA 90210, USA

Christel Larsson and Florian Beuer
Department of Prosthodontics, Faculty of Odontology, Malmö University, 20506 Malmö, Sweden

Bruno Chrcanovic
Department of Prosthodontics, Faculty of Odontology, Malmö University, Malmö 205 06, Sweden

Pentti Tengvall
Department of Biomaterials, Institute of Clinical Sciences, Sahlgrenska Academy, Gothenburg University, Gothenburg 405 30, Sweden

Michele Stocchero, Yohei Jinno, Marco Toia, Marianne Ahmad and Jonas P. Becktor
Department of Oral & Maxillofacial Surgery and Oral Medicine, Faculty of Odontology, Malmö University, 20506 Malmö, Sweden

Evaggelia Papia
Department of Materials Science and Technology, Faculty of Odontology, Malmö University, 20506 Malmö, Sweden

Satoshi Yamaguchi
Department of Biomaterials Science, Osaka University Graduate School of Dentistry, Osaka 565-0871, Japan

Markus Schlee
Private Practice, Forchheim, Germany
Department of Maxillofacial Surgery, Goethe University, 60590 Frankfurt am Main, Germany

Loubna Naili
Private Practice, Kirchbachstraße 186, 28211 Bremen, Germany

Florian Rathe
Private Practice, Forchheim, Germany
Private Practice and Department of Prosthodontics, Danube University, 3500 Krems, Austria

Urs Brodbeck
Private Practice, 8051 Zürich, Switzerland

Chih-Hao Chen
Division of Plastic and Reconstructive Surgery, Department of Surgery, Stanford University School of Medicine, Stanford, CA 94305, USA
Craniofacial Research Center, Department of Plastic and Reconstructive Surgery, Chang Gung Memorial Hospital, Chang Gung University School of Medicine, Taoyuan 33305, Taiwan

Waldemar Hoffmann and Antony Quarry
Nobel Biocare Services AG CH-8058 Zürich-Flughafen, Switzerland

Benjamin R. Coyac, Brian Leahy, U. Serdar Tulu, Maziar Aghvami, John B. Brunski and Jill A. Helms
Division of Plastic and Reconstructive Surgery, Department of Surgery, Stanford University School of Medicine, Stanford, CA 94305, USA

Masaki Arioka
Division of Plastic and Reconstructive Surgery, Department of Surgery, Stanford University School of Medicine, Stanford, CA 94305, USA
Department of Clinical Pharmacology, Faculty of Medical Sciences, Kyushu University, Fukuoka 812-8582, Japan

Stefan Holst
Nobel Biocare Services AG CH-8058 Zürich-Flughafen, Switzerland
Department of Prosthodontics, School of Dentistry, Johann-Wolfgang Goethe University, 60438 Frankfurt, Germany

Dirk Henrich
Department of Trauma, Hand & Reconstructive Surgery, Goethe University, 60590 Frankfurt am Main, Germany

Benjamin Salmon
Paris Descartes-Sorbonne Paris Cité University, EA2496 Montrouge, France
Dental Medicine Department, Bretonneau Hospital, HUPNVS, AP-HP, 75018 Paris, France

Felix Koch and Markus Schlee
Department of Maxillofacial Surgery, Goethe University, 60590 Frankfurt am Main, Germany

Holger Zipprich, Paul Weigl and Christoph Ratka
Department of Prosthodontics, Faculty of Oral and Dental Medicine at Goethe University, 60590 Frankfurt am Main, Germany

Eugenie König
Private Practice, 60385 Frankfurt am Main, Germany

Alexandra Toderas
Private Practice, 60313 Frankfurt am Main, Germany

Ümniye Balaban
Institute of Biostatistics and Mathematical Modelling at Goethe University, 60590 Frankfurt am Main, Germany

Index

www.ingramcontent.com/pod-product-compliance
Lightning Source LLC
LaVergne TN
LVHW081037210926
848485LV00004B/1045